傳統

泰式按摩

手法技巧圖解

DIAGRAMS ON TRADITIONAL THAI MASSAGE MANIPULATION TECHNIQUE

主編　王金柱
Editor-in-Chief　Wang Jinzhu

傳統泰式按摩手法技巧圖解

主　　編　王金柱
副 主 編　秦振　黃婉瑩
執　　筆（以姓氏筆劃為序）
王小萍　王金柱　閻立　羅傑　秦振　黎作旭
繪　　圖　王良培　張家慶　黃婉瑩　韓劭
封面設計　李波
編　　輯　凱華　李月薇
出　　版　和平圖書有限公司
發　　行　和平圖書有限公司
香港柴灣嘉業街12號百樂門大廈17樓　電話：2804 6687　傳真：2804 6409
台灣發行　貿騰發賣股份有限公司
台北縣永和市永和路1段69號8樓　電話：02-22313503　傳真：02-22313384
承　　印　開益出版印刷有限公司
香港葵涌華星街8號華達工業中心A座8樓15室
版　　次　2003年3月第三版
定　　價　港幣80元／台幣320元

Diagrams on Traditional Thai Massage Manipulation Technique

Editor-in-Chief	Wang Jinzhu
Deputy Editors-in-Chief	Qin Zhen　Huang Wanying
Writers	Wang Xiaoping　Wang Jinzhu　Yan Li Luo Jie　Qin Zhen　Li Zuoxu
Drawings by	Wang Liangpei　Zhang Jiaqing Huang Wanying　Han Shao
Cover Designed by	Paul Lee
Edition Editors	Kai Hua　Li Yuet Mei
Published by	Peace Book Co., Ltd.
Distributed by	Peace Book Co., Ltd. 17/F., Paramount Building, 12 Ka Yip Street, Chai Wan, Hong Kong Tel: 2804 6687　Fax: 2804 6409 Modren Professional Distribution Co., Ltd. 8/F., No. 69, Section 1, Yung Ho Road, Yung Ho City, Taipei Hsien, Taiwan Tel: 02-22313503　Fax: 02-22313384
Printed by	Editions Quaille Ltd. Rm.15, 8/F, Block A, Wha Tat Industrial Centre, 8-10 Wah Sing Street, Kwai Chung, Hong Kong
Price	HK$80.00 / NT$320.00
Third Edition 2003	

ISBN 962-238-309-2
PB-017-P

作者簡介

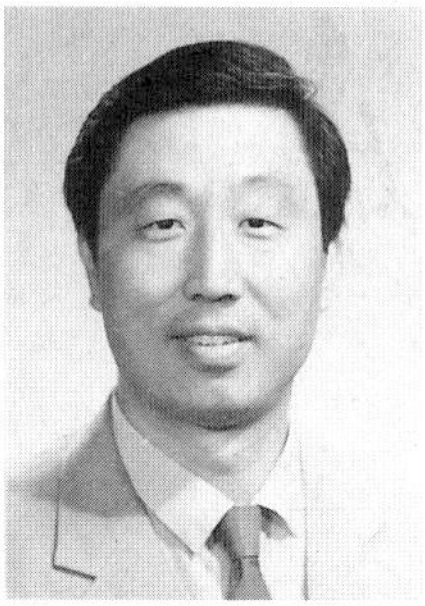

王金柱，男，51歲。副主任醫師。

1976年畢業於北京中醫藥大學（原北京中醫學院）中醫系，同年分配到中國中醫研究院廣安門醫院骨科，91年調往骨傷科研究所。曾任廣安門醫院副院長、骨傷科研究所副所長等職。

從事專業工作以來，潛心研究中國各流派推拿療法的操作技巧，學習、繼承和整理段勝如、張濤、李祖謨等老專家的臨床經驗，熟練掌握中醫傳統推拿手法，對急慢性軟組織損傷，如頸椎病、腰腿病、肩周炎、骨關節病的治療有獨到之處。能運用中醫及中西醫結合的專業理論，講授骨傷科知識，介紹推拿及康復保健的手法，特別是通過對中國31家流派推拿治療特點的分析歸納，結合自己二十多年的臨床經驗，總結出一套集各派精萃於一帙的系統手法並公諸於世。

近幾年來，在關注中醫推拿按摩療效的同時，又認真研究來自異國的泰式按摩手法的操作技巧，重點對其在保健和疾病的治療作用方面進行了深入的探討。曾主編《醫院管理知識問答》、《推拿手法技巧圖解》等著作，在國內外發表專業論文及科普文章數十篇。還多次赴國外講學、會議並進行學術交流。十餘年來始終擔任中國領導人及聯合國官員的保健工作。

About the Author

The Author, Wang Jinzhu, male, 51, deputy head doctor, graduated from the Traditional Chinese Medicine Department of the Beijing Traditional Chinese Medicine University in 1976, was formerly deputy director of the Guanganmen Hospital and deputy director of the Orthopedics Research Institute.

Since being engaged in professional work, he diligently studied the manipulation of various Chinese schools of massotherapy, learned, inherited and arranged clinic experience of Duan Shengru, Zhang Tao, Li Zumo and other veteran experts, skillfully mastered traditional Chinese medicine massotherapy and has originality in treating acute and chronic soft tissue injuries such as cervical spondylosis, lumbocrural disease, periarthritis of the shoulder and osteoarthrosis. Particularly, by analysing and summing up massotherapeutic characteristics of 31 Chinese schools and combining over 20 years of personal clinic experience, he has summed up a set of systematic manipulations integrating the essence of various schools and published them for the public.

Over the recent years, while paying attention to Chinese medical massotherapy, he has seriously studied in depth Thai massage, particularly its function in keeping fit and treatment of diseases. He has edited the *Questionnaire on Hospital Management Knowledge*, *Diagrams on Massotherapeutic Manipulations* and other works and published dozens of professional essays and popularization of scientific articles at home and abroad. He has given lectures, held group consultations and carried out academic exchanges abroad. Over the past dozen years, he has often undertaken the health care work for Chinese leaders and UN officials.

内容提要

《傳統泰式按摩手法技巧圖解》是在筆者認真學習、努力掌握、反復實踐的基礎上，參閱同類書籍編撰集成。該書系統地介紹了泰國式按摩操作技巧之精華，是一部介紹泰國文化衛生方面的專著之一。

本書以泰國式按摩的順序為主線，各種手法均以照片和圖示等富於動感的形式表現出來，並用精練的語言闡明操作技巧。全書圖文並茂，化深奧為簡明，手法技巧靜中有動、深入淺出，一目了然，使讀者易懂、易學、便於掌握使用。

全書文字洗練，附有**227**張照片，**196**幅圖示，內容新穎，豐富實用。本書主要供專業人員及業餘愛好者學習應用，也可供從事教學、科研等人員參考。

Summary of Content

The Diagrams on Traditional Thai Massage Manipulation Technique is compiled by the author on the basis of seriously learning, striving to master through repeated practice and by referring to similar books. The book systematically introduces the essence of Thai massage manipulation technique and is one of the professional works introducing Thai culture and health.

With Thai massage order as the main theme, the book illustrates manipulations with photos, figures and forms rich in movement and expounds manipulation technique with succinct language. All the pictures and their accompanying articles are excellent. They explain the profound in simple terms and are clear to understand at a glance, so that readers can easily understand, learn, master and apply.

The book is succinct in style, contains 227 photos and 196 figures, with novel contents, rich and practical. It is mainly for professional personnel and amateur lovers to learn and apply, as well as reference for teaching, scientific research and other personnel.

前言

泰國式按摩是一種傳統的治療方法，具有悠久的歷史。它的起源，可追溯至二千五百年前的古印度西部，創始人是印度國王的御醫吉瓦科·庫瑪，他的傳統醫藥和按摩知識、技法通過第一批傳教的僧人帶入泰國，經流傳和發展，至二十世紀末，泰式按摩在泰國民間廣泛採用，並有專人從事此項工作的研究和開發，而吉瓦科·庫瑪仍被泰國人民奉為醫學之父。在十八世紀，尼科洛王或瑞瑪三世執政期間，為繼承和發展傳統醫學理論的真諦，印度國王召集當時健在的傳統業醫們，廣泛吸取他們的傳統醫藥及按摩的寶貴經驗，並整理成文，銘刻在大理石碑上、鑲嵌於瓦特波臥佛寺的遊廊壁上。至今人們仍能目睹這些銘文，由此瓦特波也成了一個訓練傳統泰國式按摩的重要基地。

泰國式按摩曾是古代泰國國王招待皇家貴賓的最高禮節。現在，在泰國各地，尤其在旅遊勝地，泰國式按摩場所舉目可見。從事這項工作的人員遠比其他國家人數為多，其中以女性為主，亦有男士和殘疾人。泰國式按摩的特點係採用細膩的指壓、掌壓、肘壓、足壓等手法，着重對人體四肢及各部肌群進行重復拉、抻、推、捏，使各部位關節活動度儘量達到正常或超正常範圍，將手部的力量均勻滲透到肌肉深處，以達到疏通經絡、調和氣血的作用。特別在對脊柱和四肢關節的蹬壓和旋轉扭動及面部美容按摩過程中，令人有輕鬆愉悦、神態一新之感。

泰國式按摩進行一次約需兩小時。很多當地人都喜歡這種按摩，凡去泰國的觀光者大都願意體會一下泰國式按摩的特殊滋味，因為它不僅能使人消除疲勞，而且還對人體肌肉損傷、痛風、炎症有明顯的治療作用。

筆者為探索泰國式按摩的操作技巧及治療範圍，曾專程赴泰國考察，並在按摩師指導下，經過數年的理論學習和實踐，深深體會到其獨到之處。經系統總結，他將傳統泰國式按摩的手法，依按摩的順序全部用照片展現出來，其中既有反映整體姿式的大體照片，也有突出手法技巧的細部影像，動靜結合，圖文並茂，將這一特色按摩技巧形象地展現在廣大愛好者及專業人員面前。

為具體、清晰地展現按摩的每一個動作，筆者特地讓本書照片中的操作人員及被按摩者均以泳裝出現。

在諸多推拿按摩的著作中，介紹泰國式按摩手法並不多見。鑑於泰國式按摩的特殊療效，筆者願將其多年來潛心研究和實踐的經驗通過本著作獻給廣大讀者。

Introduction

Thai massage is a kind of traditional therapy with a long history. Its origin can be traced as far back to ancient west India 2,500 years ago and the founder was Jiwako Koma, court doctor to the Indian king. His traditional medicine, massage knowledge and technique were introduced to Thailand by the first group of missionary monks who spread and developed it. By the end of the 20th century, their experience widely existed among the people and professionals who were engaged in this work. Today, Jiwako Koma is still respected as the father of medicine by the Thai people. In the 18th century, during the rule of King Nikolo or Rama the 3rd, in order to inherit and develop the true essence of traditional medicine theory, the king called together the then traditional doctors and widely absorbed their traditional medicine and valuable massage experiences, transcribed them into words, inscribed them on marble tablets and inlaid them on a corridor wall in the Temple of the Sleeping Buddha in Watapo. Today, people can still see these inscriptions, and Watapo has become an important base for training traditional Thai massage.

Thai massage was the highest rite for Thai kings in ancient times to receive distinguished imperial guests. At present, in Thailand, particularly in tourist regions, massage centers can be seen everywhere. The number of people engaged in this work is far more than that in other countries, who are mainly females as well as males and the handicapped. The characteristics of Thai massage adopt exquisite finger, palm, elbow and foot pressing and other manipulations with stress on carrying out repeated pulling, stretching, pushing, and grasping of four limbs and various muscles in the human body to make the movement of various joints normal or super normal, and make hand strength evenly penetrate into the depths of muscles and circulate meridians and collaterals and regulating qi (life force or vital energy) and blood. In particular, stamping, rolling and swinging of spine and four limb joints and massage beautifying of face make people feel happy and relaxed and fresh looking. Thai massage requires about two hours each time. Most local people enjoy this massage and all who tour Thailand like to experience it because it not only eliminates fatigue, but also has obvious curative effect to human muscle injury, gout and inflammation.

In order to probe the manipulation technique and treatment of Thai massage, the author has specially gone to Thailand to investigate and practice under massage masters for a few years and gradually experience its originality. After systematic summing up and sorting out, he shows all the traditional Thai massage manipulations with photos according to massage order, of which are photos reflecting the whole postures as well as photos in detail stressing manipulation technique combining movement and quiet feeling showing this characteristic massage technique to all who have great interest in massage and for professional personnel.

For showing clearly in detail each massage movement, the author has specially shown the massagist and patient in bathing costumes.

Among many massotherapy and massage books, very few introduce Thai massage manipulations. In view of the special curative effect of Thai massage, the author wishes to contribute to all readers his studies applied by personal practice and experience over many years in this book.

目錄
CONTENTS

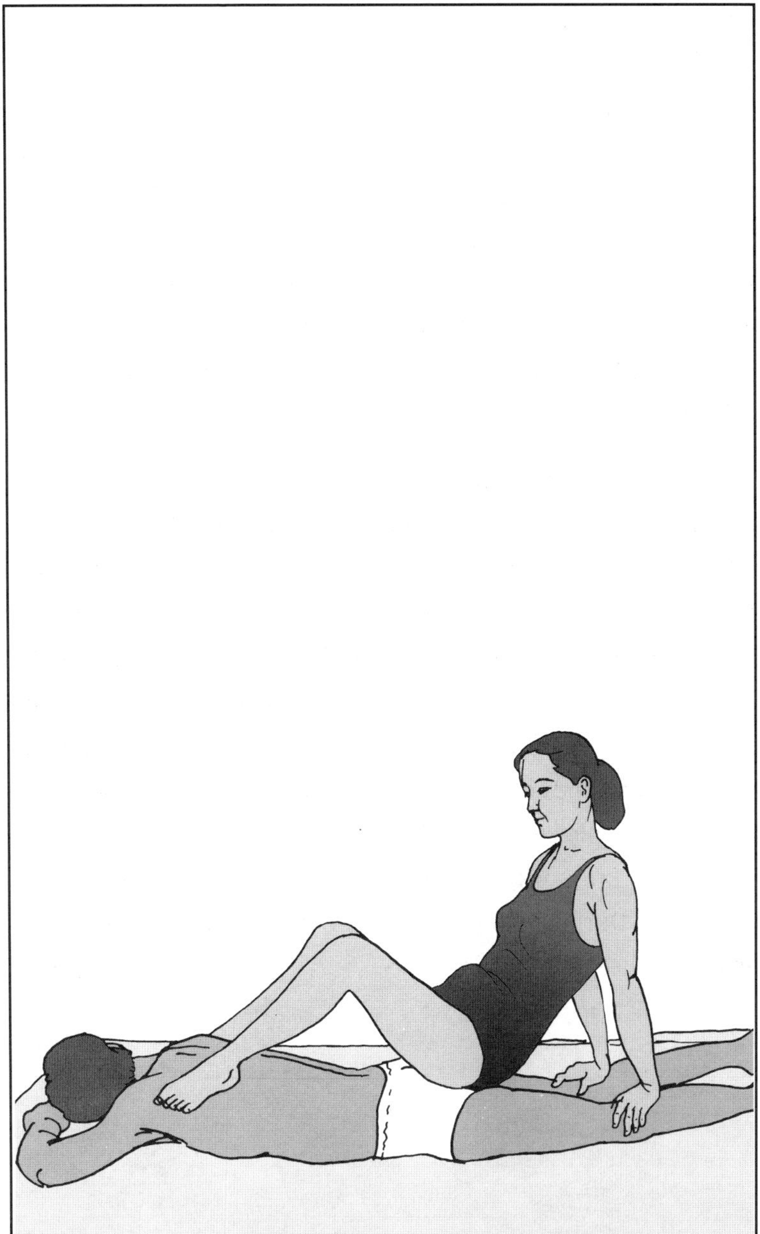

1 屈踝法：

被按摩者仰臥位，雙上肢置於軀體兩側，雙下肢外展，中立位，與肩同寬；按摩者屈髖屈膝、跪坐臥者兩內踝之間，雙手拇指放於足拇指內緣，其餘四指自然地放在足背，略呈扇形，掌心和掌根向下按壓雙足足趾遠端的背側，使踝關節、跖跗關節、跖趾關節處於屈曲狀態（見照片**1**、**2** 和圖示**1**）。左右手交替用力，反復按壓**2－4**次。操作時，用力不宜過猛，以免造成不必要的損傷。

Ankle bending method:

The patient lies flat on back with both upper limbs down the sides of the body, and both lower limbs astride the same width as the shoulders. The massagist bends hip and knees and kneels between both inner ankles of the patient with thumbs of both hands on the inner ends of big toes and other four fingers naturally on the dorsum of feet, slightly in a fan shape, and palm centers and roots pressing the back of far ends of both feet toes so that ankle joints, sole instep and metatarsophalangeal joints are in a bent state (see Photos 1, 2 and Fig.1). Press with left and right hands 2-4 times with force alternately. During manipulation, note not to use too strong force that may cause unnecessary injury.

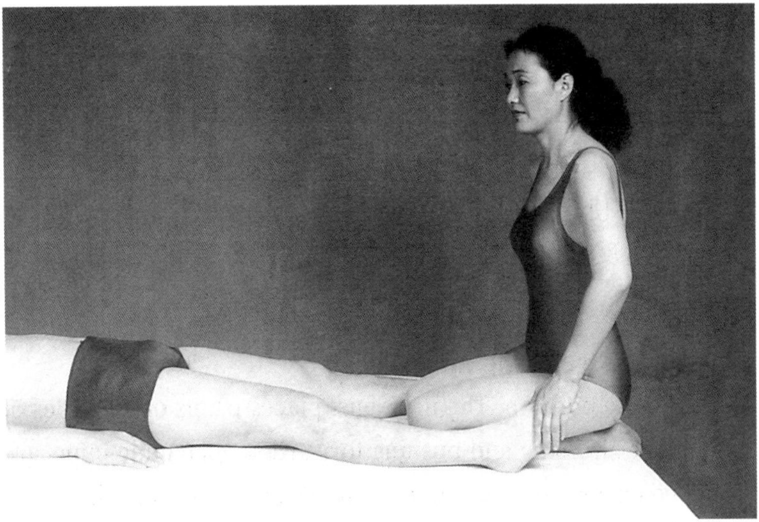

照片 (Photo) 1

照片 (Photo) 2

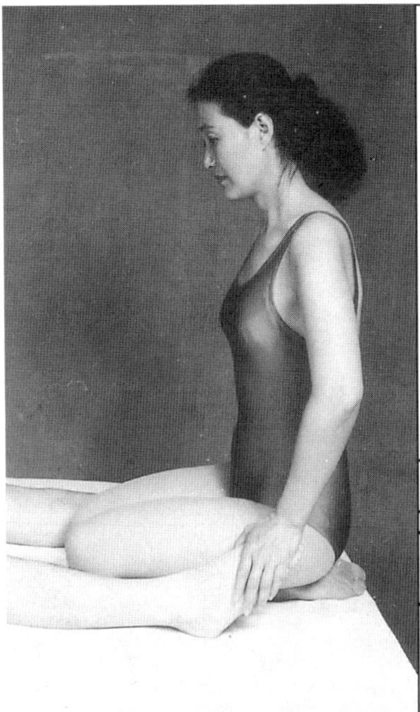

圖示 (Fig.) 1

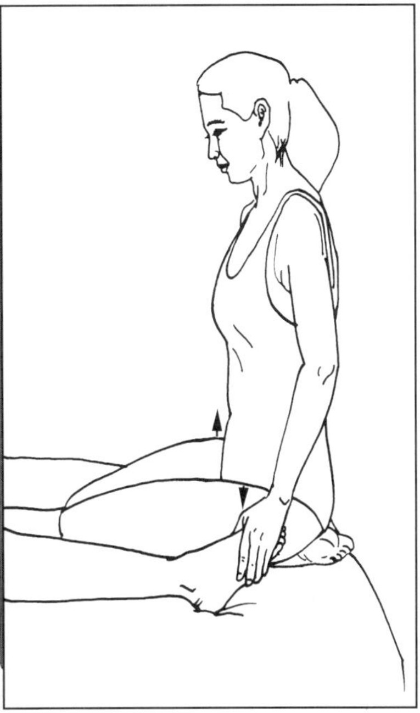

2 伸踝法：

體位同上。按摩者雙手掌置於被按摩者雙足底跖部，向前方按推，使踝關節極度背伸，左右手交替進行（見照片3 和圖示2），反復操作2－4次。此法要求用力適中，防止造成跟腱拉傷。

Ankle stretching method:

In same position. The massagist places palms on the soles of the patient, pressing and pushing forward so that ankle joints are stretched backward to the utmost with left and right hand alternately (see Photo 3 and Fig. 2). Repeat the manipulation 2-4 times. Moderate force should be used to prevent injury of heel tendons.

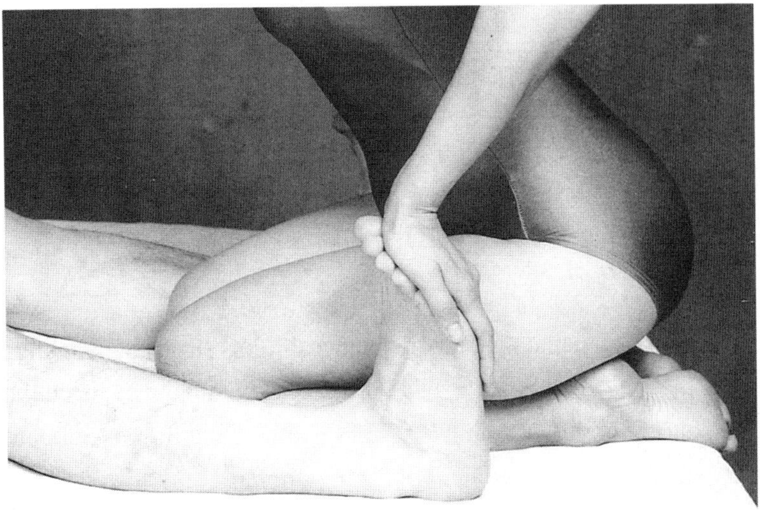

照片 (Photo) 3

圖示 (Fig.) 2

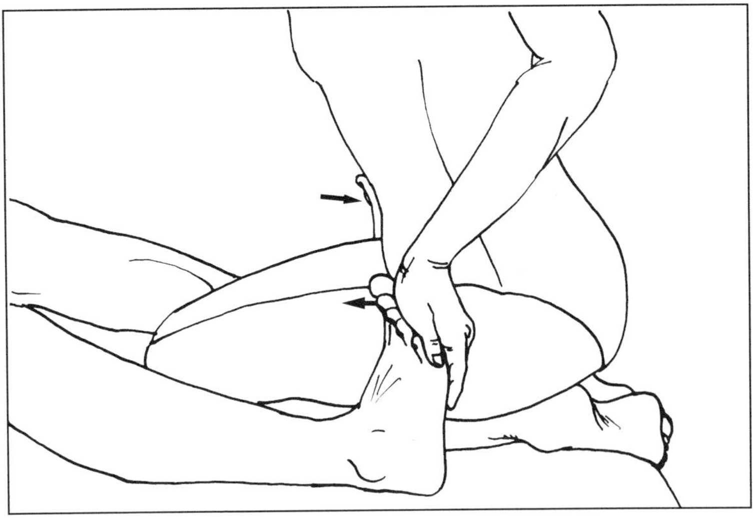

3 伸跖跗及跖趾關節法：

體位同上。按摩者雙手掌根置於雙足足趾的跖側，五指扣住被按摩者雙足五趾，向前下方按推，使其背伸跖跗關節及跖趾關節，反復操作**2 －4** 次（見照片**4** 和圖示**3** ）。注意用力應由輕到重，不宜過猛。

Sole instep and metatarsophalangeal joints stretching method:

In same position. The massagist places both palm roots on the toe soles of both feet with five fingers buckling the five toes of both the patient's feet, pressing and pushing forward and downward so that sole instep and metatarsophalangeal joints stretch backward. Repeat the manipulation 2-4 times (see Photo 4 and Fig. 3). Note, force should be used from light to heavy but not too fierce.

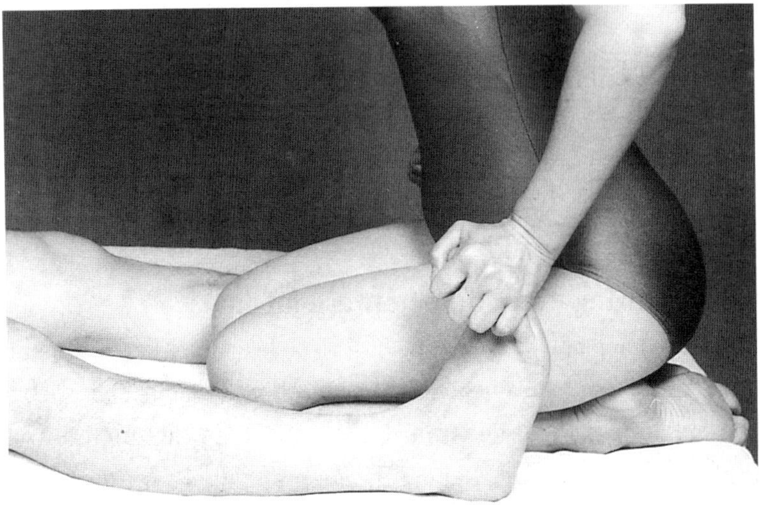

照片 (Photo) 4

圖示 (Fig.) 3

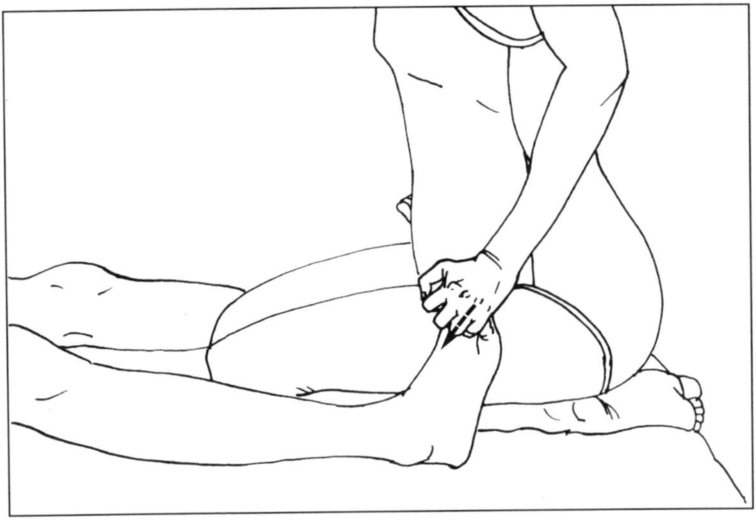

4 外旋下肢法：

體位同上。按摩者上肢伸直，雙手置於被按摩者雙足前內側，交替向外下方按壓，使雙下肢外旋，反復操作2－4次（見照片5和圖示4）。

Revolving lower limb outward method:

In same position. The massagist stretches upper limbs straight and places both hands inside the front of both of the patient's feet, pressing outside and downward alternatively so that both lower limbs revolve outward. Repeat the manipulation 2-4 times (see Photo 5 and Fig. 4).

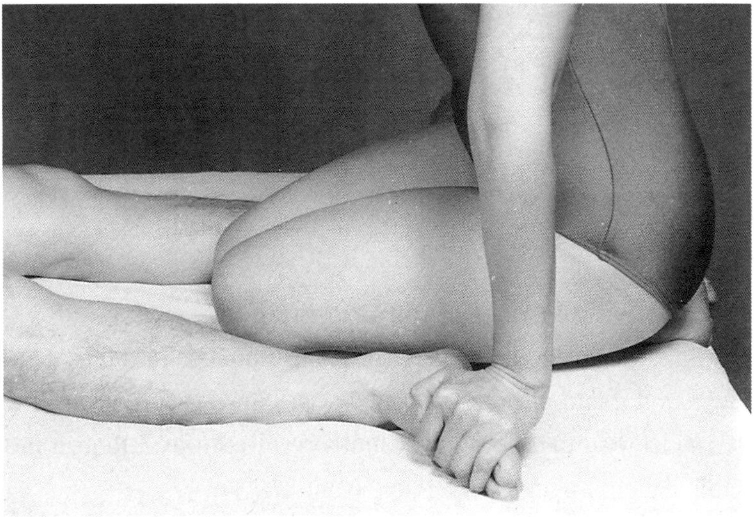

照片 (Photo) 5

圖示 (Fig.) 4

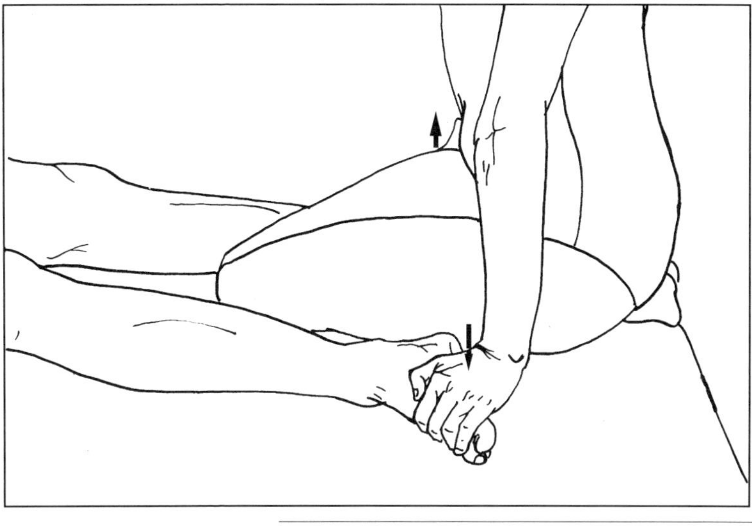

5 內旋下肢法：

體位同上。按摩者雙手掌置於被按摩者雙足背外側，交替向內下方按壓，使雙下肢內旋，反復操作2－4次（見照片6和圖示5）。

Revolving lower limb inward method:

In same position. The massagist places both palms outside the patient's dorsum of both feet and presses inward and downward alternatively so that both lower limbs revolve inward. Repeat the manipulation 2-4 times (see Photo 6 and Fig. 5).

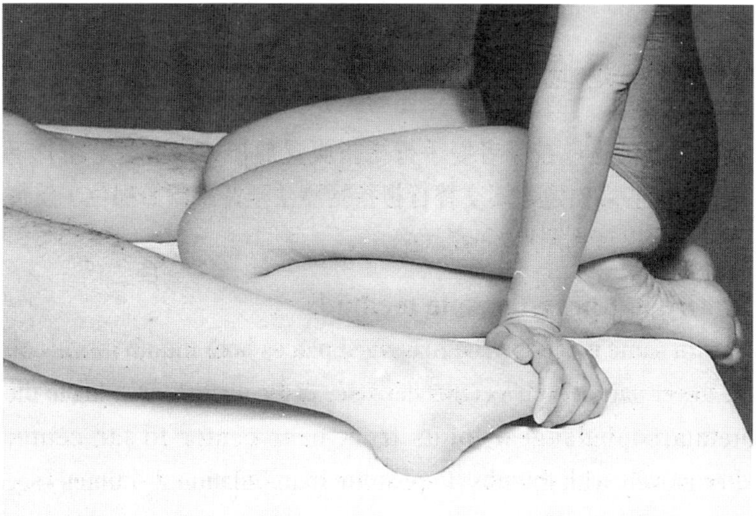

照片 (Photo) 6

圖示 (Fig.) 5

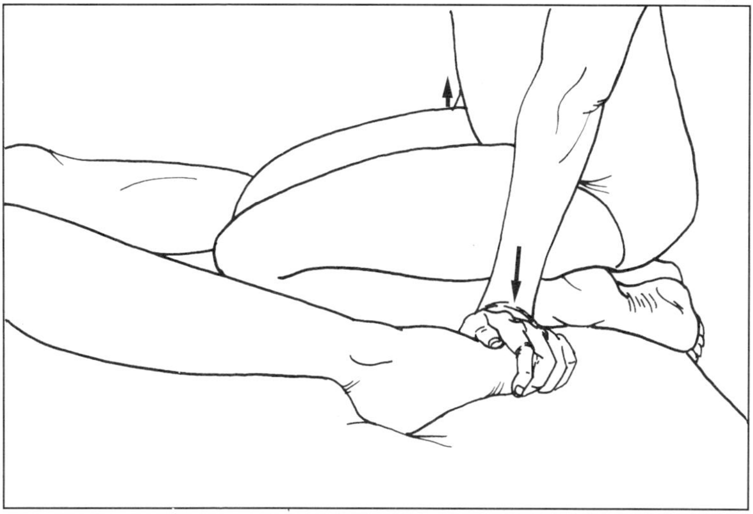

6 指壓足底法：

體位同上。按摩者雙手拇指指腹置於被按摩者雙足距骨下方，由近心端向遠心端交替行拇指指壓法至跖趾關節部位，反復操作2－4次（見照片7和圖示6）。

Digital-pressing sole method:

In same position. The massagist places both thumb insides on the lower part of both feet metatarsuses of the patient, pressing to the metatarsophalangeal joints from near center to far center alternatively with thumbs. Repeat the manipulation 2-4 times (see Photo 7 and Fig. 6).

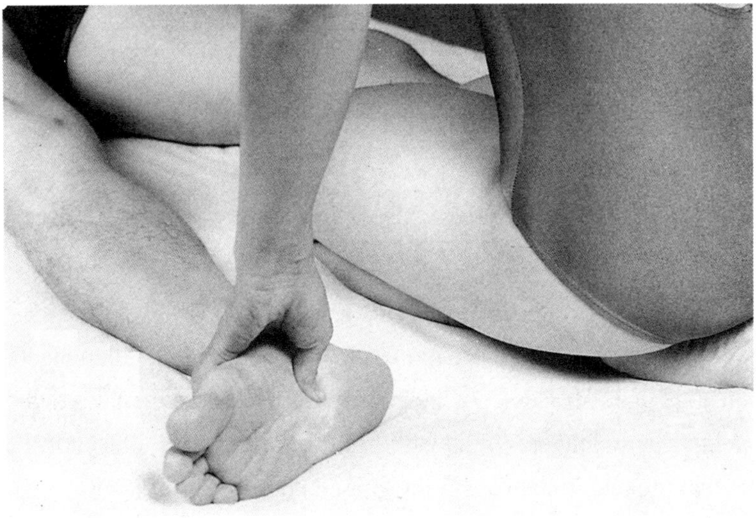

照片 (Photo) 7

圖示 (Fig.) 6

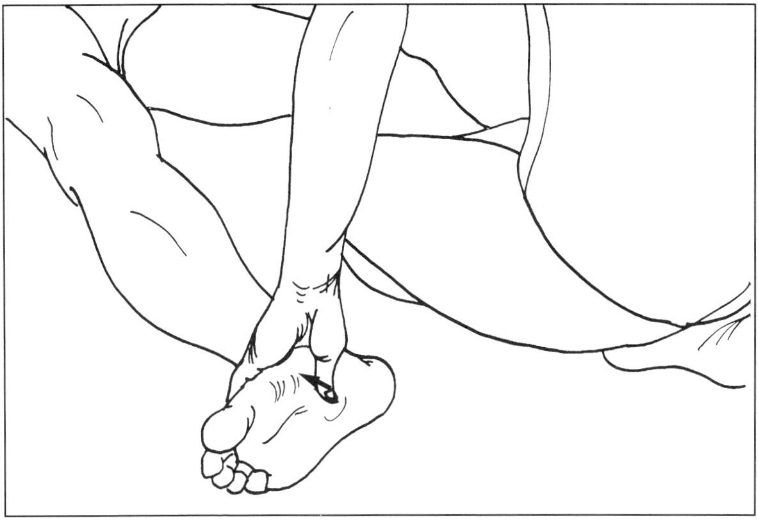

7 指壓內踝法：

體位同上，操作技巧不變。被按摩部位係從雙內踝下方，按摩者用雙手拇指指腹交替按至跖趾關節處，反復操作**2－4**次（見照片**8**和圖示**7**）。

Digital-pressing inner ankle method:

In same position. The manipulation technique is unchanged. The massagist presses from the lower part of both inner ankles to the metatarsophalangeal joints with both thumb insides alternatively. Repeat the manipulation 2-4 times (see Photo 8 and Fig. 7).

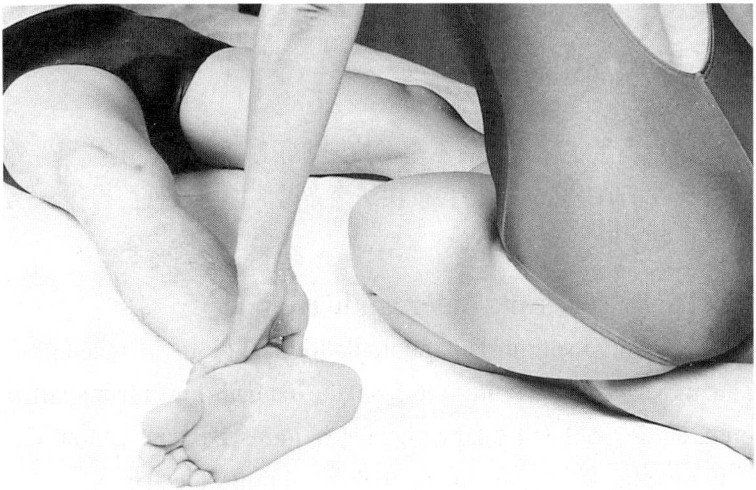

照片 (Photo) 8

圖示 (Fig.) 7

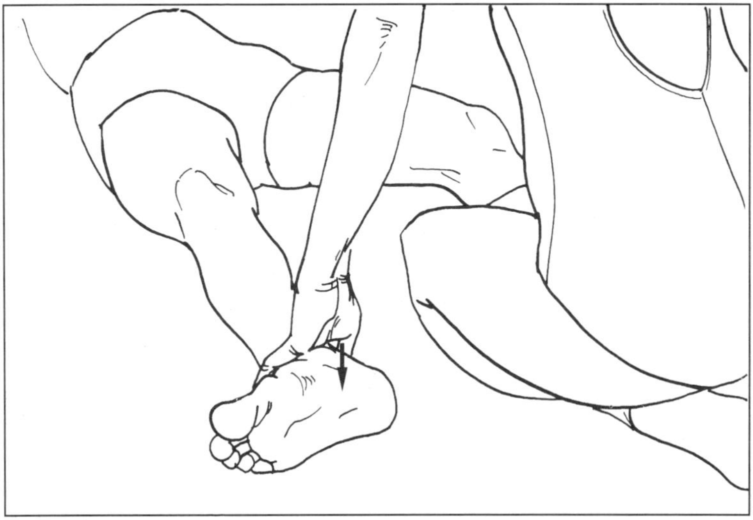

8 指壓外踝法：

體位同上，操作技巧不變。按摩者用雙手拇指從被按摩者外踝前下方，向遠心端行拇指按揉法至跖趾關節處，反復操作**2－4**次（見圖示**8**）。

Digital-pressing outer ankle method:

In same position. The manipulation technique is unchanged. The massagist presses and rubs from the patient's lower front part of outer ankles to the metatarsophalangeal joints at the far center with both thumbs. Repeat the manipulation 2-4 times (see Fig. 8).

圖示 (Fig.) 8

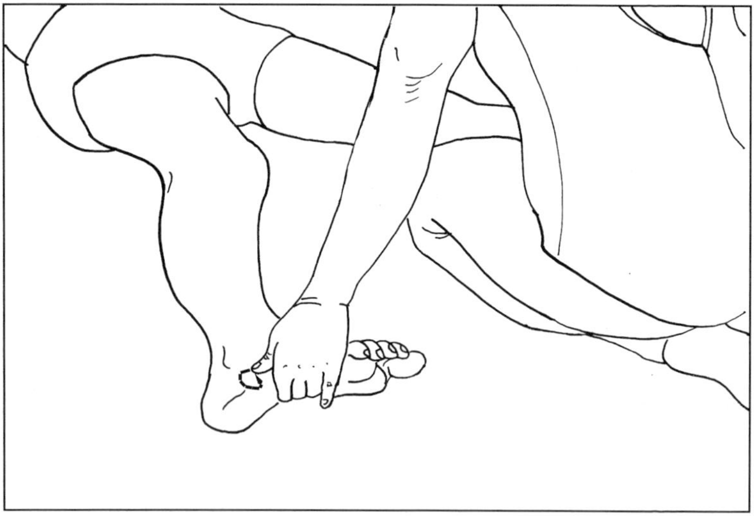

9 指揉跖趾關節法：

體位同上。按摩者用雙手拇指指腹分別置於被按摩者雙足小趾跖趾關節背側，同時由外向內側行環轉按揉法至拇趾跖趾關節背側（見照片**9**和圖示**9**），再由內向外側按揉至小趾跖趾關節處（見照片**10**），反復操作**2－4**次。

Digital-rubbing metatarsophalangeal joints method:

In same position. The massagist places both thumb insides on the back of both little toe metatarsophalangeal joints of the patient and rolls and rubs to the back of 1st toe metatarsophalangeal joints from outside to inside (see Photo 9 and Fig. 9) and then to the little toe metatarsophalangeal joints from inside to outside (see Photo 10). Repeat the manipulation 2-4 times.

照片 (Photo) 9

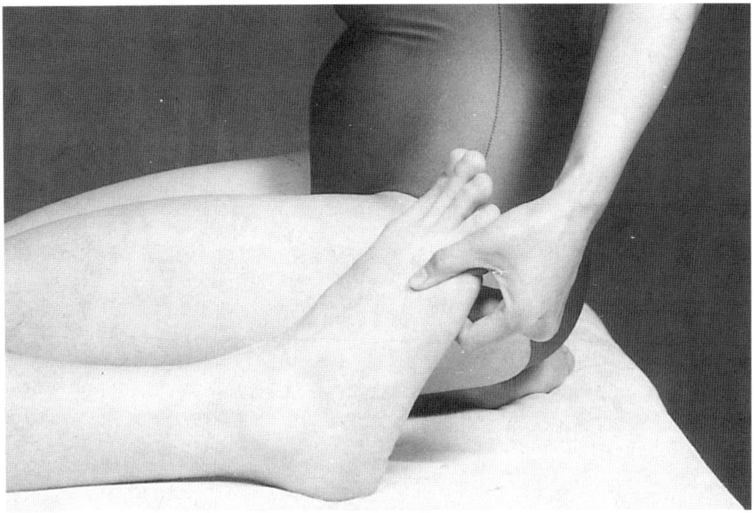

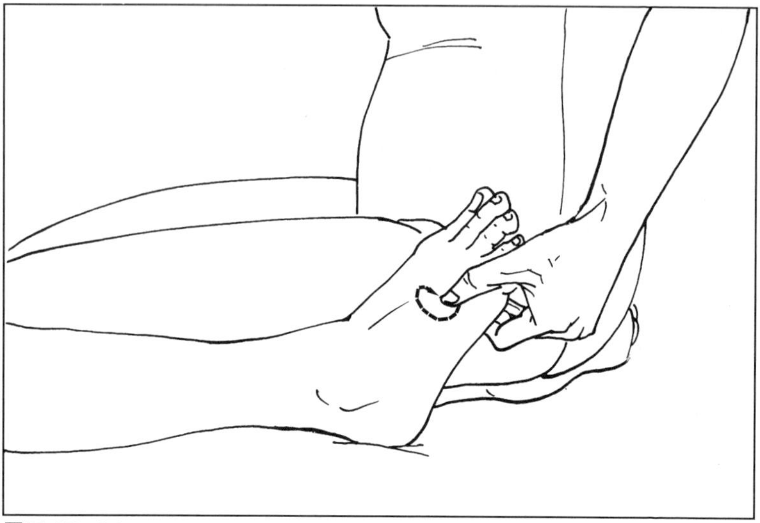

圖示 (Fig.) 9

照片 (Photo) 10

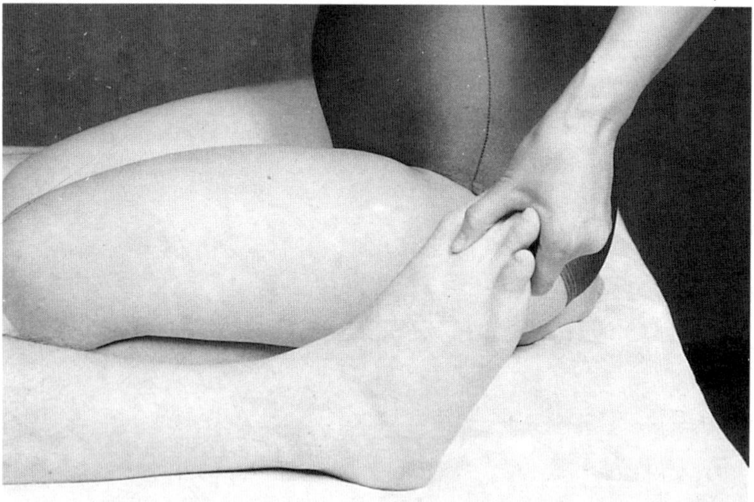

10 指揉趾腹法：

體位同上。按摩者雙手拇指指腹分別捻揉被按摩者雙足趾腹部，由拇趾至小趾，反復操作**2－4**次（見照片**11**和圖示**10**）。

Digital-rubbing toe inside method:

In same position. The massagist rubs the toe inside of the patient's two feet with both inside of thumbs respectively from 1st toes to little toes. Repeat the manipulation 2-4 times (see Photo 11 and Fig. 10).

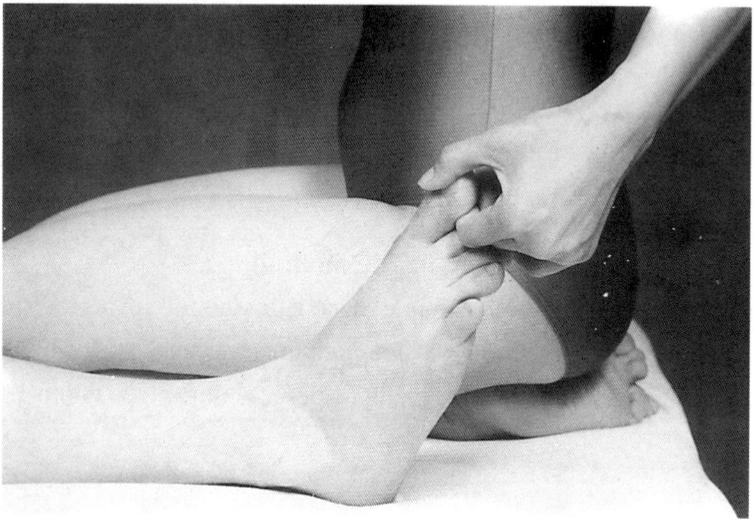

照片 (Photo) 11

圖示 (Fig.) 10

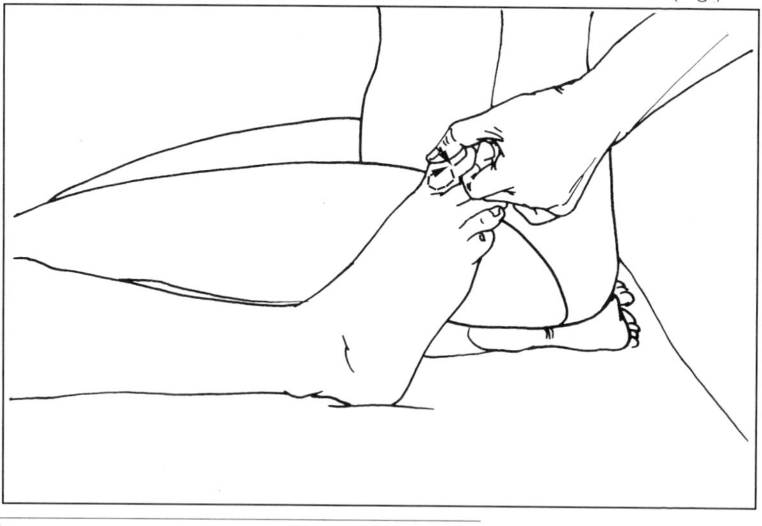

11 足趾拔伸法：

體位同上。按摩者雙手拇指略屈，食指屈曲，分別置於被按摩者雙足小趾的背側和跖側遠端，向遠心端屈趾拔伸，從小趾至拇指，各拔伸一次（見照片12和圖示11）。

Toe pulling and stretching method:

In same position. The massagist places slightly-bent thumbs and other bent forefingers of both hands on the back of patient's little toes and the far end of soles of both feet, pulling and stretching toward the far center and from little toes to 1st toes each one once (see Photo 12 and Fig. 11).

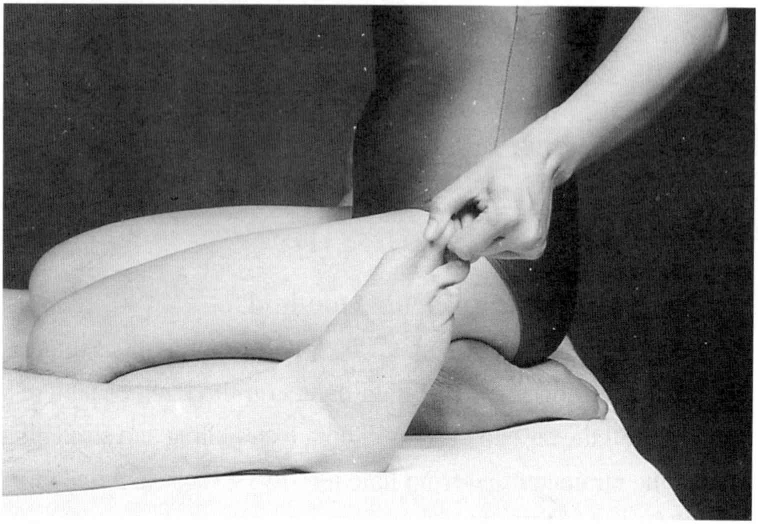

照片 (Photo) 12

圖示 (Fig.) 11

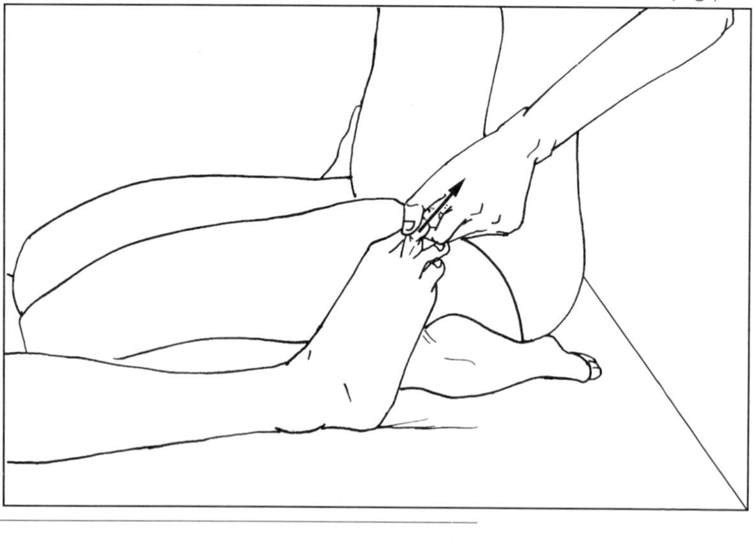

12 點壓足底法：

體位同上。按摩者雙手四指並攏、微屈、置於被按摩者足背側，拇指置於其跖側，用拇指指端點壓足底諸穴，邊點按邊外旋雙下肢，借上身重心左右移動，交替加重對足部點按的力量（見照片**13**和圖示**12**）。

Sole pointing and pressing method:

In same position. The massagist close four fingers of both hands together, slightly bends, and places them on the dorsum of both feet of the patient with thumbs on soles and presses all acupoints on soles with thumb tips, pressing while revolving outward both lower limbs and moving left and right with the gravity of upper body and alternately increasing the force of pointing and pressing the feet (see Photo 13 and Fig. 12).

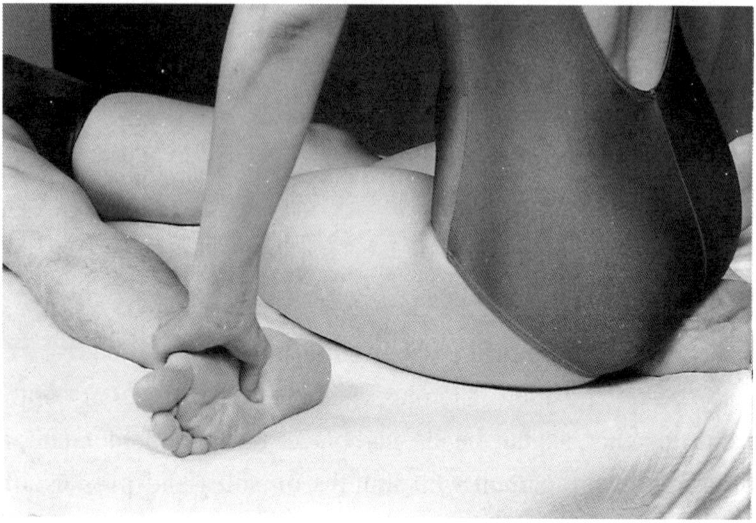

照片 (Photo) 13

圖示 (Fig.) 12

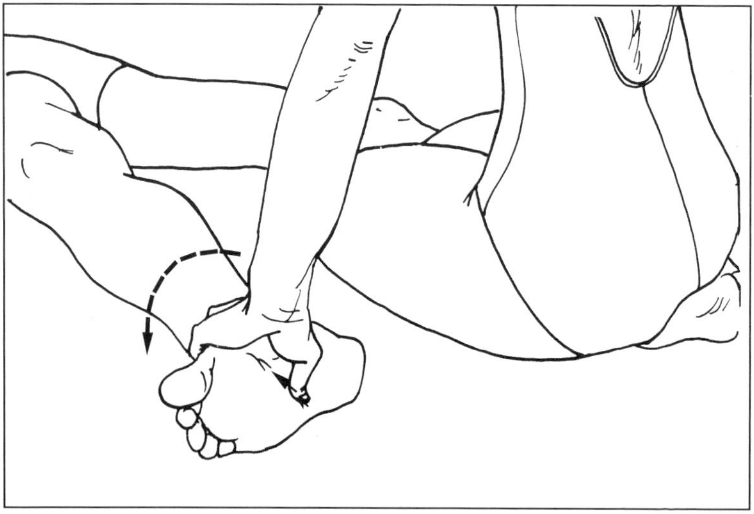

13 點壓下肢內側法：

體位同上。按摩者雙手拇指分別置於被按摩者內踝後方（見照片**14**），做上身重心左右轉移動作，並依據其頻率，由遠心端向近心端按壓小腿（見照片**15**）及大腿內側肌群至腹股溝部（見照片**16**和圖示**13**），按壓間距以**3**公分左右為宜，反復操作**2－4**次。

Pointing and pressing lower inside of limb method:

In same position. The massagist places both thumbs on the rear of patient's inner ankles respectively (see Photo 14), making the gravity of the upper body move from left to right and pressing the inner muscles of shanks (see Photo 15) and thighs to groin (see Photo 16 and Fig. 13) from far center toward near center according to the frequency . The distance between pressing is around 3 cm. Repeat the manipulation 2-4 times.

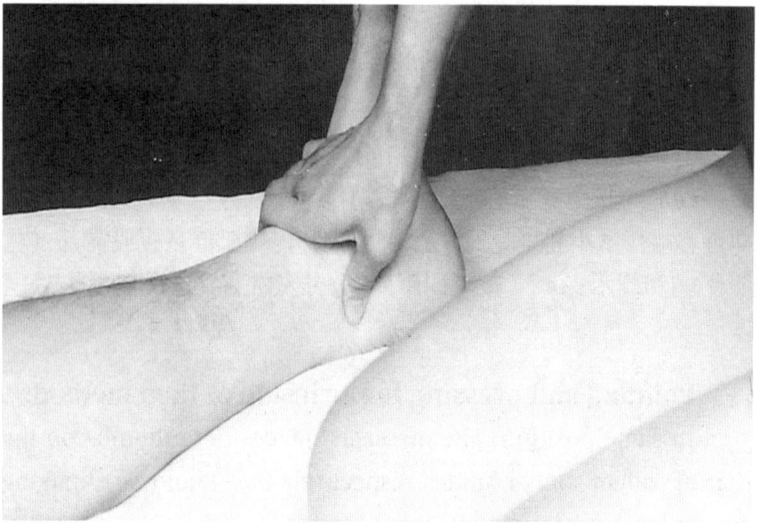

照片 (Photo) 14

照片 (Photo) 15

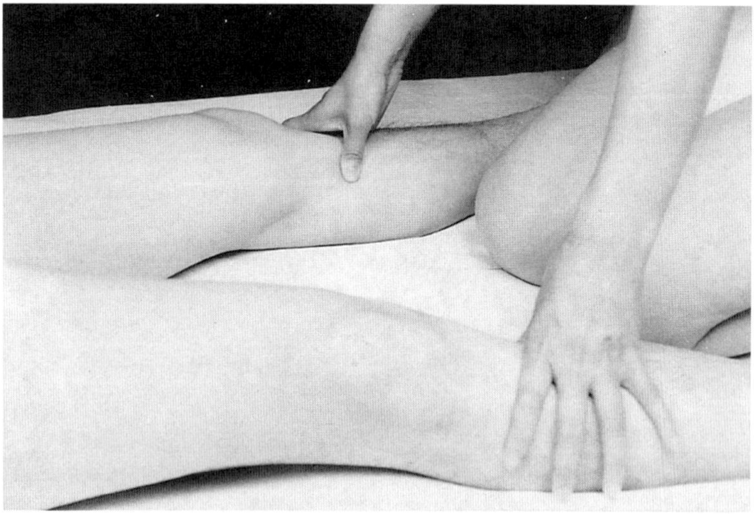

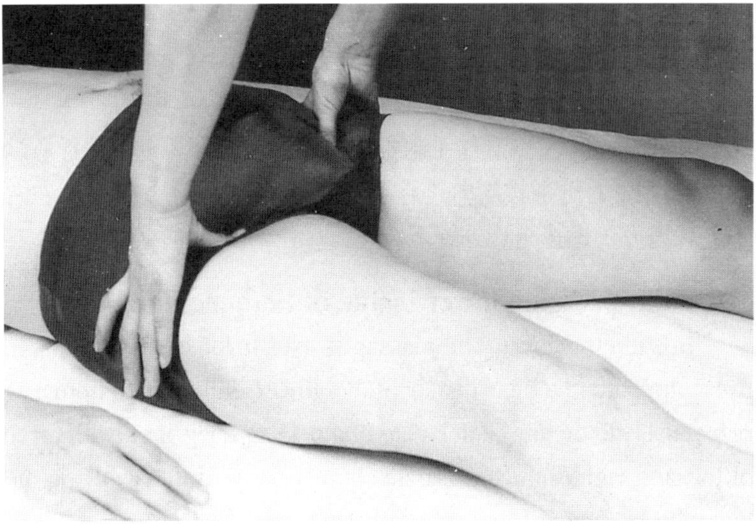

照片 (Photo) 16

圖示 (Fig.) 13

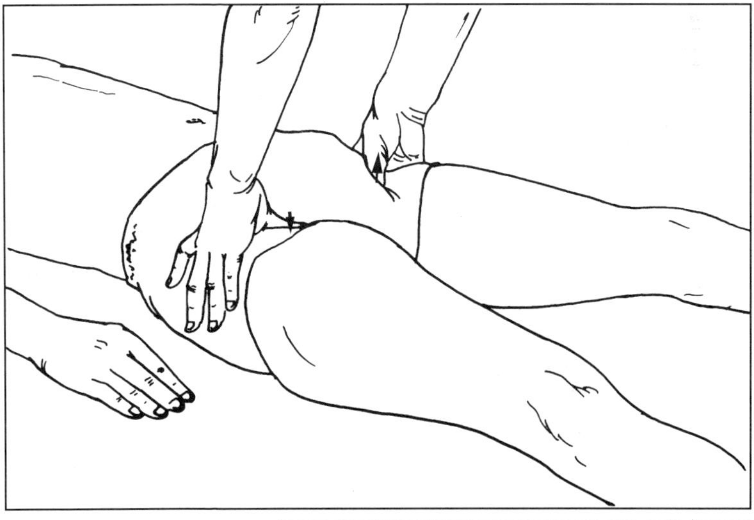

14 掌壓下肢內側法：

體位同上。按摩者雙手掌根着力，從被按摩者雙下肢近心端（見照片**17**）分別按壓向遠心端（見照片**18**和圖示**14**），左右手交替施力，邊按壓邊外旋下肢。

Palm-pressing lower inside of limb method:

In same position. The massagist uses force of both palms to press the patient's near center of two lower limbs (see Photo 17) respectively to the far center (see Photo 18 and Fig. 14), with force of left and right hands alternatively, pressing while revolving the lower limbs outward.

照片 (Photo) 17

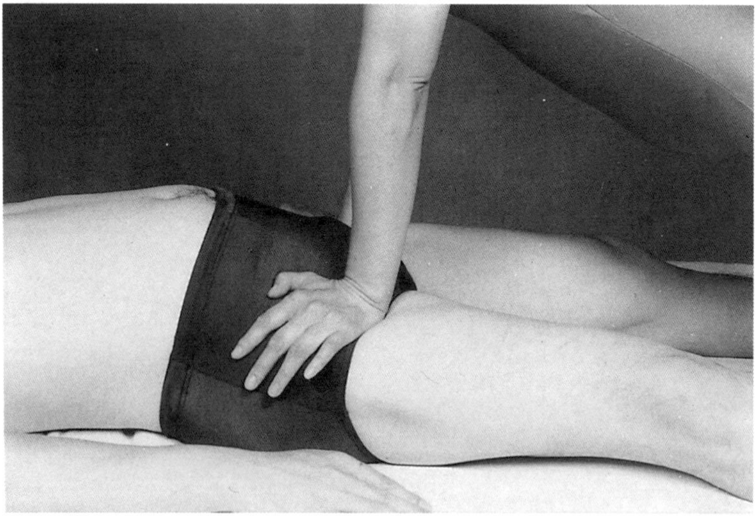

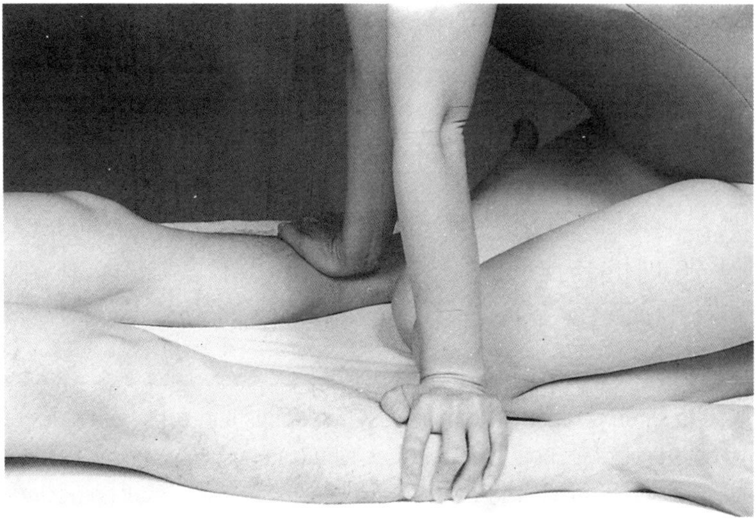

照片 (Photo) 18

圖示 (Fig.) 14

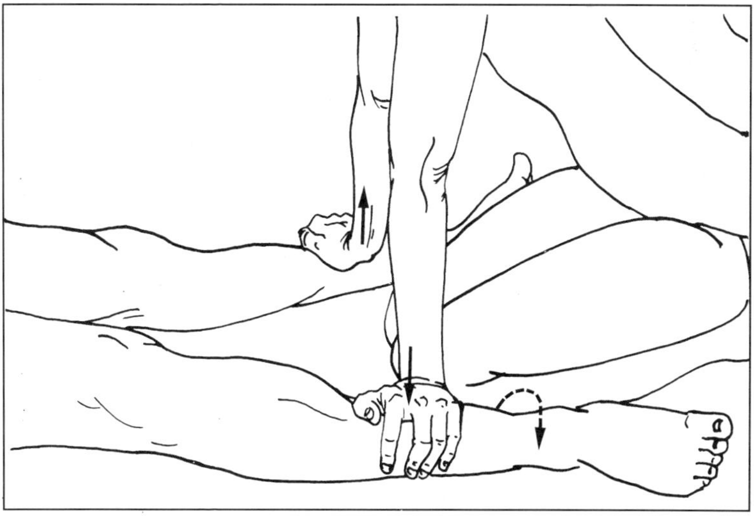

15 掌根按壓法：

體位同上。按摩者先用雙手拇指指腹同時點揉被按摩者雙側腹股溝部（見照片19），再改用雙手大魚際肌及掌根部用力按壓其股動脈。為增加所施力的強度，按摩者上半身略向前傾以借其力（見照片20和圖示15）。按壓時間為1－2分鐘。然後迅速抬手，使股動脈中的血液下行，以被按摩者雙下肢有蟻行感和熱感為宜。

Palm-root pressing method:

In same position. The massagist first points and rubs both sides of patient's groin with both thumb insides simultaneously (see Photo 19) and then presses the groin artery with force of big thenar muscles of both hands and palm roots. To increase the force, the massagist slightly inclines the upper body forward for force (see Photo 20 and Fig. 15). The time for pressing is 1-2 minutes and then rapidly lifts hands away so that the blood in groin artery flows downward. The patient should have ants running and hot feeling on both lower limbs.

照片 (Photo) 19

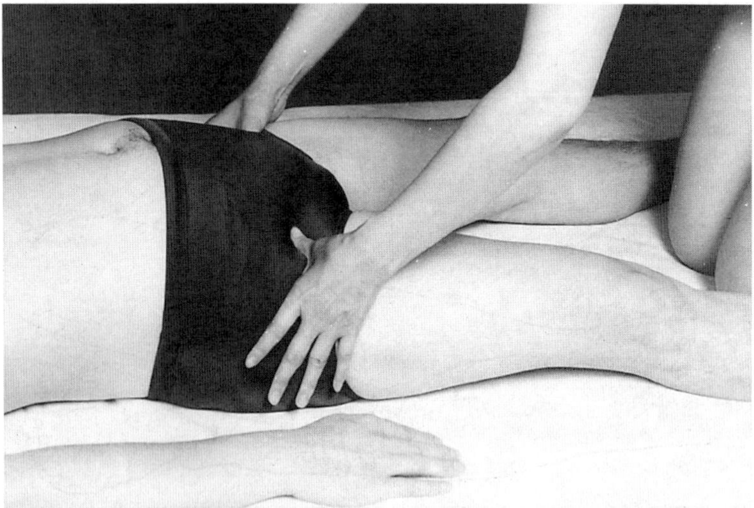

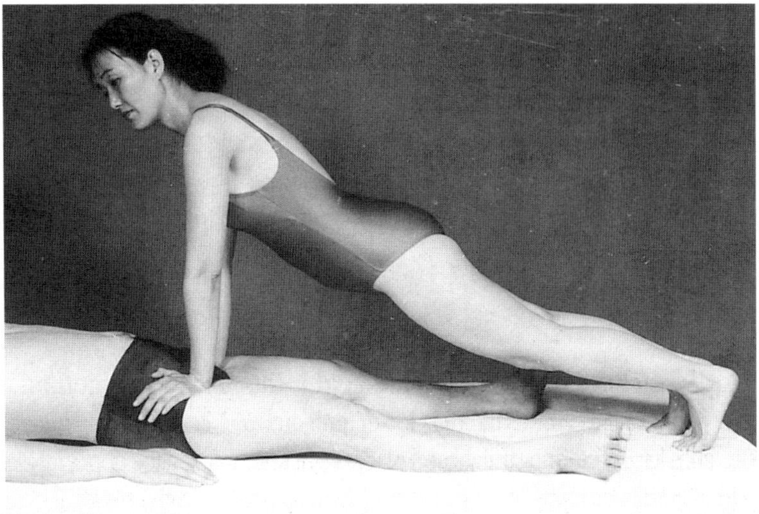

照片 (Photo) 20

圖示 (Fig.) 15

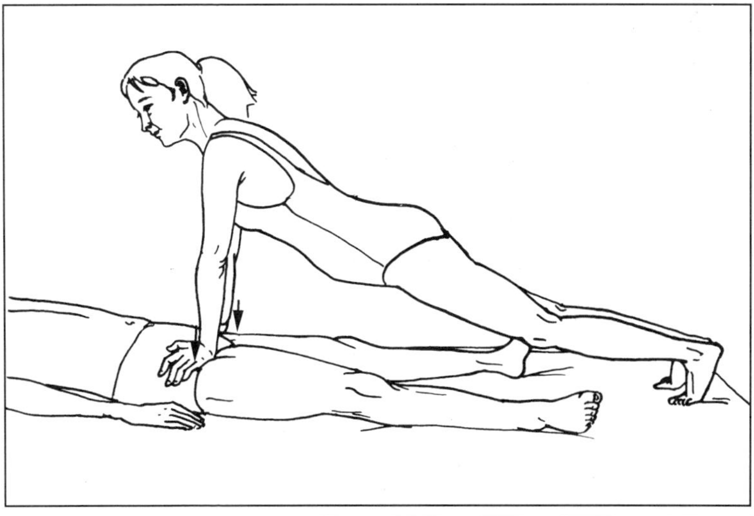

16 背伸跖趾關節法：

被按摩者右下肢外旋屈髖屈膝位，左下肢伸直，將右膝關節置於按摩者雙膝關節內上方，按摩者盤坐於足側，左手2、3、4、5指置其前足背側，掌根置於同水平跖側，以屈指之力使足跖趾關節極度背伸（見照片21、22和圖示16），反復操作4－6次。一側完畢更換另一側。

Stretching metatarsophalangeal joints backward method:

The patient revolves the right lower limb outward, bends hip and knees, stretches left lower limb straight and places right knee joint on the upper inside part of both knee joints of the massagist. The massagist sits with crossed legs at the side of foot, places the 2nd, 3rd, 4th and 5th fingers of left hand on the dorsum of the patient's front foot and the palm root on the sole at the same level, and uses the force of bent fingers to stretch the metatarsophalangeal joints backward to the utmost (see Photos 21, 22 and Fig. 16). Repeat the manipulation 4-6 times. Do one side, then the other.

照片 (Photo) 21

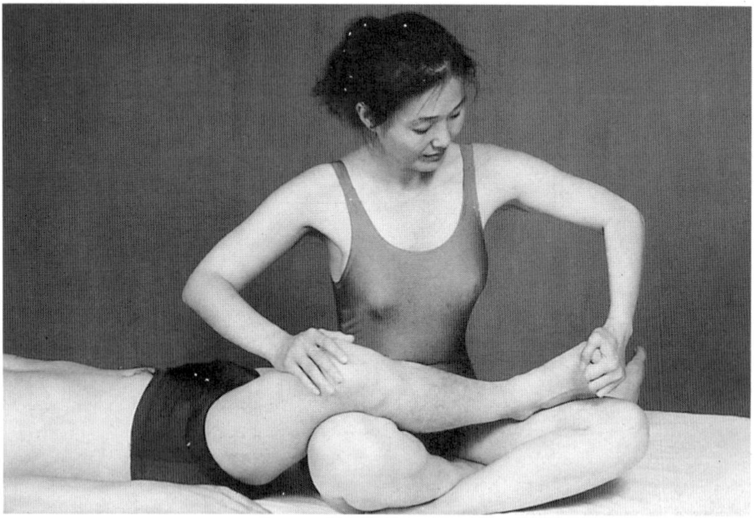

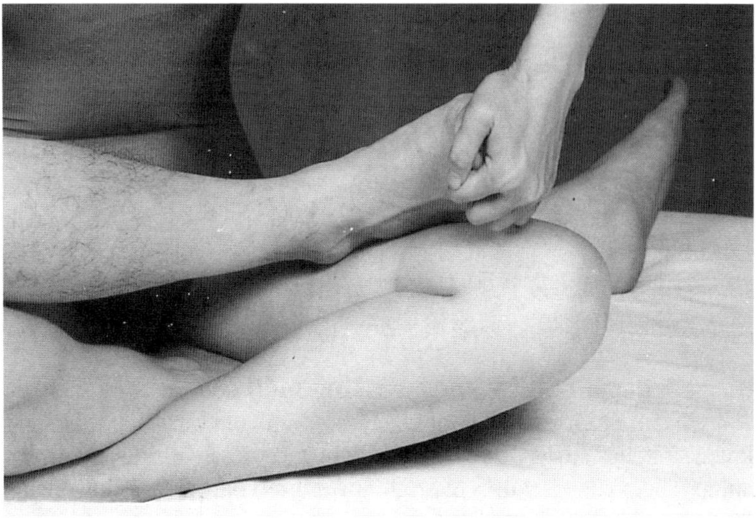

照片 (Photo) 22

圖示 (Fig.) 16

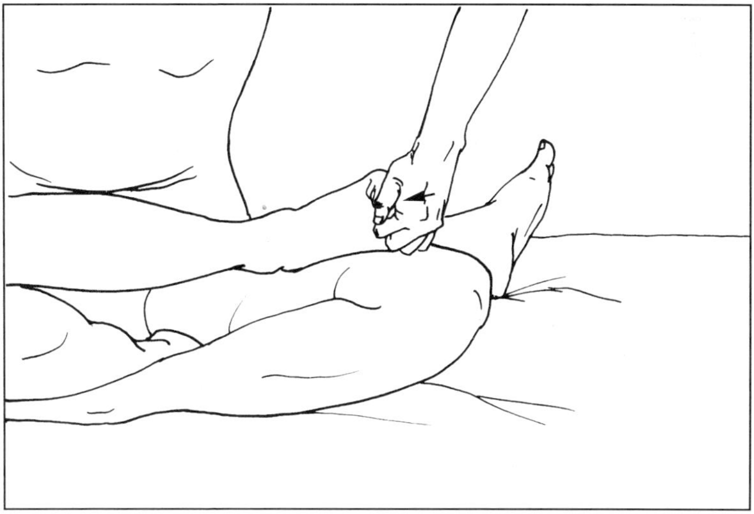

17 前臂滾按法：

按摩者右下肢外旋並屈髖屈膝，左下肢伸直壓於被按摩者的前踝部，被按摩者右下肢外旋，稍屈髖、膝關節，並置於按摩者右下肢之上。按摩者先用右肘按壓腹股溝，按壓時間以30秒為宜（見照片23和圖示17）。而後改用前臂的近端從大腿內側開始行前臂滾按法，至膝關節內上方（見照片24、圖示18和照片25）。滾按部位主要是大腿前內側肌群。反復滾按2－4次。一側完畢更換另一側。

Forearm rolling and pressing method:

The massagist revolves the right lower limb outward, bends hip and knee, stretches the left lower limb straight and presses the patient's front ankle. The patient revolves the right lower limb outward, slightly bends the hip and knee joints and places them on the massagist's right lower limb. The massagist first presses the groin with right elbow, best for 30 seconds (see Photo 23 and Fig. 17) and then rolls and presses from the inside of the thigh to the inside upper part of knee joint (see Photo 24, Fig. 18 and photo 25) with near end of front arm. Rolling mainly the front inside muscles of the thigh. Repeat the manipulation 2-4 times.Do one side, then the other.

照片 (Photo) 23

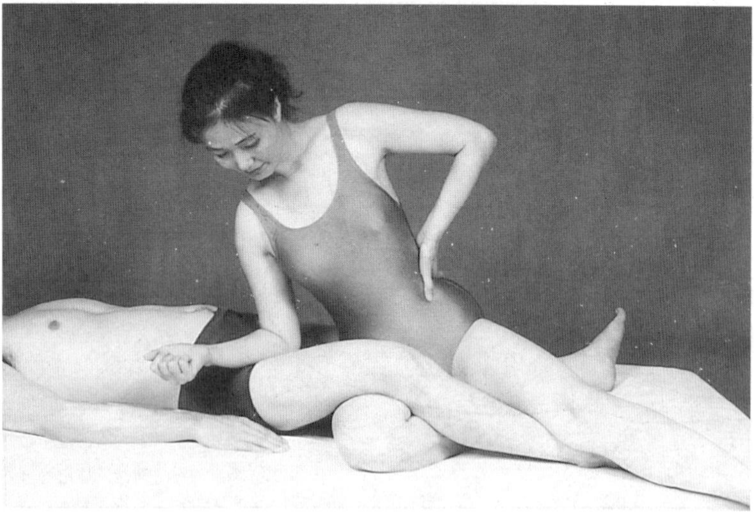

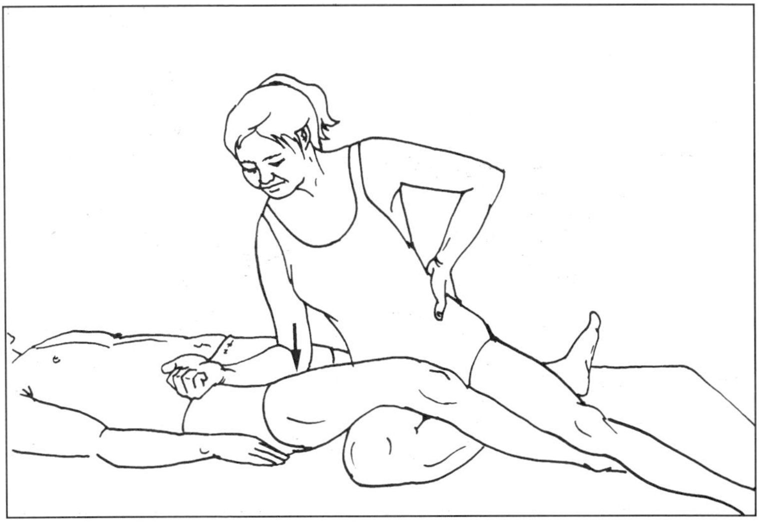

圖示 (Fig.) 17

照片 (Photo) 24

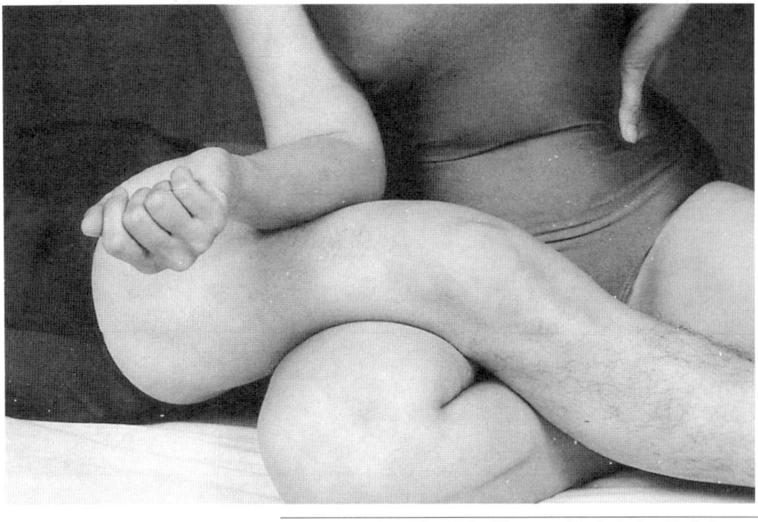

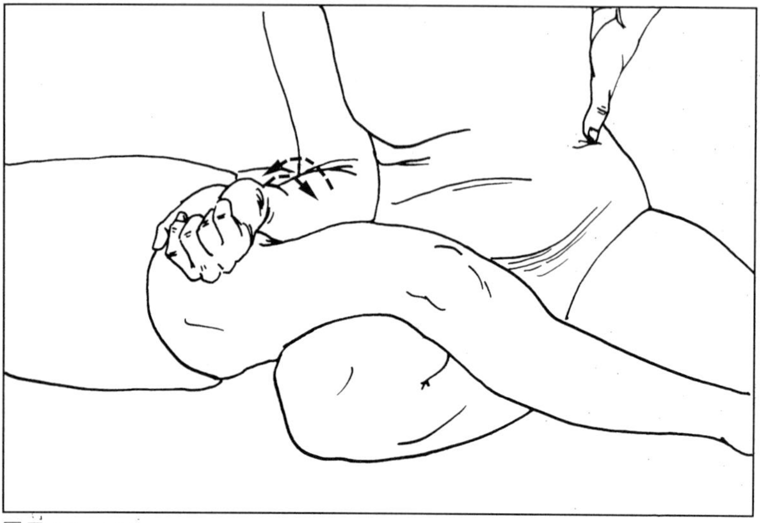
圖示 (Fig.) 18

照片 (Photo) 25
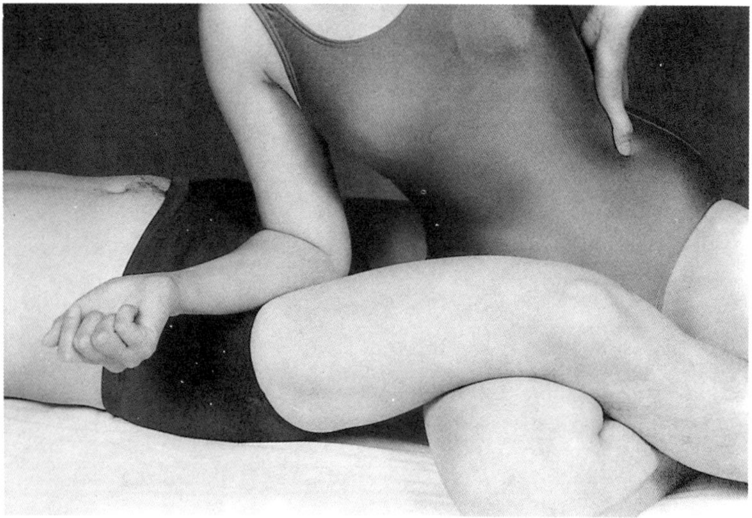

18 肘按揉法：

體位同上，被按摩者右下肢改稍內旋；按摩者用右肘後方依次從大腿外側按揉至膝關節外上方，反復操作2－4次（見照片26、27和圖示19）。一側完畢更換另一側。

Elbow-pressing and rubbing method:

In same position, the paient with right lower limb slightly revolving inward. The massagist rubs from the outside of thigh to the outside upper part of knee joint with the back of right elbow. Repeat the manipulation 2-4 times (see Photos 26, 27 and Fig. 19). Do one side, then the other.

照片 (Photo) 26

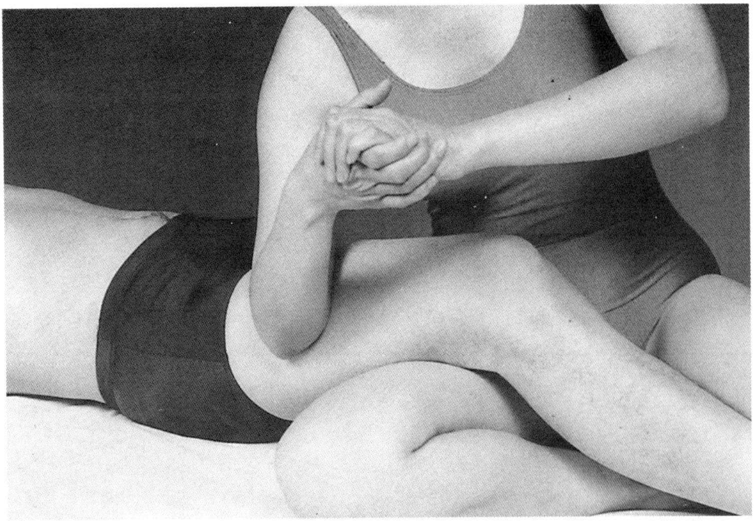

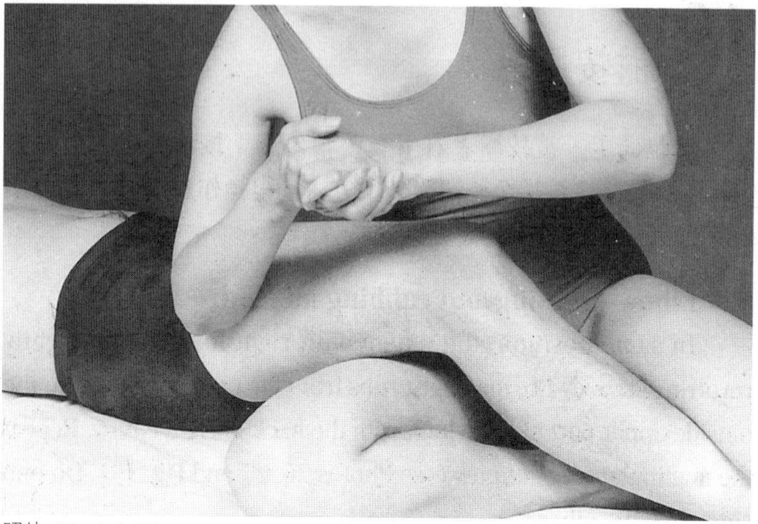
照片 (Photo) 27

圖示 (Fig.) 19
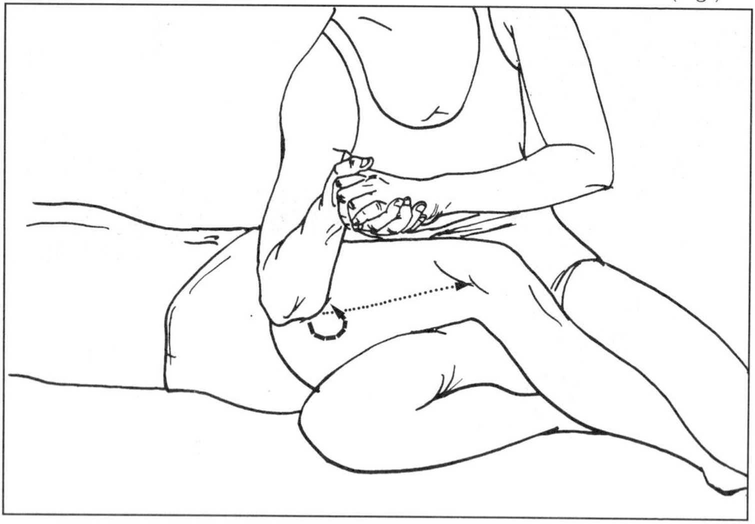

19 提搓法：

體位同上。按摩者用右肘後方從被按摩者下肢近端外側開始，由下向上提搓外側肌群至膝關節外上方處，反復操作2－4次（見照片28、29和圖示20）。一側完畢更換另一側。

Lifting and kneading method:

In same position. The massagist uses the back of right elbow to lift and knead the outside muscles downward to upward from the outside of the patient's lower limb near end to the outside upper part of knee joint. Repeat the manipulation 2-4 times (see Photos 28, 29 and Fig. 20). Do one side, then the other.

照片 (Photo) 28

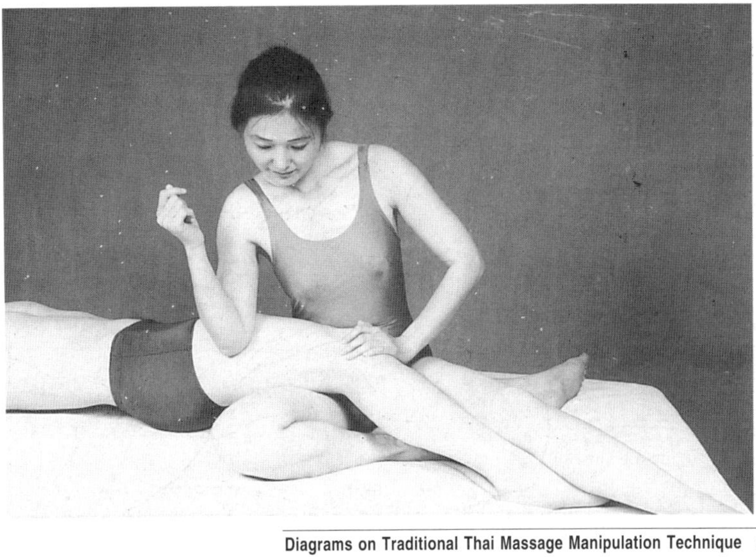

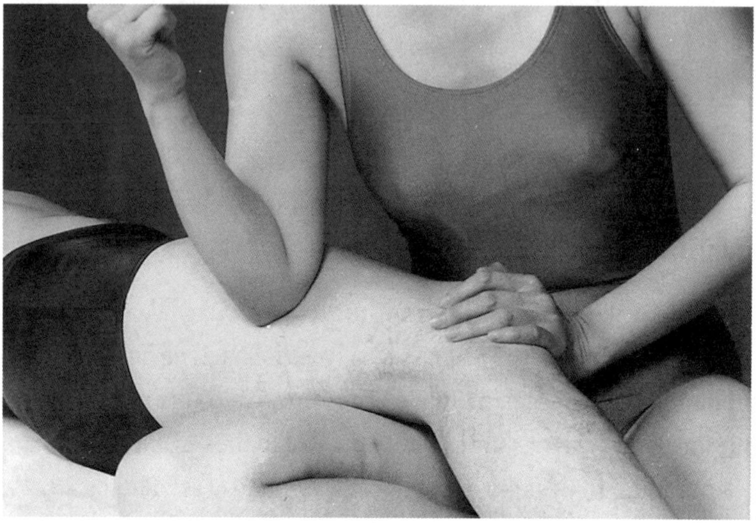

照片 (Photo) 29

圖示 (Fig.) 20

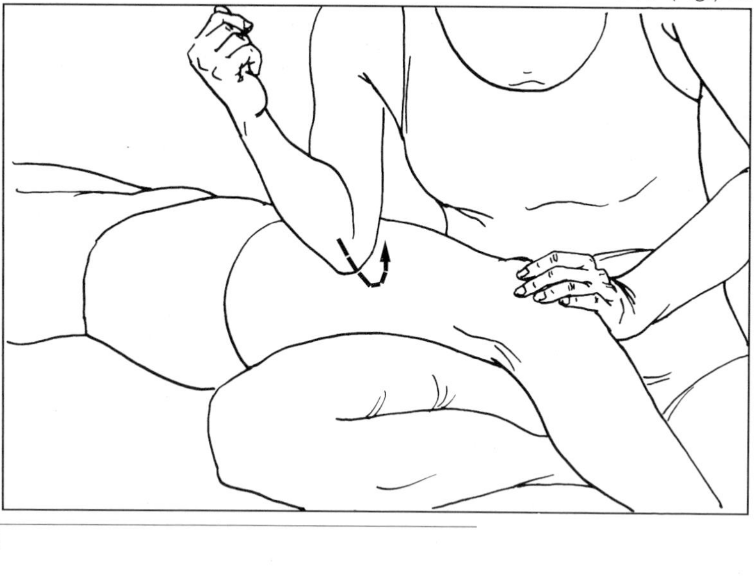

20 刮筋法：

體位同上。按摩者雙手拇指與其餘四指的指端分別置於被按摩者髕骨的內外緣，以五指的對合之力，沿髕骨兩側做按揉動作（見照片**30**和圖示**21**），力量的輕重，應以患者能忍受為度。順逆時針各操作**4－6**次。一側完畢更換另一側。

Muscle scraping method:

In same position. The massagist places thumbs and other four finger tips of both hands on the patient's inside and outside of kneecap and presses and rubs along both sides of kneecap with the joint force of five fingers (see Photo 30 and Fig. 21). The patient should be able to bear the force. Repeat the manipulation 4-6 times in both clockwise and counter-clockwise respectively. Do one side, then the other.

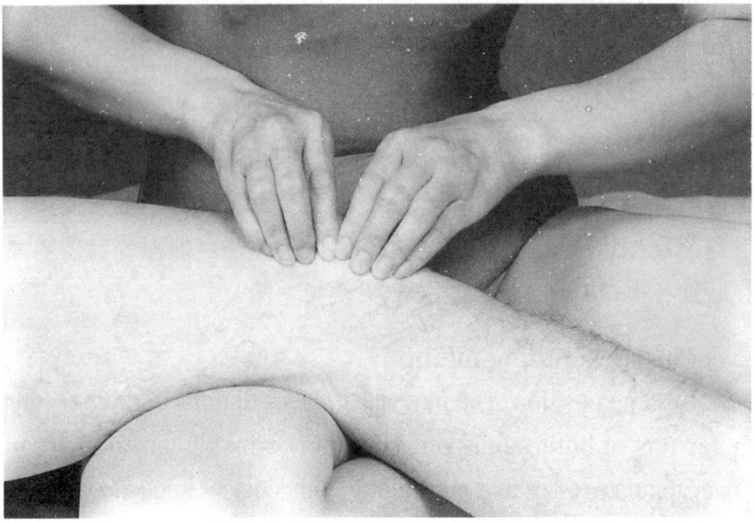

照片 (Photo) 30

圖示 (Fig.) 21

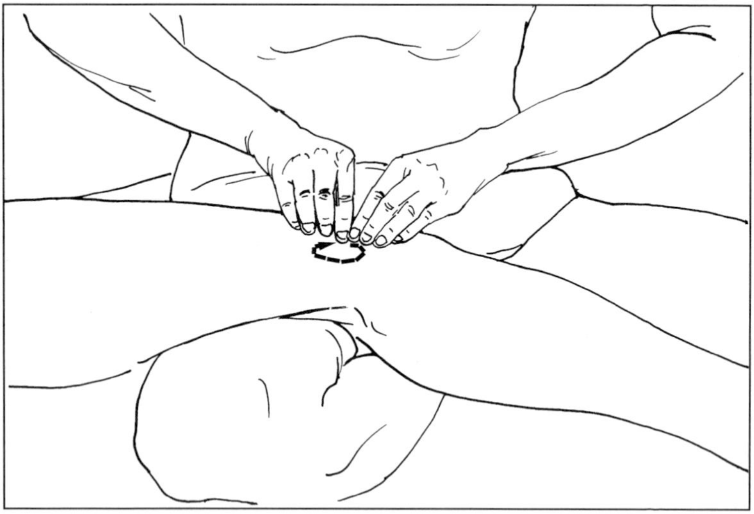

21 按提法：

體位同上。按摩者一側上肢屈肘，用尺骨鷹嘴部位從被按摩者膝關節外下方開始沿脛前肌走行向肢體遠端按提。先用尺骨鷹嘴部位向下按壓1－2秒鐘（見照片31和圖示22），再用肘後上方由下向上提搓小腿外側肌群，如此邊按提（見照片32和圖示23），邊向肢體遠端移動至踝關節上方止，反復操作2－4次。一側完畢更換另一側。

Pressing and lifting method:

In same position. The massagist bends the upper limb at one side and presses and lifts from the outside lower part of the patient's knee joint along the front shin muscle to the far end of limb with the ulna hawk beak. First press downward with the ulna hawk beak for 1-2 seconds (see Photo 31 and Fig. 22) and then lift and knead the outside muscles of shank from downward to upward with the rear upside of elbow. Press and lift in this way (see Photo 32 and Fig. 23) while moving to the far end of limb and stop on the upper part of ankle joint. Repeat the manipulation 2-4 times. Do one side, then the other.

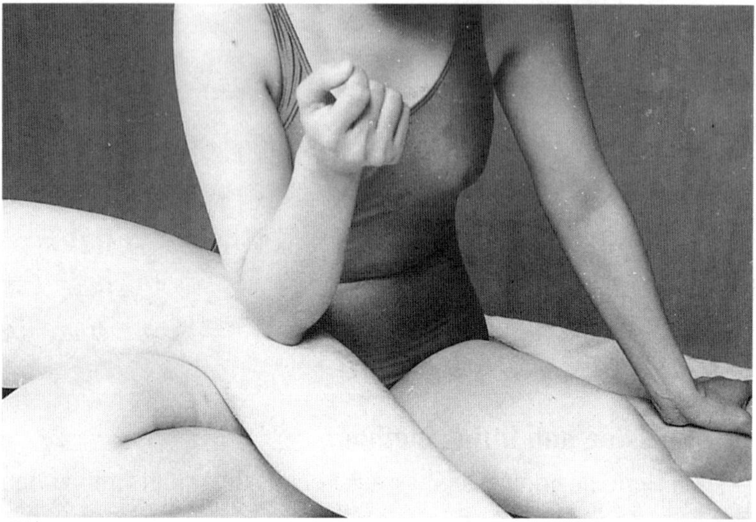
照片 (Photo) 31

圖示 (Fig.) 22
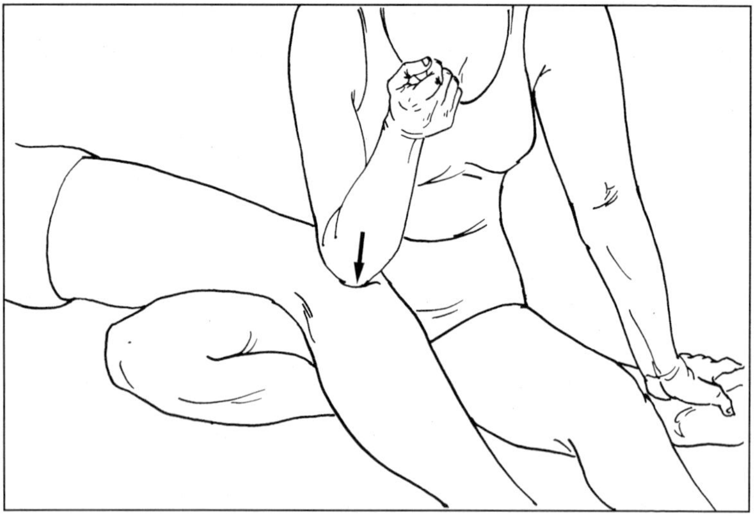

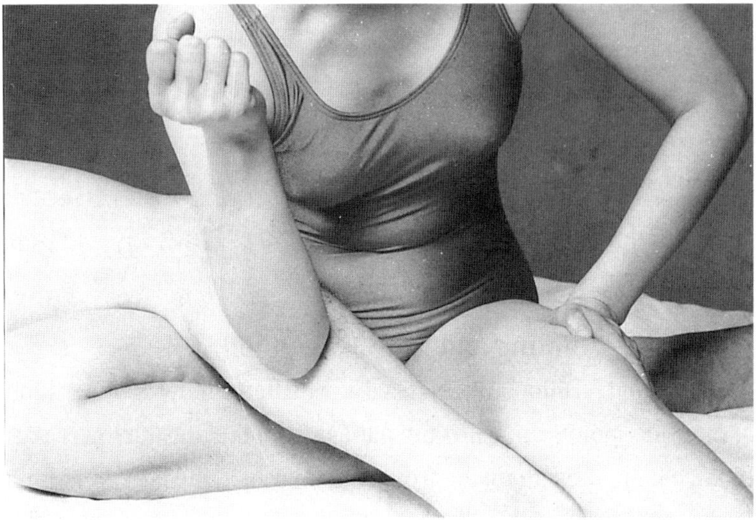

照片 (Photo) 32

圖示 (Fig.) 23

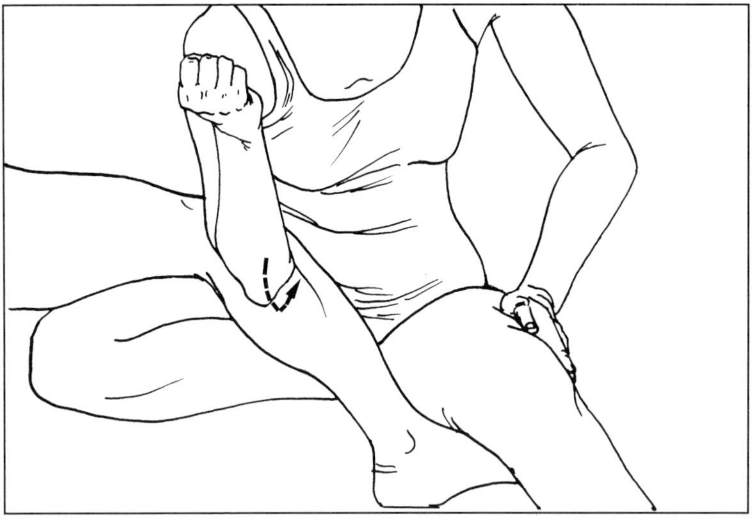

22 肘點揉法：

體位同上。按摩者一側上肢屈肘，用尺骨鷹嘴部位從被按摩者膝關節外下方開始，沿脛前肌走行，向肢體遠端邊點邊揉至踝關節上方止，反復操作2－4次（見照片33和圖示24）。一側完畢更換另一側。

Elbow-pointing and rubbing method:

In same position. The massagist, with bent elbow of upper limb at one side, points and rubs the patient from the outside lower part of knee joint, then along the front shin muscle to the far end of limb and stops at the upper part of the ankle joint. Repeat the manipulation 2-4 times (see Photo 33 and Fig. 24). Do one side, then the other.

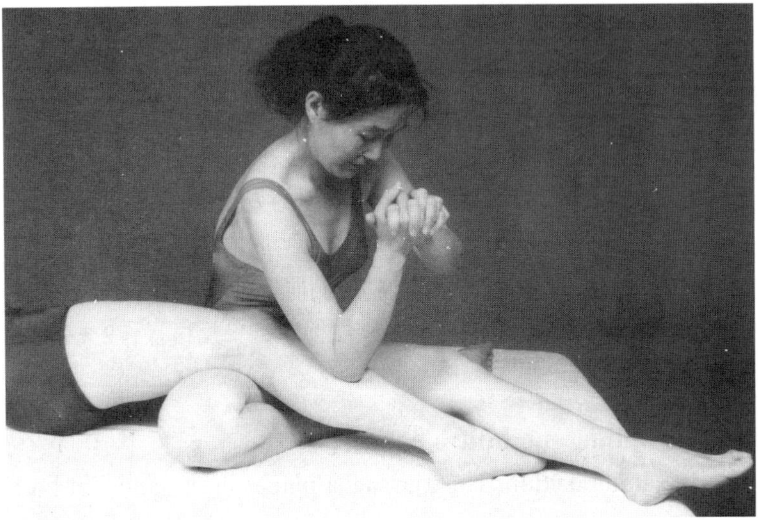

照片 (Photo) 33

圖示 (Fig.) 24

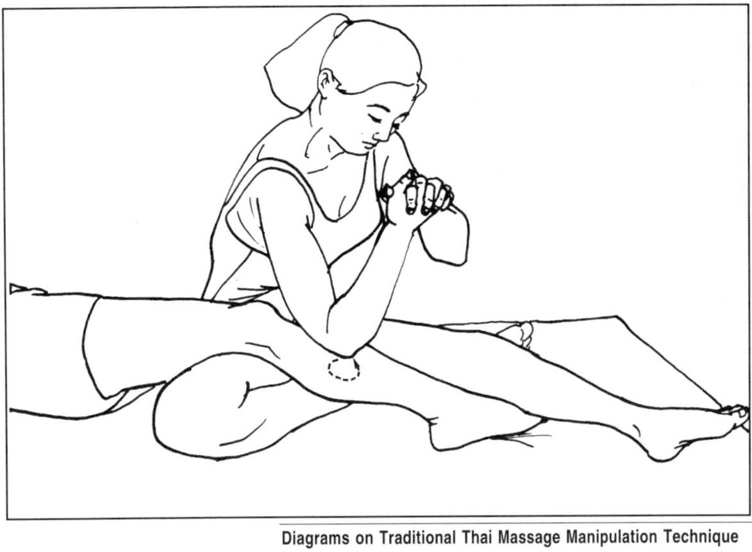

23 捏拿法：

體位同上。按摩者雙手分別置於被按摩者膝關節前下方的兩側，2、3、4、5指指端相對，置於小腿的後正中線部位，拇指置於小腿前方，先後捏拿小腿後方的內外側肌群，先將外側肌肉外旋（見照片34和圖示25），再將內側肌肉內旋（見照片35和圖示26），由此自上而下，捏拿至踝關節上方，反復操作2－4次。一側完畢更換另一側。

Kneading method:

In same position. The massagist places both hands on both sides on the lower front part of a knee joint of the patient respectively. The 2nd, 3rd, 4th and 5th finger tips of both hands touch each other and are placed on the rear central line of shank and thumbs placed on the front of shank. Knead the inside and outside muscles of rear shank. First revolve the outside muscle outward (see Photo 34 and Fig. 25) and then revolve the inside muscle inward (see Photo 35 and Fig. 26) and knead from upward to downward to the upper part of ankle joint. Repeat the manipulation 2-4 times. Do one side, then the other.

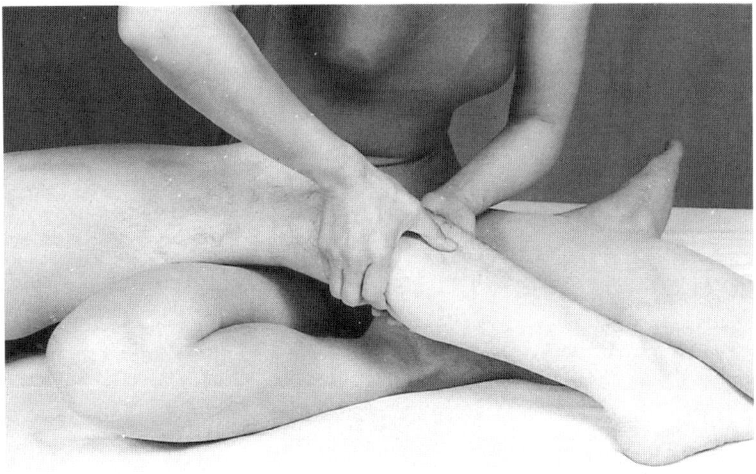

照片 (Photo) 34

圖示 (Fig.) 25

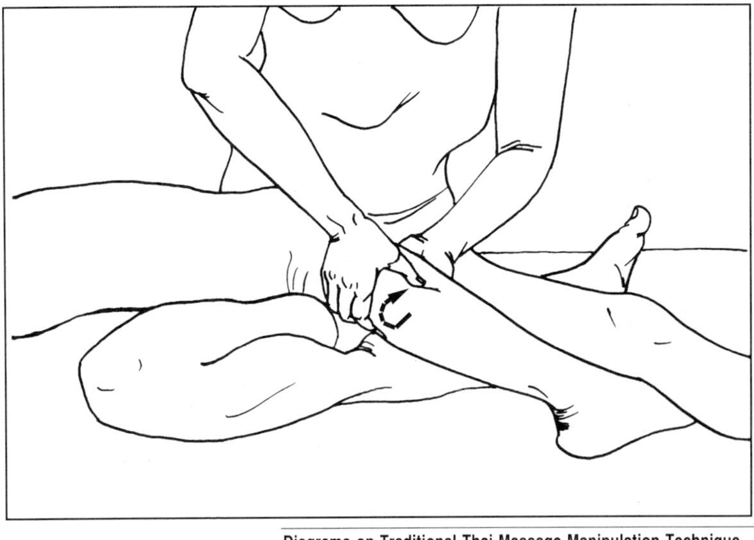

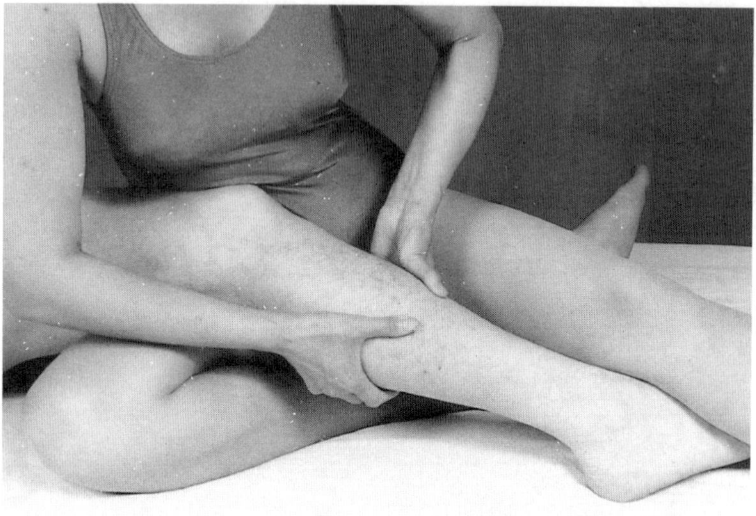

照片 (Photo) 35

圖示 (Fig.) 26

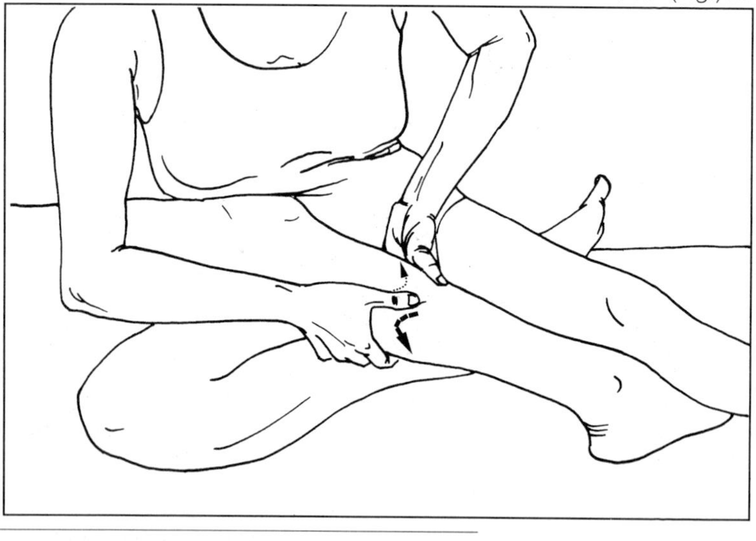

24 指按揉法：

體位同上。按摩者一手拇指置於被按摩者膝關節外下方，**2**、**3**、**4**、**5**指置於同水平的小腿後側肌群處，用拇指及其餘四指指腹按揉小腿前後方（見照片**36**和圖示**27**），邊按揉邊向遠端移動至踝關節上方，如此往返按揉，反復操作**2－4**次。一側完畢更換另一側。

Digital-pressing and rubbing method:

In same position. The massagist places a thumb on the lower outside part of the patient's knee joint and the 2nd, 3rd, 4th and 5th fingers on the muscles at rear shank at the same level. Use the thumb and other four finger insides to press and rub the front and rear part of shank (see Photo 36 and Fig. 27) to the upper part of ankle joint at the far end to and fro for 2-4 times. Do one side, then the other.

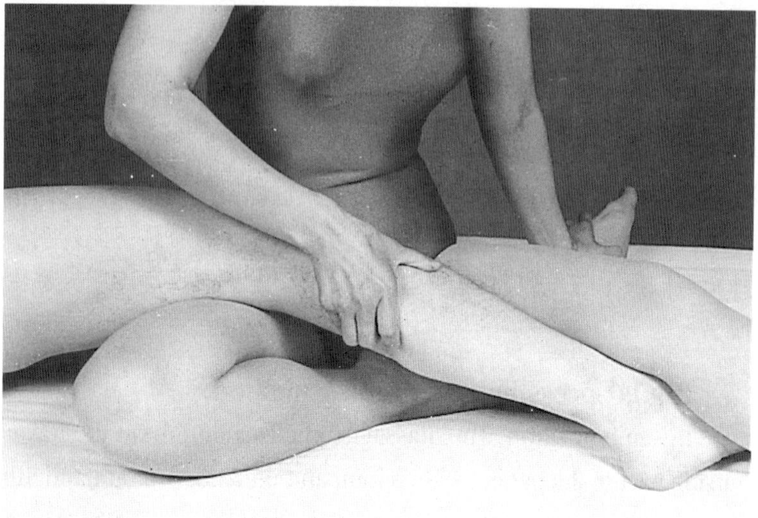

照片 (Photo) 36

圖示 (Fig.) 27

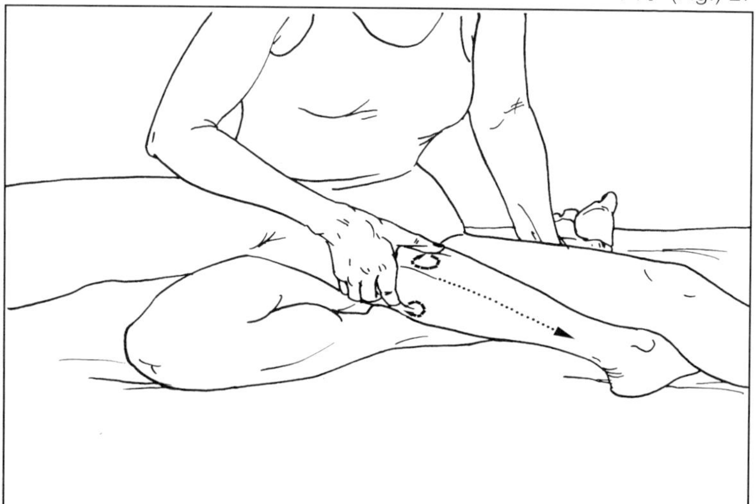

25 肘揉足底法：

按摩者雙下肢外旋、屈髖屈膝、小腿交叉盤坐位；而被按摩者外旋一側下肢，略屈髖屈膝，置於按摩者大腿之上（見照片**37**）。按摩者左上肢屈肘，用尺骨鷹嘴部位從足跟部按揉至足遠端的跖側，反復操作**2－4**次（見照片**38**和圖示**28**）。一側完畢更換另一側。

Elbow-rubbing sole method:

The massagist revolves both lower limbs outward, bends hip and knees and sits cross-legged. The patient revolves the lower limb at one side outward, slightly bends hip and knee and places them on the massagist's thigh (see Photo 37). The massagist bends the elbow of left upper limb and presses and rubs from the heel of foot to the sole at the far end with the ulna hawk beak. Repeat the manipulation 2-4 times (see Photo 38 and Fig. 28). Do one side, then the other.

照片 (Photo) 37

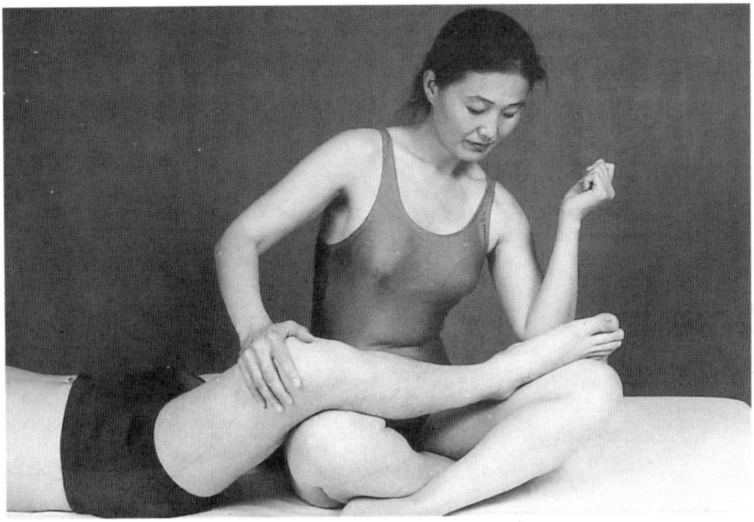

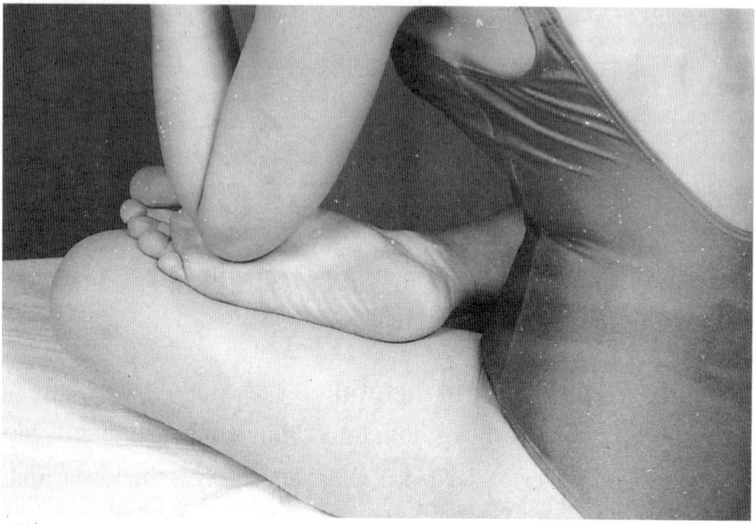

照片 (Photo) 38

圖示 (Fig.) 28

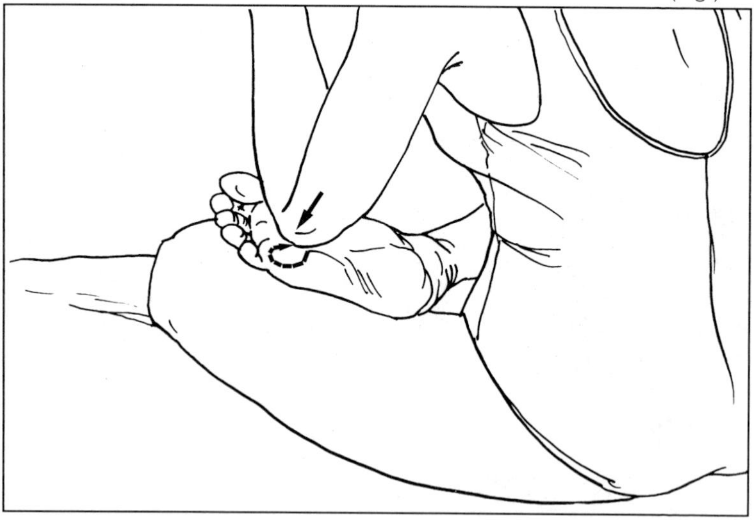

26 按揉趾腹法：

體位同上。按摩者用左手拇指依次從被按摩者足拇趾趾腹按揉至第五趾趾腹，反復操作**2－4**次（見照片**39**和圖示**29**）。一側完畢更換另一側。

Pressing and rubbing toe inside method:

In same position. The massagist using left thumb presses and rubs the inside of the patient's 1st toe to the 5th toe in proper order. Repeat the manipulation 2-4 times (see Photo 39 and Fig. 29). Do one side, then the other.

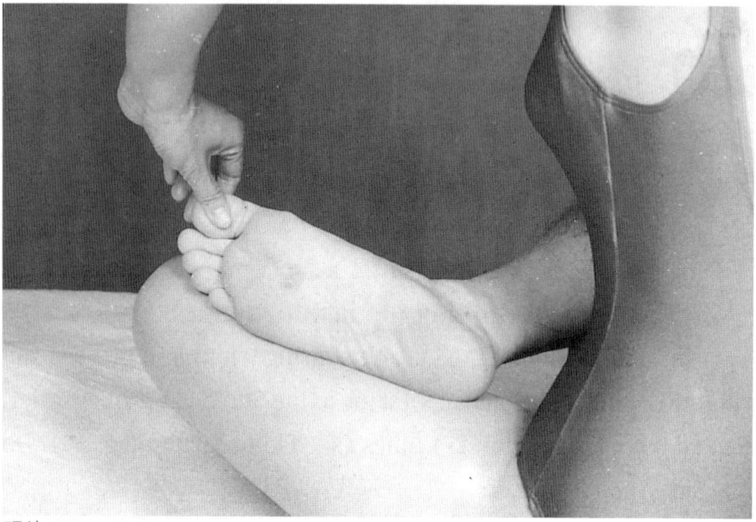
照片 (Photo) 39

圖示 (Fig.) 29

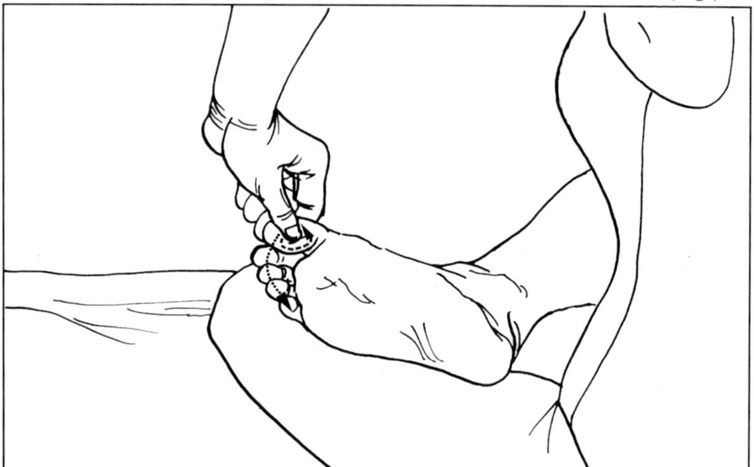

27 按揉跖趾關節法：

體位同上。按摩者用左手拇指依次從被按摩者足第一趾跖趾關節的跖側向足背側施力，按揉至第五趾跖趾關節的跖側，反復操作**2－4**次（見照片**40**和圖示**30**）。一側完畢更換另一側。

Pressing and rubbing metatarsophalangeal joints method:

In same position. The massagist presses and rubs with the force of left thumb from the patient's 1st toe metatarsophalangeal joint sole to the 5th toe metatarsophalangeal joint sole. Repeat the manipulation 2-4 times (see Photo 40 and Fig. 30). Do one side, then the other.

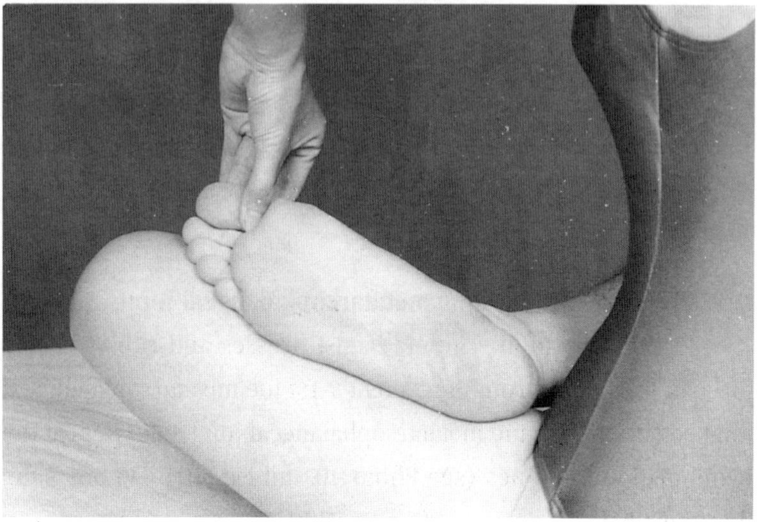

照片 (Photo) 40

圖示 (Fig.) 30

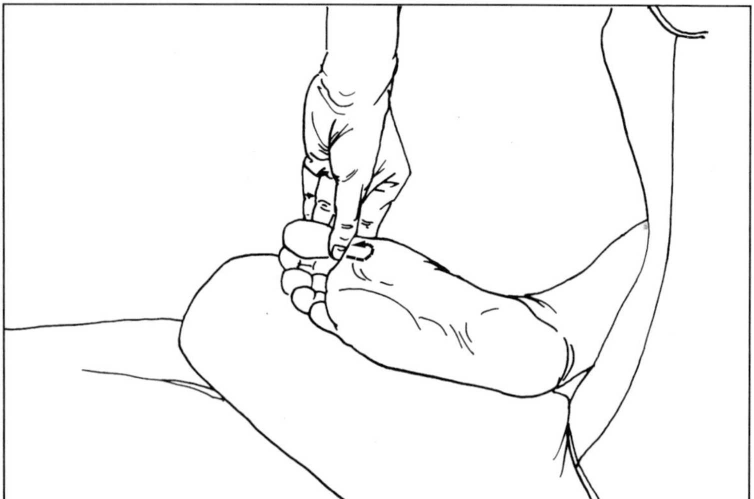

28 按壓足底法：

體位同上。按摩者左手拇指指腹置於被按摩者足的跖側，其餘四指扶於背側，以第一跖趾關節、第五跖趾關節和兩者之間為起點，分三條刺激線依次用拇指指腹按壓至足跟部，反復操作2－4次（見照片41和圖示31）。一側完畢更換另一側。

Sole pressing method:

In same position. The massagist places left thumb inside on the patient's sole and the other four fingers on the dorsum of foot. Starting from the place between the 1st and 5th toe metatarsophalangeal joints and the two, and dividing into three stimulating lines, press to heel in proper order. Repeat the manipulation 2-4 times (see Photo 41 and Fig. 31). Do one side, then the other.

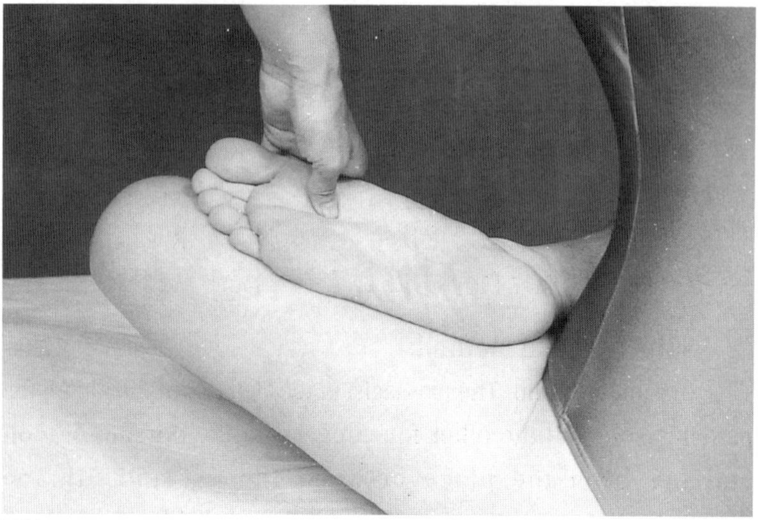

照片 (Photo) 41

圖示 (Fig.) 31

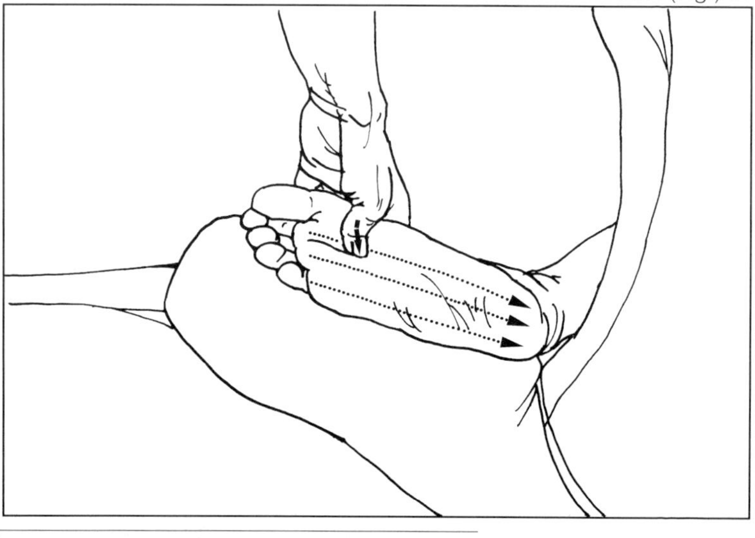

29 拳壓足底法：

體位同上。按摩者手握實拳，以2、3、4、5指近端指間關節的背側為着力點，旋轉按揉被按摩者足底（見照片42）。從前足的跖側按揉至足根部（見照片43和圖示32），反復操作2－4次。一側完畢更換另一側。

Fist-pressing sole method:

In same position. The massagist clenches a fist, and with the force of near end backs of 2nd, 3rd, 4th and 5th finger joints, rolls, presses and rubs the patient's sole (see photo 42) from the sole of front foot to heel (see Photo 43 and Fig. 32). Repeat the manipulation 2-4 times. Do one side, then the other.

照片 (Photo) 42

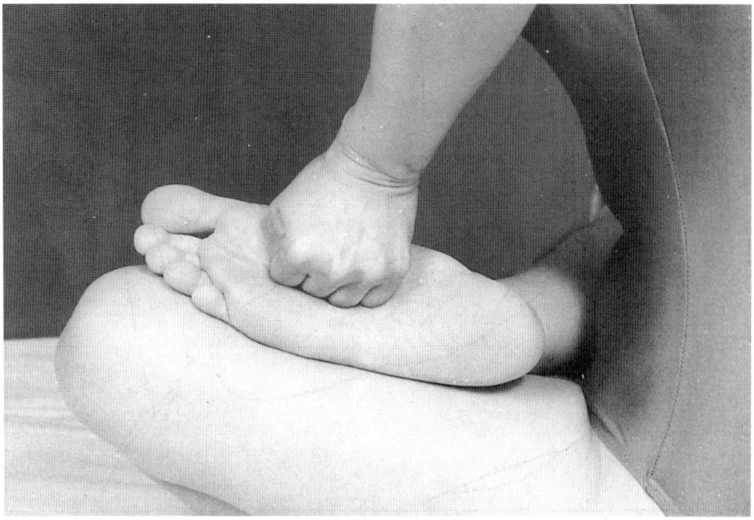

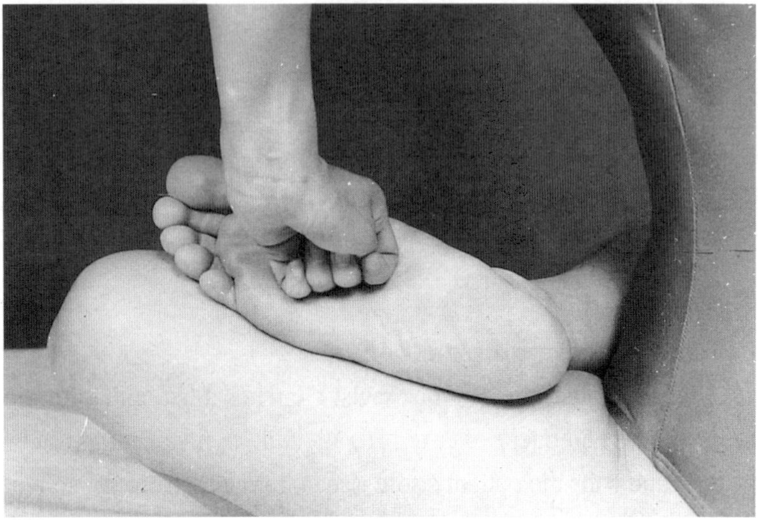

照片 (Photo) 43

圖示 (Fig.) 32

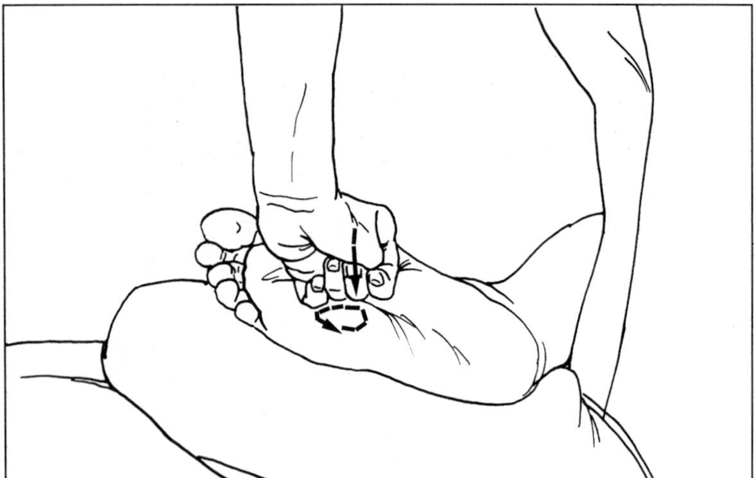

30 叩擊法：

體位同上。按摩者手握實拳，用小指及小魚際尺側面為着力點，從被按摩者前足跖側均勻施力向足跟部叩擊，反復操作**2－4**次（見照片**44**、**45**和圖示**33**）。一側完畢更換另一側。

Tapping method:

In same position. The massagist clenches a fist, and with the force of the little finger and small thenar ulna side, taps the sole of the patient's front foot to heel with even force. Repeat the manipulation2-4 times (see Photos 44, 45 and Fig.33). Do one side, the n the other.

照片 (Photo) 44

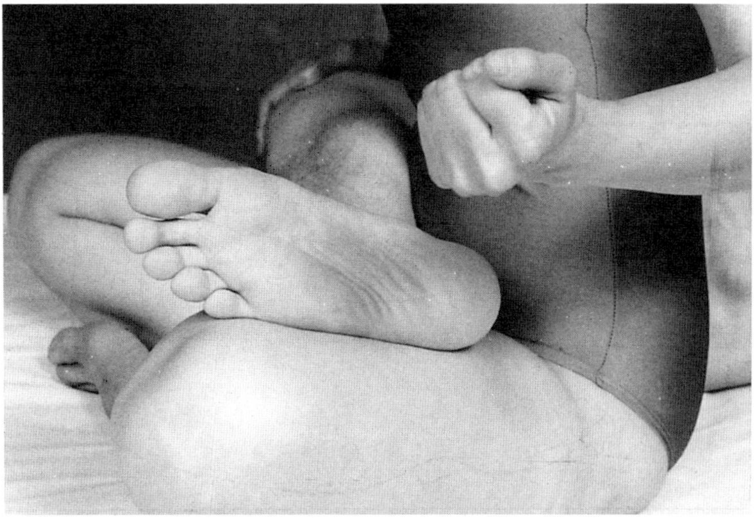

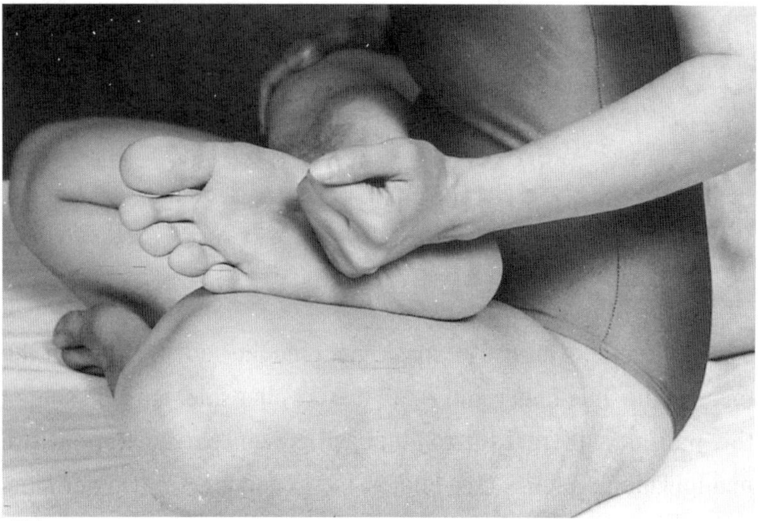

照片 (Photo) 45

圖示 (Fig.) 33

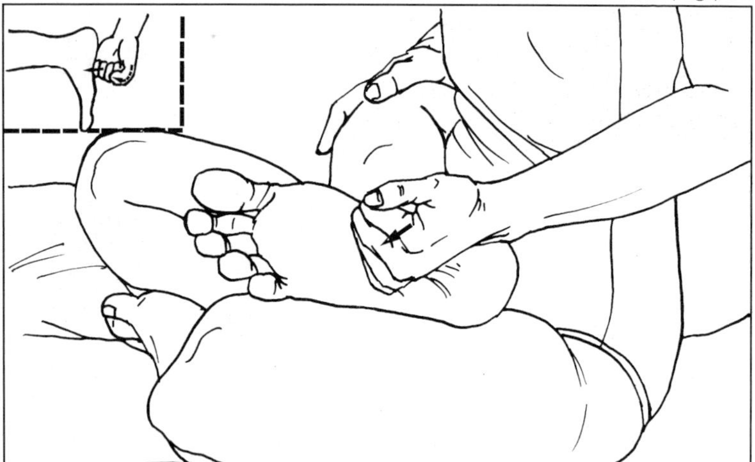

31 指壓小腿內側法：

體位同上。按摩者雙手拇指伸直，以指腹為着力點，從被按摩者內踝後上方開始，沿脛骨內側緣向肢體近端行指腹按壓法，至膝關節內下方，反復操作**2－4**次（見照片**46**和圖示**34**）。一側完畢更換另一側。

Digital-pressing inside of shank method:

In same position. The massagist stretches both thumbs straight. With the force of thumb inside, press from the patient's rear upper side of inner ankle, along the inside of shin bone to the lower inside part of knee joint at the near end of limb. Repeat the manipulation 2-4 times (see Photo 46 and Fig. 34). Do one side, then the other.

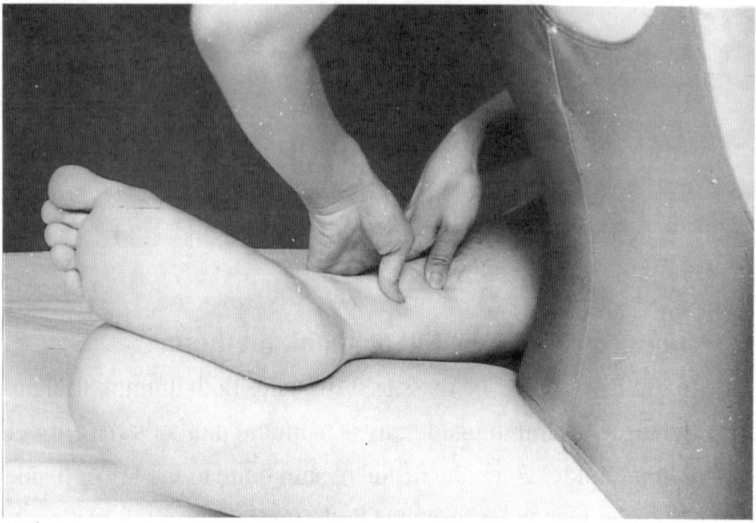

照片 (Photo) 46

圖示 (Fig.) 34

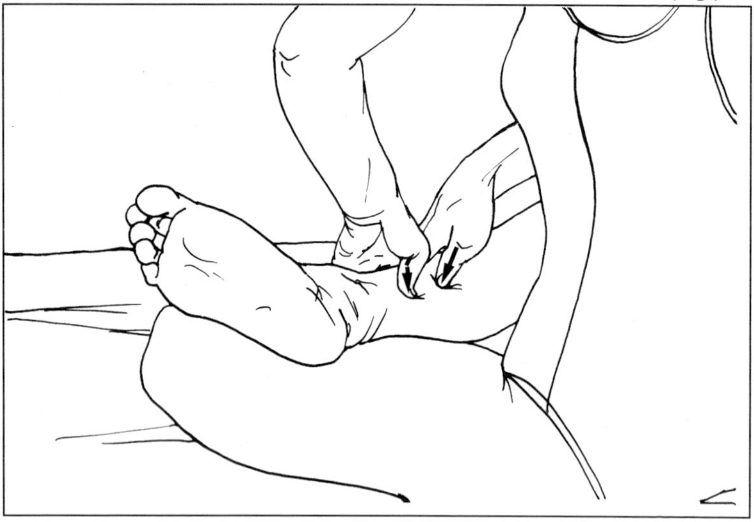

32 內旋小腿三頭肌：

體位同上。按摩者的雙手2、3、4、5指置於被按摩者膝關節前下方，拇指置於同水平的小腿後方肌群近端，屈五指遠端指間關節，以對指之力將小腿三頭肌向內前方旋起，反復操作2－4次（見照片47和圖示35）。一側完畢更換另一側。

Revolving shank triceps inward:

In same position. The massagist places the 2nd, 3rd, 4th and 5th fingers of both hands on the lower front side of the patient's knee joint and the thumbs on the near end of back muscles of shank at the same level, bends the far end joints of five fingers and revolves the shank triceps inward and forward with the force of fingers. Repeat the manipulation 2-4 times (see Photo 47 and Fig. 35). Do one side, then the other.

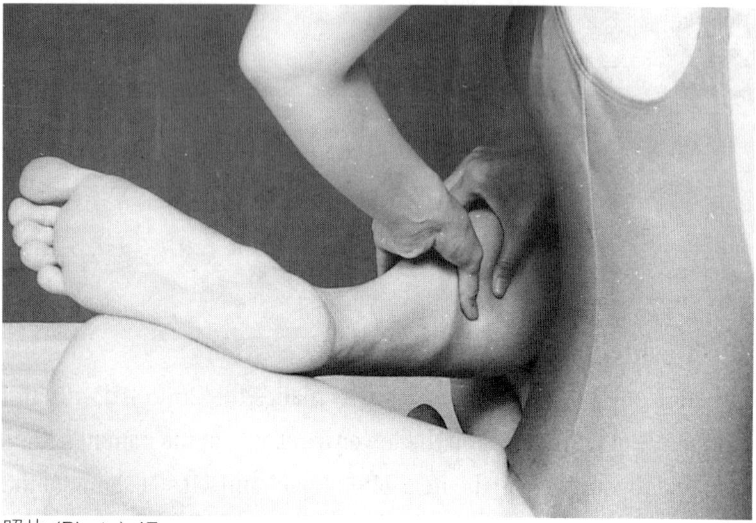
照片 (Photo) 47

圖示 (Fig.) 35
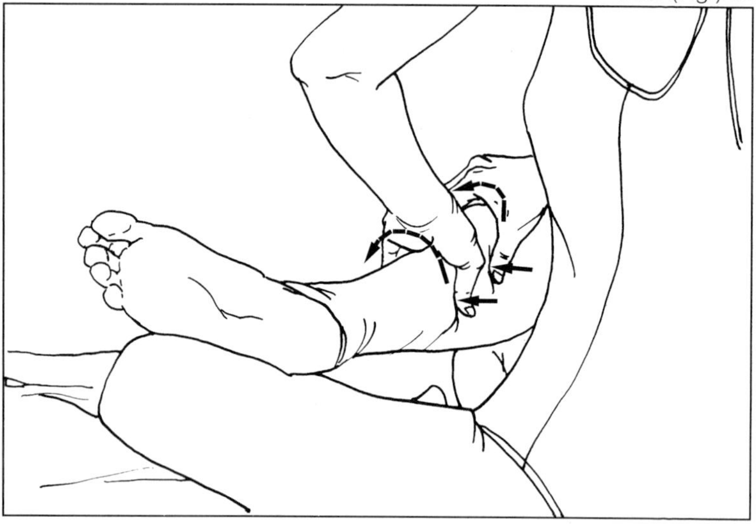

33 提拉點壓法：

體位同上。按摩者雙手掌心向上，拇指置於被按摩者膝關節前下方內側，**2**、**3**、**4**、**5**指併攏，置於同水平的小腿後側，以五指對合之力，邊將小腿三頭肌向內前方提拉，邊用拇指指端點壓小腿內側緣，至踝關節上方，反復操作**2－4**次（見照片**48**和圖示**36**）。一側完畢更換另一側。

Lifting, pulling, pointing and pressing method:

In same position. The massagist turns both palms upward and places both thumbs on the inside of the lower front part of the patient's knee joint, closes together the 2nd, 3rd, 4th and 5th fingers and places them on the back of shank at the same level. With the joint force of five fingers, lift and pull the shank triceps inward and forward while pointing and pressing the inside of shank with thumb tips to the upper part of ankle joint. Repeat the manipulation 2-4 times (see Photo 48 and Fig. 36). Do one side, then the other.

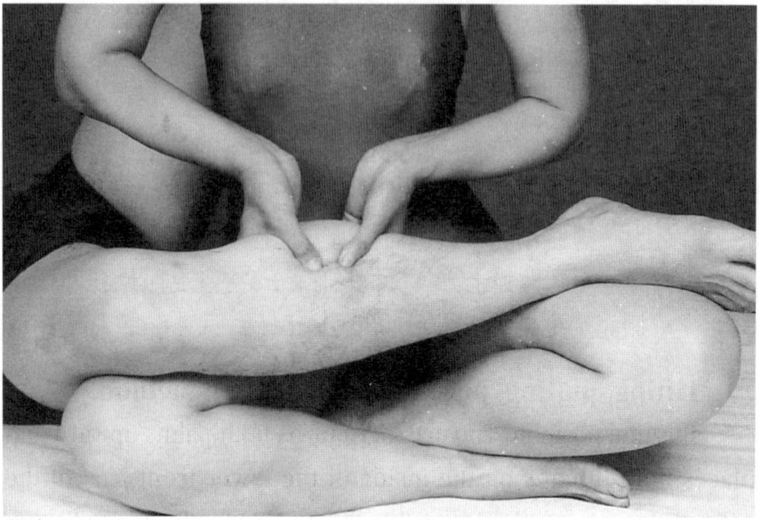
照片 (Photo) 48

圖示 (Fig.) 36
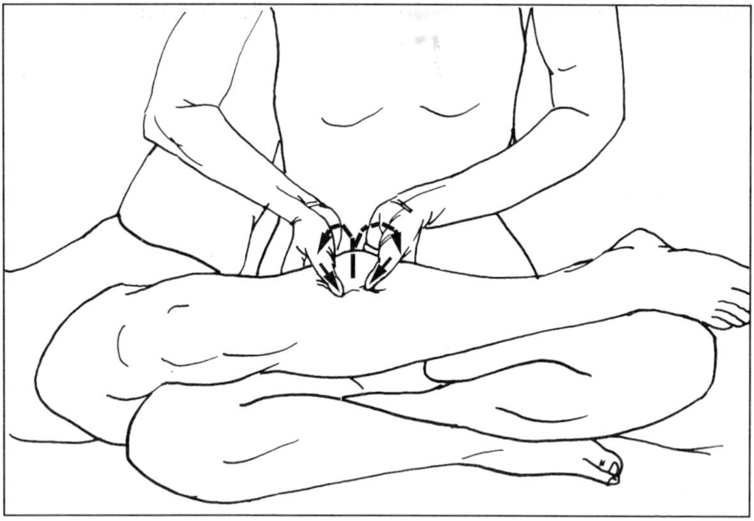

34 內旋大腿後方肌群：

體位同上。按摩者右手拇指置於被按摩者膕窩後上方，**2**、**3**、**4**、**5**指併攏微屈，置於同水平的大腿內側肌群處，以五指對指之力將大腿後側肌肉向內前方旋推，反復操作**2－4**次（見照片**49**和圖示**37**）。一側完畢更換另一側。

Revolving rear muscles of thigh inward:

In same position. The massagist places right thumb at the back upper part of the patient's hollow of knee and closes together and slightly bends 2nd, 3rd, 4th and 5th fingers and places them on the inside muscles of thigh at the same level. With the joint force of five fingers, revolve and push the rear muscle of thigh inward and forward. Repeat the manipulation 2-4 times (see Photo 49 and Fig. 37). Do one side, then the other.

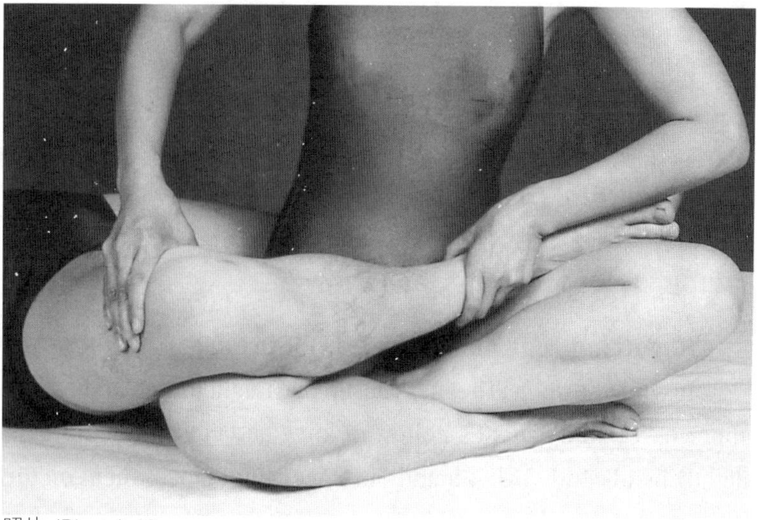

照片 (Photo) 49

圖示 (Fig.) 37

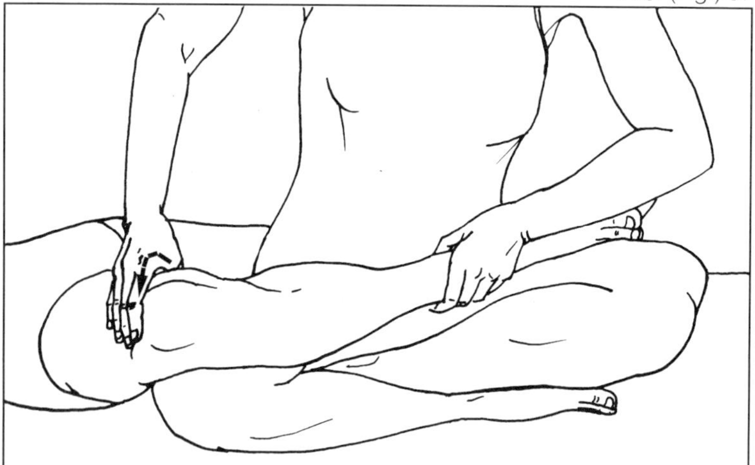

35 拇指按壓法：

被按摩者右下肢外旋並屈髖屈膝位，將足置於按摩者的左側腹股溝處，按摩者為跪位，左手握被按摩者踝關節前方，右手置其膕窩內上方，用拇指指腹按壓大腿後內側肌群（見照片**50**），依次從膕窩內上方按壓至大腿根部（見照片**51**和圖示**38**），反復操作**2－4**次。一側完畢更換另一側。

Thumb-pressing method:

The patient revolves the right lower limb outward, bends hip and knee, and places the foot on the left groin of the massagist. The massagist kneels with the left hand holding the front of the patient's ankle joint and right hand on the upper inside of the hollow of knee. Use the inside of thumb to press rear inside muscles of thigh (see Photo 50) from the upper inside of the hollow of knee to the thigh root in an orderly way (see Photo 51 and Fig. 38). Repeat the manipulation 2-4 times. Do one side, then the other.

照片 (Photo) 50

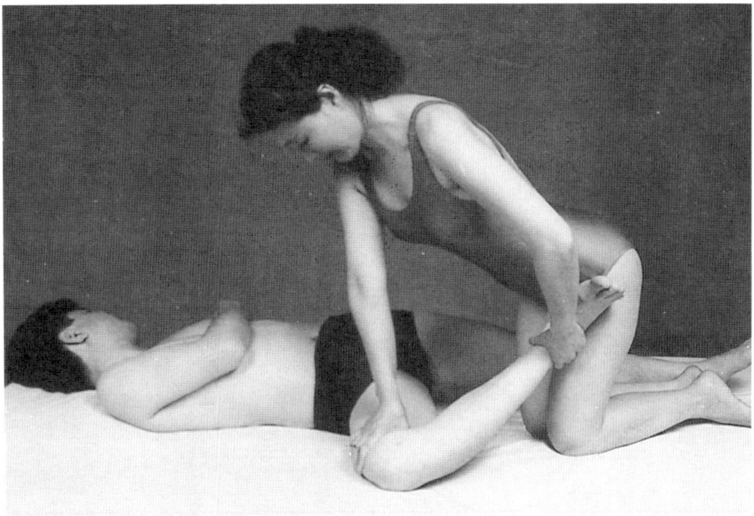

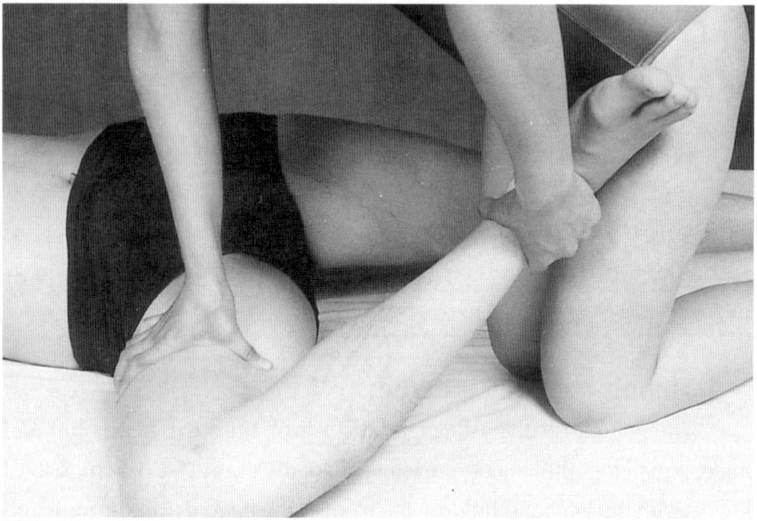

照片 (Photo) 51

圖示 (Fig.) 38

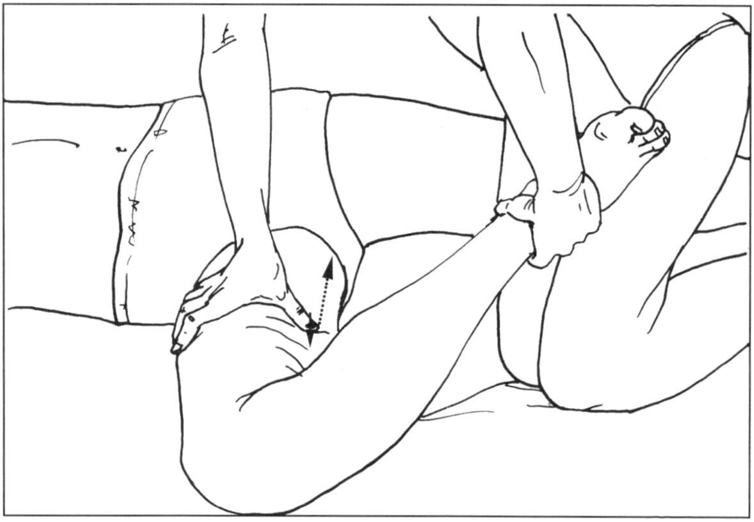

36 提拉法：

體位同上。按摩者右手拇指置於被按摩者膕窩內上方，其餘四指置於同水平的前內側，五指微屈，以對指之力，借屈腕動作將大腿內側肌群向上方提拉至腹股溝部，反復操作**2－4**次（見照片**52**和圖示**39**）。一側完畢更換另一側。

Lifting and pulling method:

In same position. The massagist places right thumb on the upper inside of the hollow of patient's knee and the other four fingers at the front inside at the same level and slightly bends five fingers. With the force of fingers and the movement of bending wrist, lift and pull the inside muscles of thigh upward to the groin. Repeat the manipulation 2-4 times (see Photo 52 and Fig. 39). Do one side, then the other.

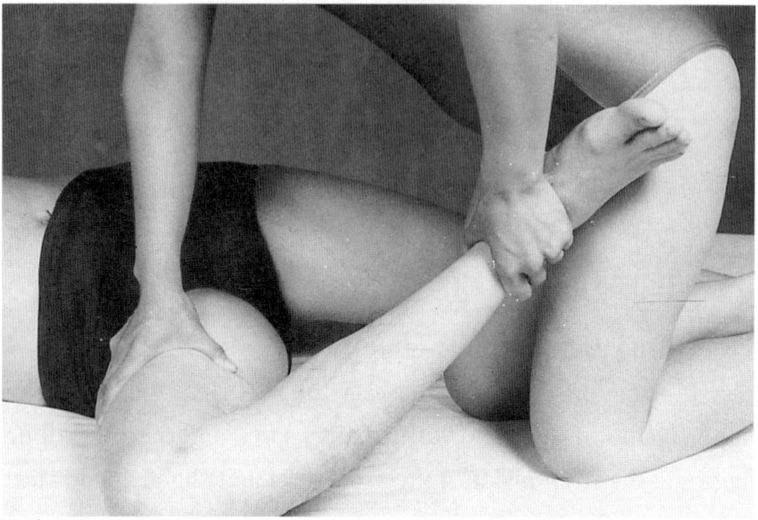
照片 (Photo) 52

圖示 (Fig.) 39
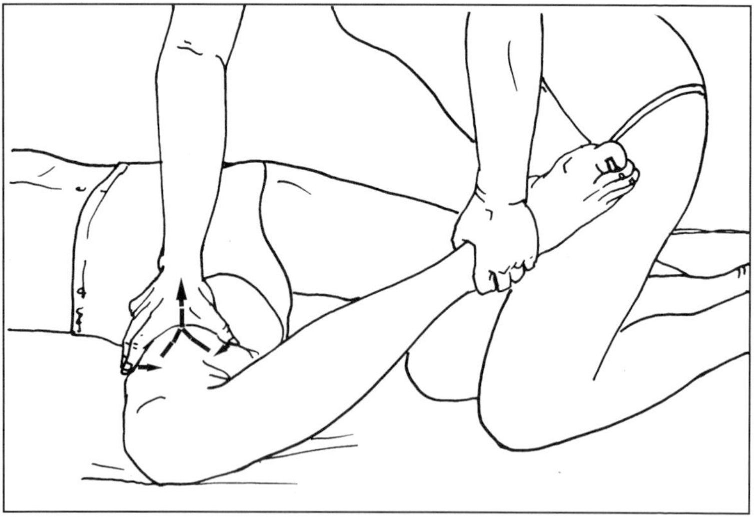

37 掌按壓法：

體位同上。按摩者左手掌根部置於被按摩者膕窩內上方，用掌按法按壓至腹股溝處，反復操作**2－4**次（見照片**53**和圖示**40**）。一側完畢更換另一側。

Palm-pressing method:

In same position. The massagist places the left palm root on the upper inside of the hollow of patient's knee. Press to the groin with the palm. Repeat the manipulation 2-4 times (see Photo 53 and Fig. 40). Do one side, then the other.

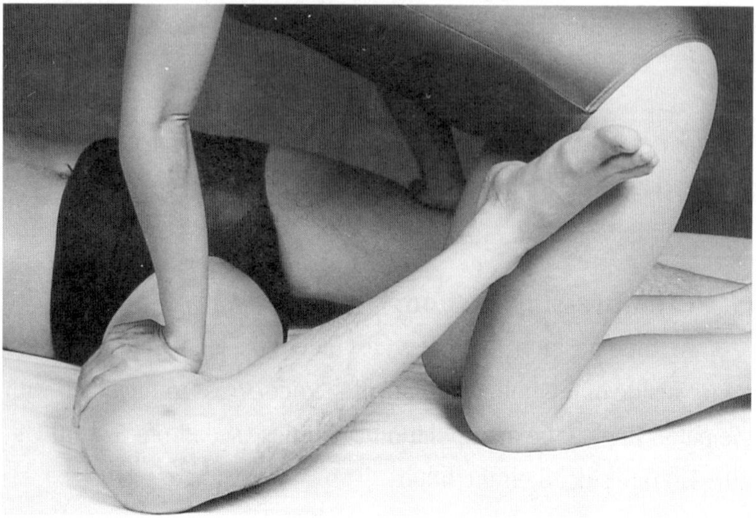

照片 (Photo) 53

圖示 (Fig.) 40

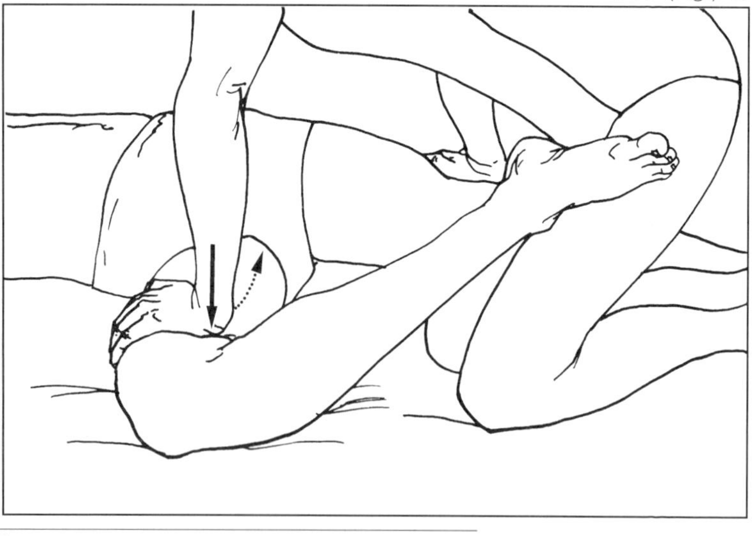

38 掌按下肢內側法：

被按摩者雙下肢外旋、屈髖屈膝位，雙足置於按摩者雙膝關節之間並被夾住（見照片**54**），按摩者用雙手掌根由膝關節的內側交替向大腿近端、再向小腿遠端行掌按法（見照片**55**和圖示**41**），反復操作**2－4**次。

Palm-pressing inside lower limb method:

The patient revolves both lower limbs outward, bends hip and knees and places both feet to be held together between both knee joints of the massagist (see Photo 54). The massagist presses from the inside of knee joints to the near end of thighs and then to the far end of shanks alternately with both palm roots (see Photo 55 and Fig. 41). Repeat the manipulation 2-4 times.

照片 (Photo) 54

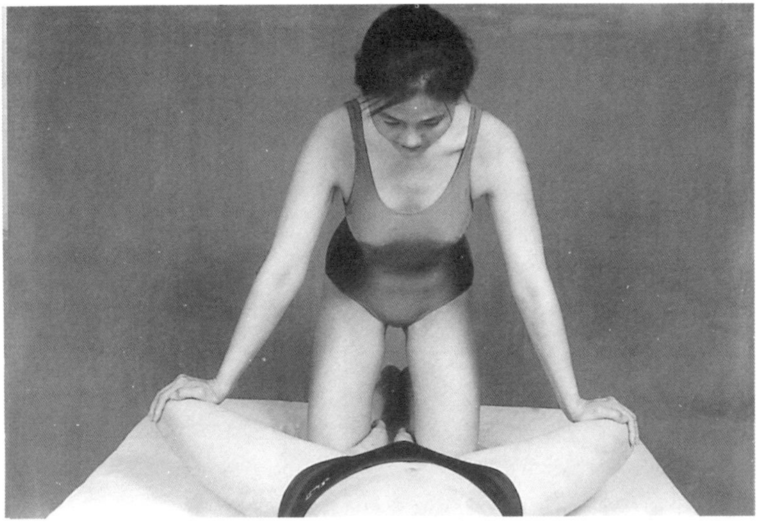

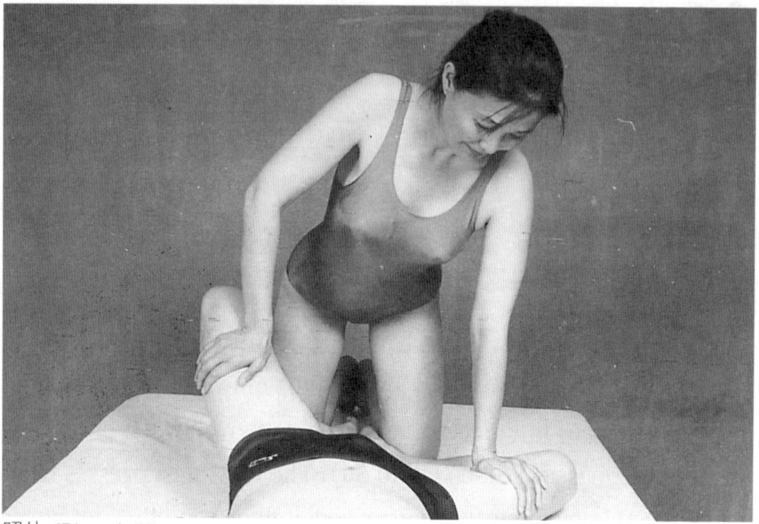

照片 (Photo) 55

圖示 (Fig.) 41

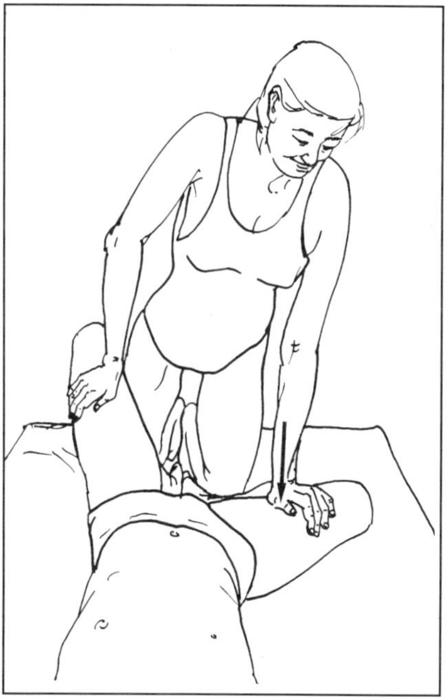

39 指揉小腿內側肌群：

體位同上。按摩者以雙手拇指及其餘四指的對合之力，按揉被按摩者小腿內側肌群，從膝關節內下方按揉至遠端（見照片**56**、**57**和圖示**42**）。

Digital-rubbing inside muscles of shank:

In same position. The massagist uses the joint force of the thumbs and other four fingers of both hands to press and rub the inside muscles of the patient's shanks from the lower inside part of knee joints to far ends (see Photos 56, 57 and Fig. 42).

照片 (Photo) 56

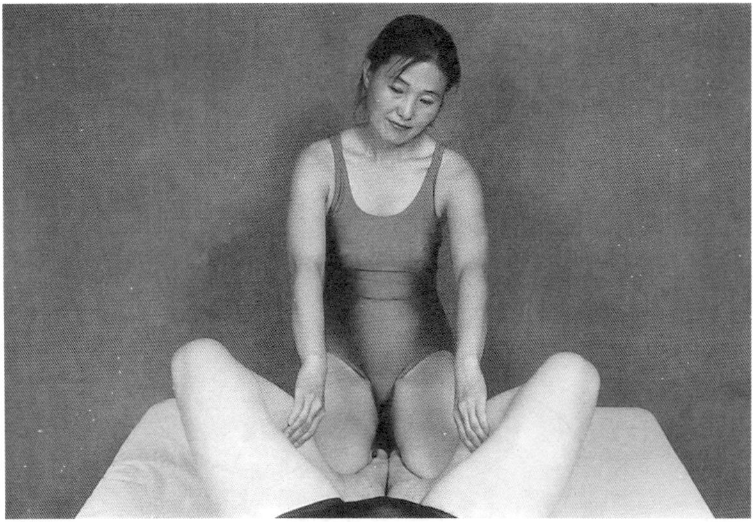

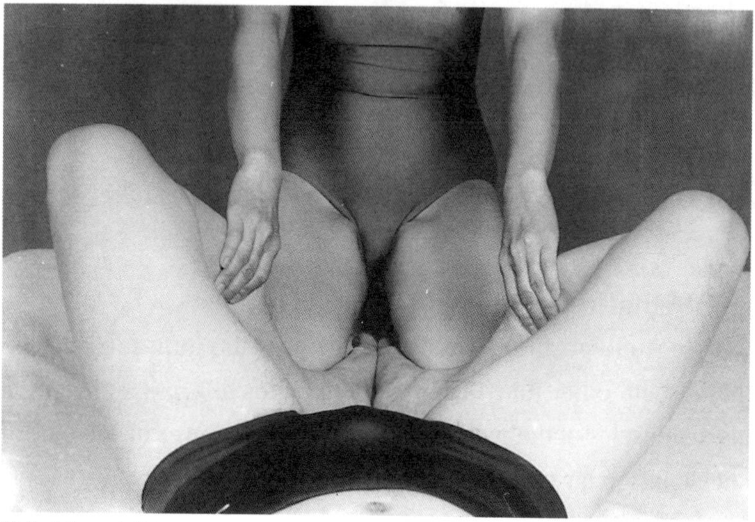

照片 (Photo) 57

圖示 (Fig.) 42

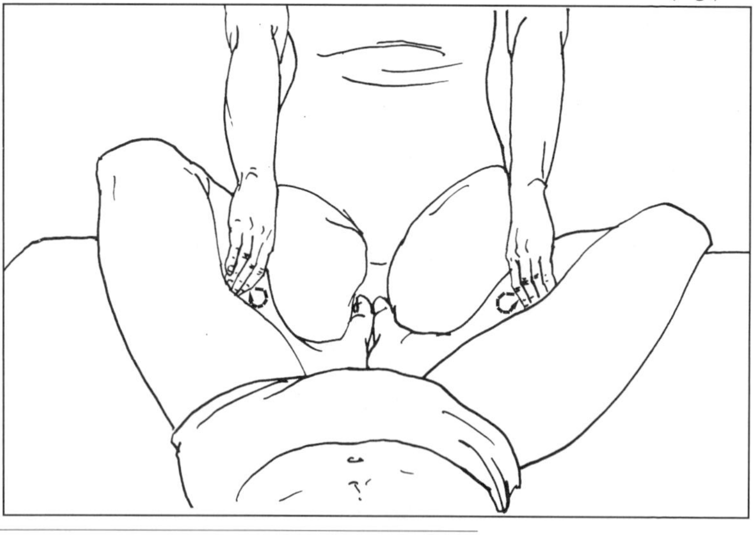

40 蹬推法：

被按摩者右側下肢外展外旋屈髖屈膝各**90**度，按摩者坐位，左手握被按摩者踝關節，雙下肢略伸直，用雙足蹬推其膝關節後上方，以雙足交替蹬推之力，依次從膝關節後上方蹬推至腹股溝處，反復操作**2－4**次（見照片**58**和圖示**43**）。一側完畢更換另一側。

Stamping and pushing method:

The patient revolves the right lower limb outward and bends both hip and knee at 90 degrees. The massagist sitting, holds the patient's ankle joint with the left hand, stretches slightly both lower limbs straight and stamps and pushes the rear upper part of knee joint with both feet. With the force of stamping and pushing both feet alternately, stamp and push from rear upper part of knee joint to groin. Repeat the manipulation 2-4 times (see Photo 58 and Fig. 43). Do one side, then the other.

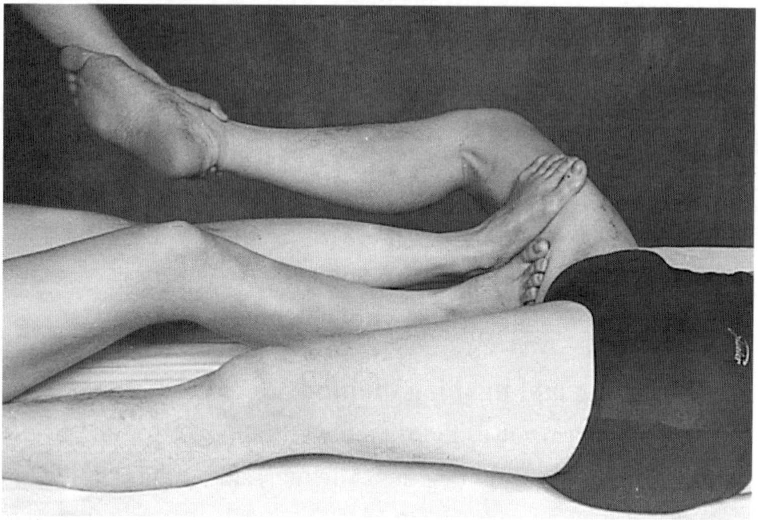

照片 (Photo) 58

圖示 (Fig.) 43

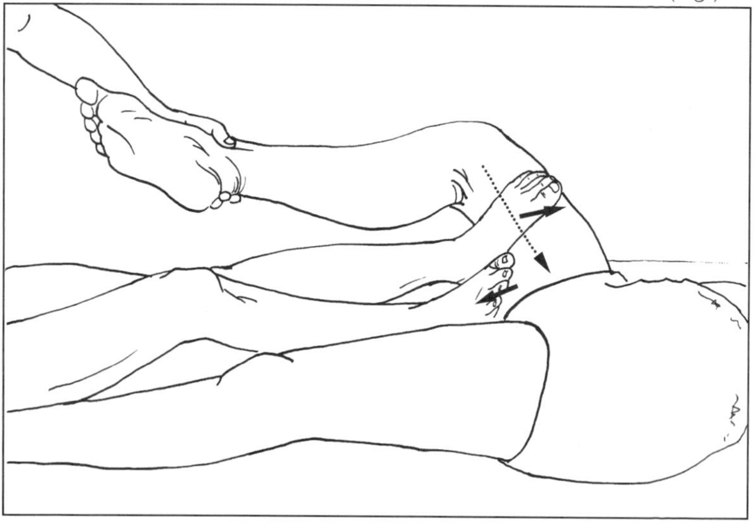

41 鈎推牽拉法：

被按摩者體位同上。按摩者左下肢置其大腿後側，以右足背伸之力鈎按大腿前側肌群，左足向前蹬推其大腿後側肌群，雙下肢交錯施力至膕窩處（見照片**59**）。與此同時，按摩者雙手緊握踝關節向肢體遠端牽拉（見照片**60**和圖示**44**）。一側完畢更換另一側。

Hooking, pushing and drawing method:

The patient in same position. The massagist places left lower limb on the patient's thigh back. Hook the front muscles of thigh with the force of stretching right foot backward and stamp and push forward the rear muscles of thigh with alternate force of both lower limbs to the hollow of knee (see Photo 59). At the same time, the massagist grasps the ankle joint with both hands and pulls it to the far end of limb (see Photo 60 and Fig. 44). Do one side, then the other.

照片 (Photo) 59

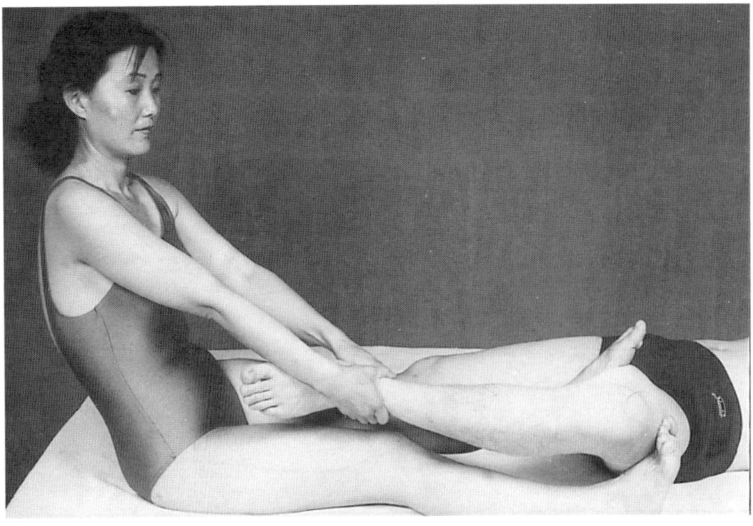

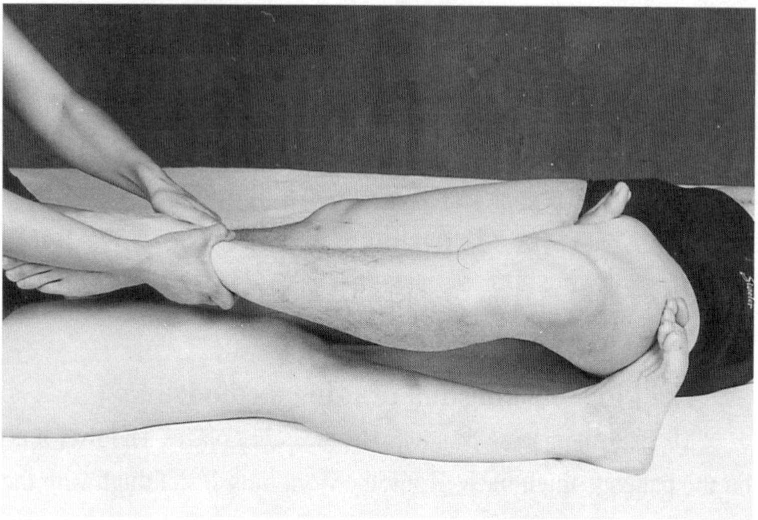

照片 (Photo) 60

圖示 (Fig.) 44

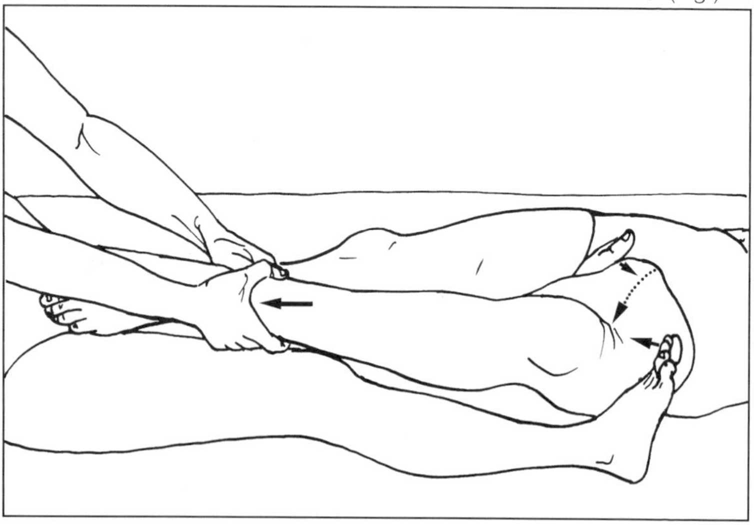

42 提拉大腿內側肌群：

被按摩者右下肢外旋屈髖屈膝，並將足背鉤住按摩者左下肢的小腿內側、膝關節下方（見照片**61**）。按摩者坐位，左足踏推患者膕窩處，雙手置於腹股溝前下方，五指略屈，以對指之力將肌肉向內側拉提，至膝關節上方，反復操作**2－4**次（見照片**62**和圖示**45**）。一側完畢更換另一側。

Lifting and pulling inside muscles of thigh:

The patient revolves right lower limb outward, bends hip and knee and uses the dorsum of foot to hook the inside of left lower limb shank and the lower part of knee joint of the massagist (see Photo 61). The massagist sits, stamps and pushes the patient's hollow of knee with left foot, places both hands on the lower front part of groin and pulls and lifts the muscle inward to the upper part of knee joint with the joint force of five slightly-bent fingers. Repeat the manipulation 2-4 times (see Photo 62 and Fig. 45). Do one side, then the other.

照片 (Photo) 61

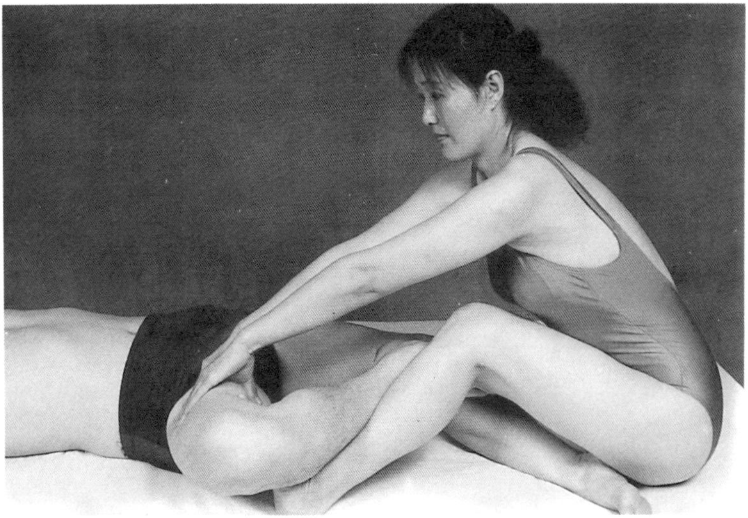

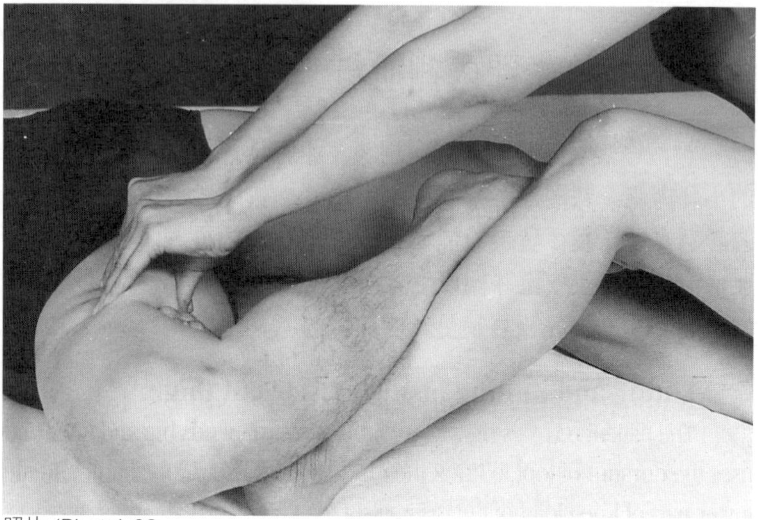

照片 (Photo) 62

圖示 (Fig.) 45

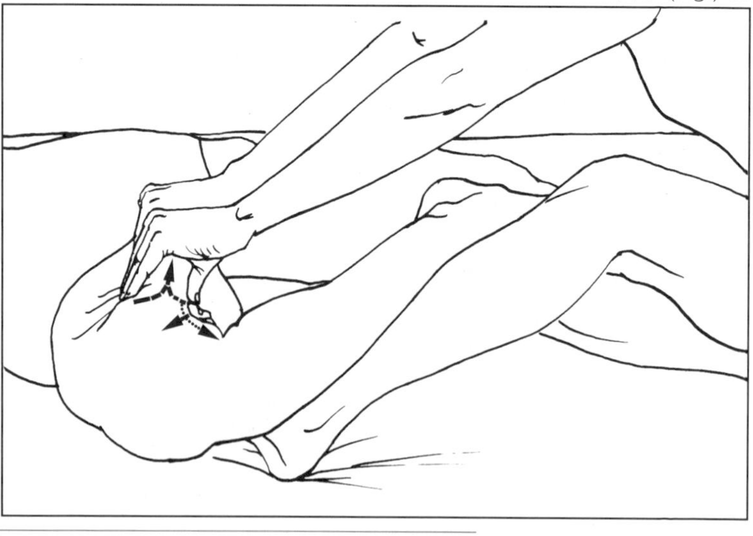

43 拉旋大腿前方肌群：

體位同上。按摩者上肢伸直，雙手掌置於被按摩者大腿近端的前側肌群，以屈指之力，將股四頭肌向內側拉旋至膝關節前上方，反復操作**2－4**次（見照片**63**和圖示**46**）。一側完畢更換另一側。

Pulling and revolving front muscles of thigh:

In same position. The massagist stretches upper limbs straight and places both palms on the front muscles of the patient's near end of thigh; with the force of bent fingers, pulls and revolves the quadriceps inward to the front upper side of knee joint. Repeat the manipulation 2-4 times (see Photo 63 and Fig. 46). Do one side, then the other.

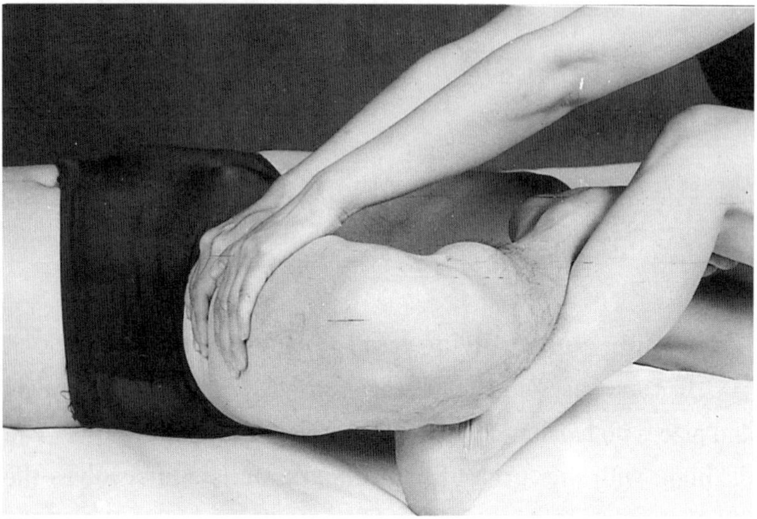

照片 (Photo) 63

圖示 (Fig.) 46

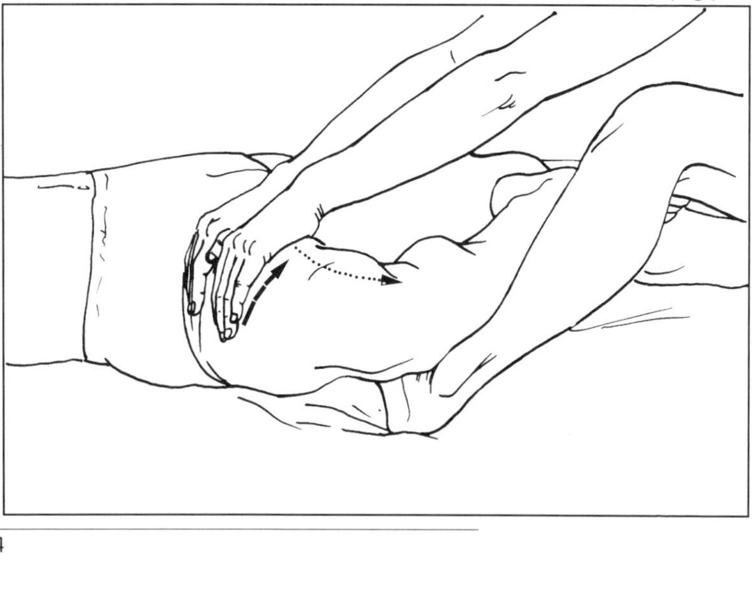

44 提拉大腿前方肌群：

被按摩者右下肢屈髖屈膝位，按摩者跪坐於被按摩者足側，並用雙膝關節夾住其前足，雙手的**2**、**3**、**4**、**5**指置其膝關節的前上方（見照片**64**），以對掌之力，將大腿前方肌群向前提拉至腹股溝部（見照片**65**和圖示**47**），反復操作**2－4**次。一側完畢更換另一側。

Lifting and pulling front muscles of thigh:

The patient bends the hip and knee of right lower limb. The massagist kneels on the side of patient's foot, clamps the front foot with both knee joints and places the 2nd, 3rd, 4th and 5th fingers of both hands on the patient's front upper part of knee joint (see Photo 64); with the force of palm-to-palm, lifts and pulls the front muscles of thigh forward to the groin (see Photo 65 and Fig. 47). Repeat the manipulation 2-4 times. Do one side, then the other.

照片 (Photo) 64

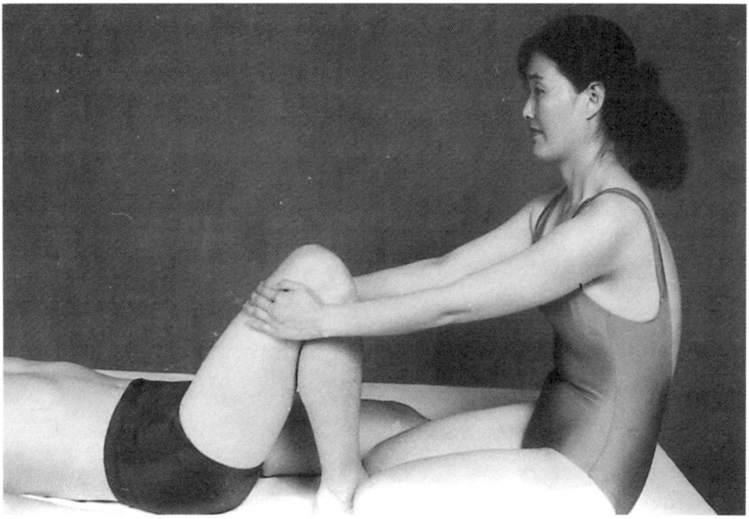

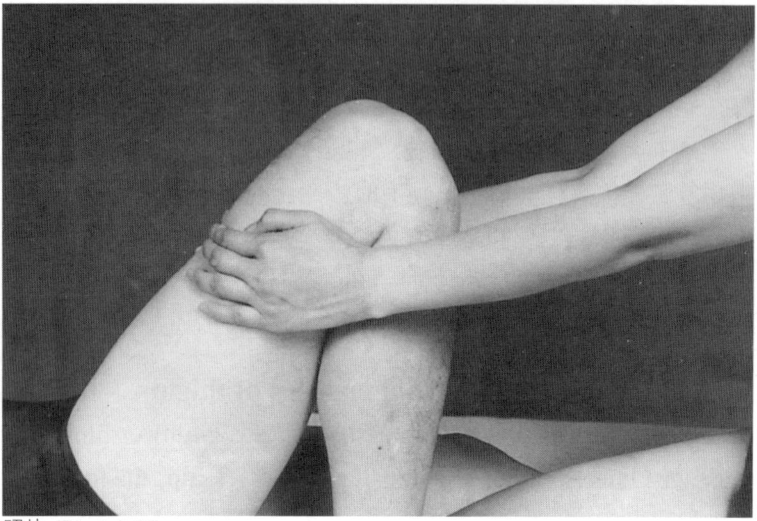

照片 (Photo) 65

圖示 (Fig.) 47

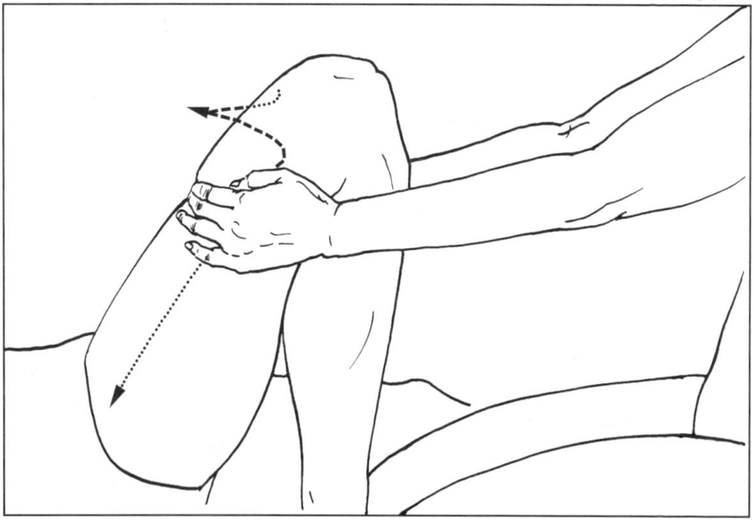

45 歸揉法：

體位同上。按摩者雙手五指交叉分別置於被按摩者膝關節內外側（見照片**66**），以雙掌根部歸揉之力，依次從膝關節歸揉至腹股溝處（見照片**67**和圖示**48**），反復操作**2－4**次。一側完畢更換另一側。

Backward rubbing method:

In same position. The massagist clasps the five fingers of both hands and places them on the inside and outside of the patient's knee joint respectively (see Photo 66); with the force of both palm roots, rubs from the knee joint backward to the groin in an orderly way (see Photo 67 and Fig. 48). Repeat the manipulation 2-4 times. Do one side, then the other.

照片 (Photo) 66

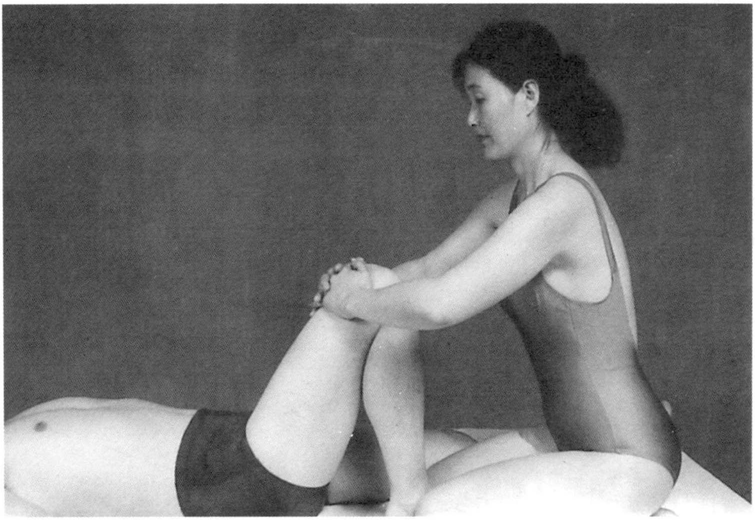

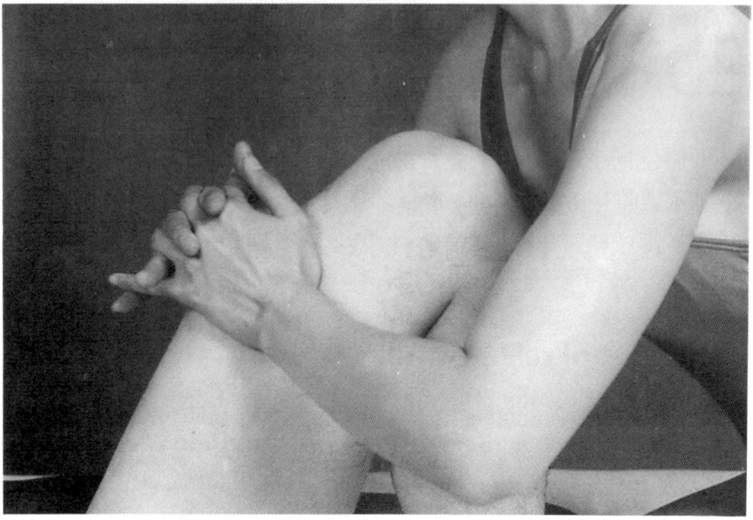

照片 (Photo) 67

圖示 (Fig.) 48

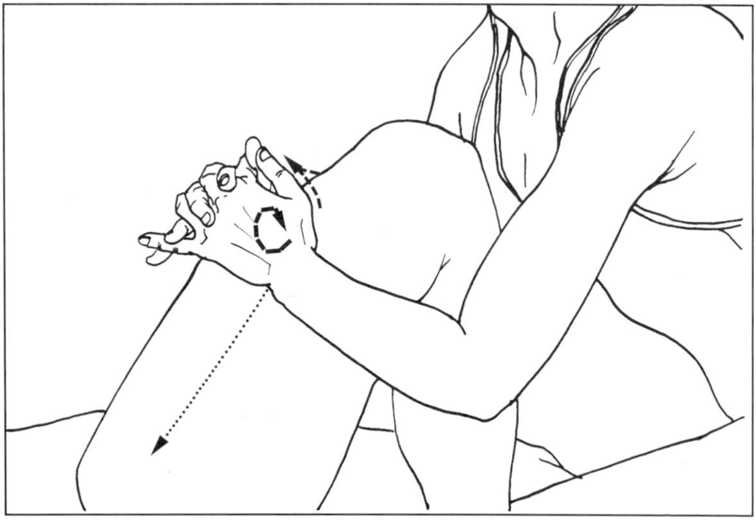

46 推拉大腿前方肌群：

體位同上。按摩者雙手分別置於被按摩者膝關節上方兩側（見照片68），將其大腿前部肌群交替向外向內側拉推（見照片69和圖示49），反復操作2－4次。一側完畢更換另一側。

Pushing and pulling front muscles of thigh:

In same position. The massagist places both hands on the two upper sides of the patient's knee joint respectively (see Photo 68) and pulls and pushes the front muscles of thigh outside and inside alternately (see Photo 69 and Fig. 49). Repeat the manipulation 2-4 times. Do one side, then the other.

照片 (Photo) 68

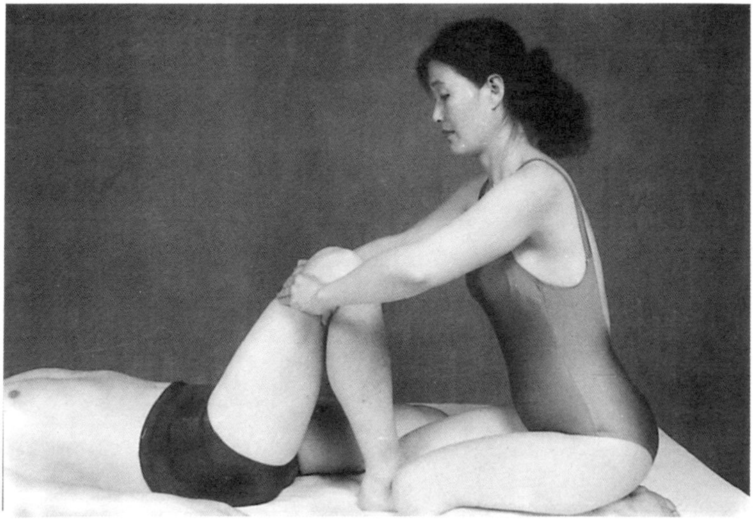

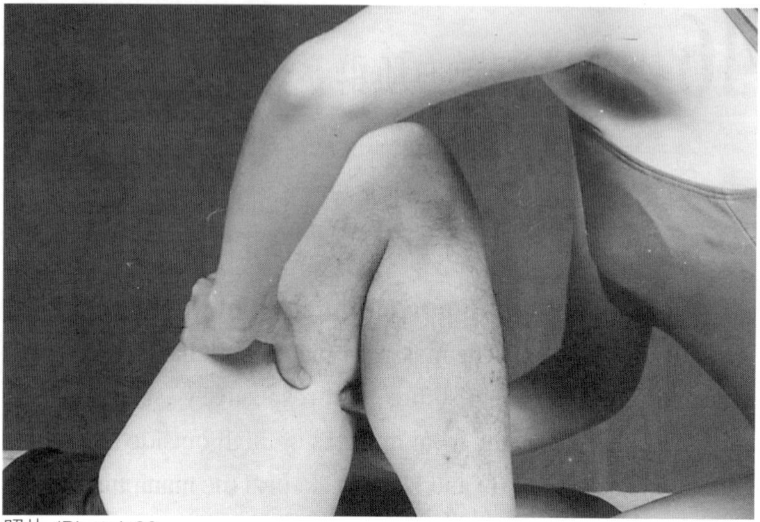

照片 (Photo) 69

圖示 (Fig.) 49

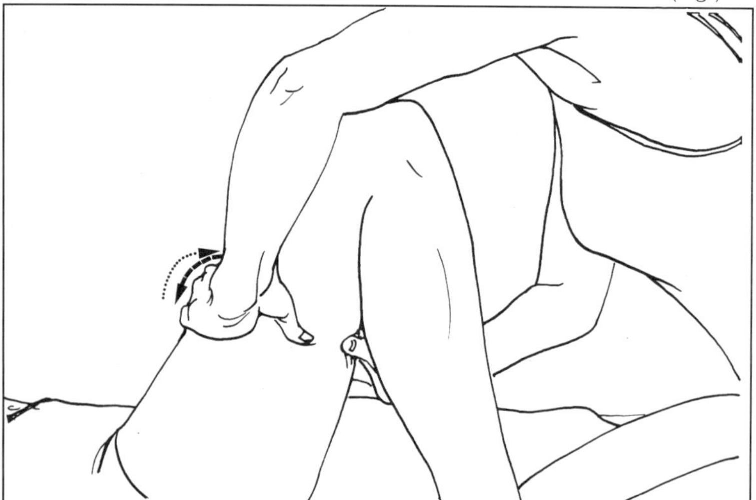

47 壓拉大腿前方肌群：

體位同上。按摩者雙手拇指與相併攏的**2**、**3**、**4**、**5**指屈掌指關節，伸指間關節，從被按摩者膝關節上方左右交替壓拉大腿前側肌群至腹股溝處，反復操作**2－4**次（見照片**70**和圖示**50**）。一側完畢更換另一側。

Pressing and pulling front muscles of thigh:

In same position. The massagist uses the thumbs, bent joints between the palm and fingers and stretched finger joints of 2nd, 3rd, 4th and 5th fingers of both hand to press and pull the front side muscles of thigh left and right from the upper side of knee joint alternately to the groin. Repeat the manipulation 2-4 times (see Photo 70 and Fig. 50). Do one side, then the other.

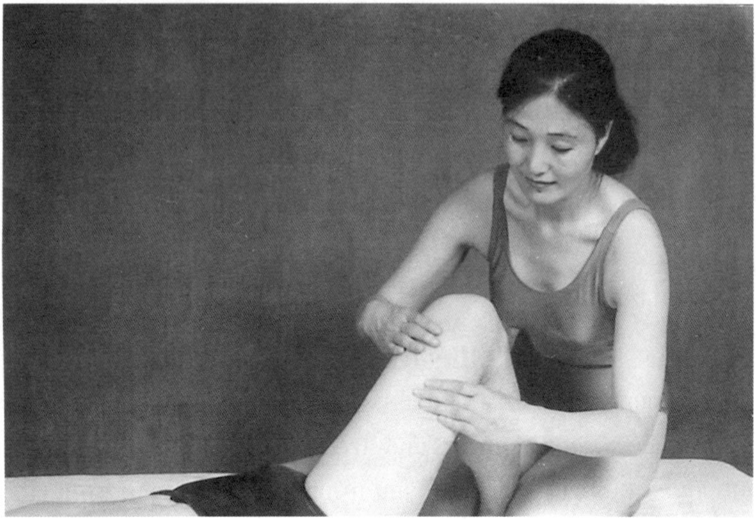

照片 (Photo) 70

圖示 (Fig.) 50

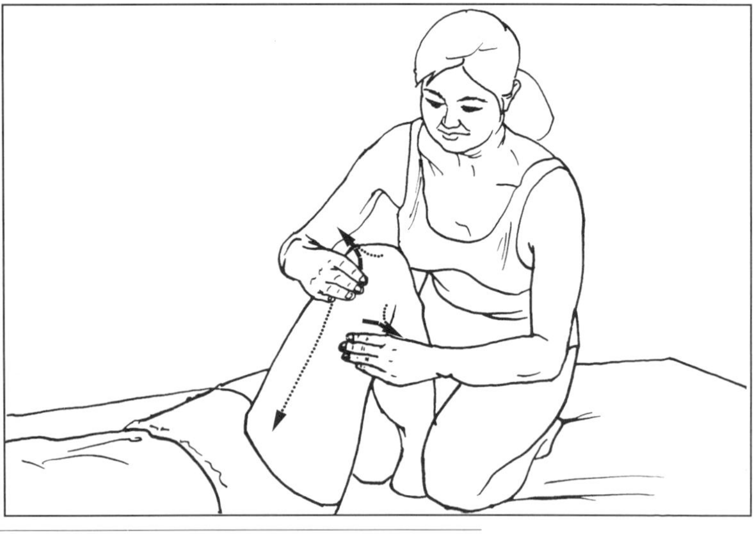

48 提拿旋肌法：

體位同上。按摩者一手以上述拿法從被按摩者膝關節上方將大腿外側肌群提拿並旋前（見照片7 1），然後以另一手將大腿內側肌群向內提拿並旋後，反復操作2－4次（見照片72和圖示51）。一側完畢更換另一側。

Lifting and revolving muscle method:

In same position. The massagist lifts and revolves forward the outside muscles of thigh from the upper part of knee joint of the patient with one hand (see Photo 71) and then lifts inward and revolves backward the inside muscles of thigh with the other hand. Repeat the manipulation 2-4 times (see Photo 72 and Fig. 51). Do one side, then the other.

照片 (Photo) 71

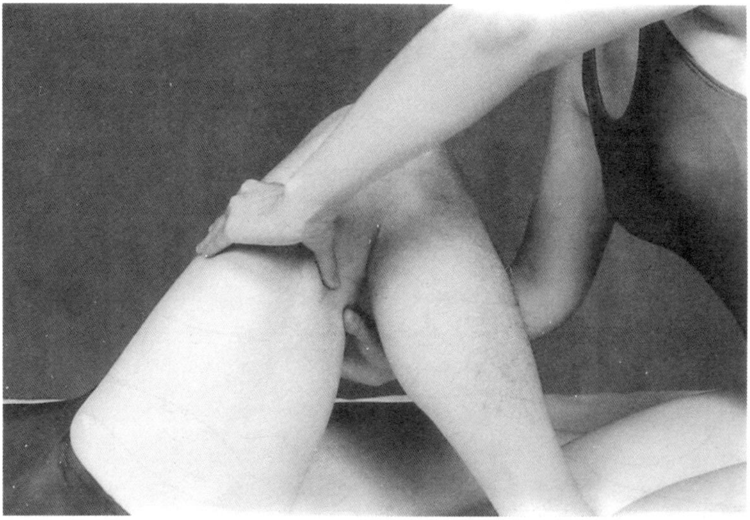

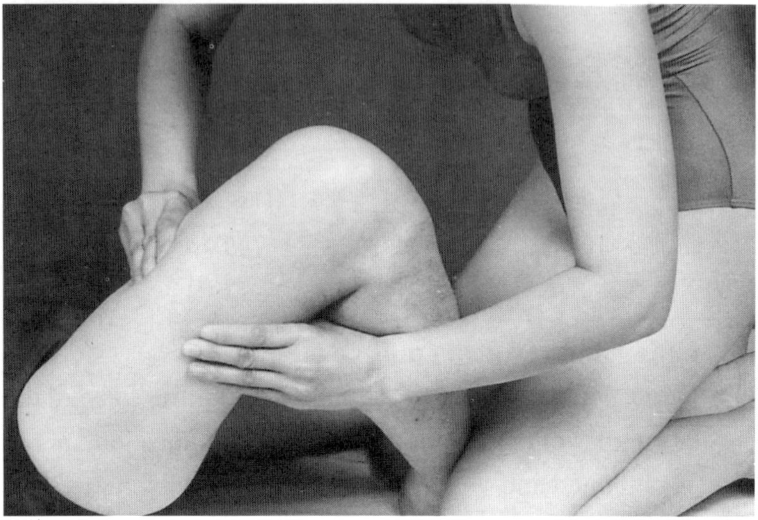
照片 (Photo) 72

圖示 (Fig.) 51
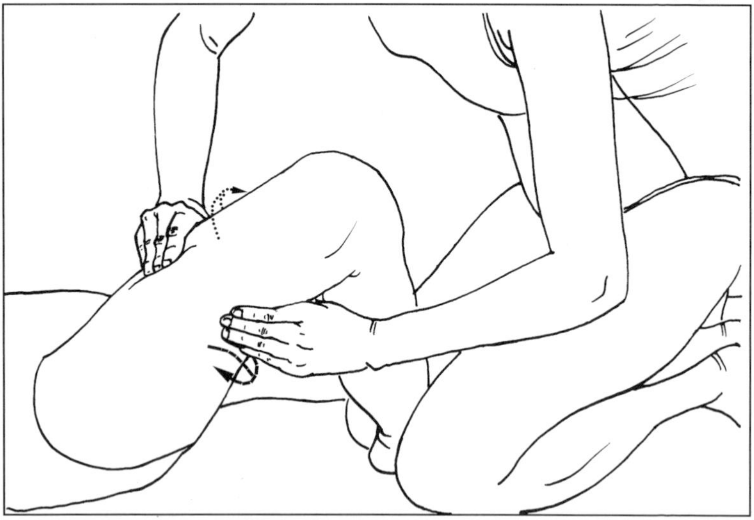

49 捋拉法：

體位同上。按摩者雙手的2、3、4、5指置於被按摩者的小腿近端後方，屈掌指及指間關節，拇指置於前方，上肢伸直，通過腰部的背伸動作，以五指對合之力將小腿後群肌肉向內前方拉起，反復操作2－4次（見照片73和圖示52）。一側完畢更換另一側。

Stroking and pulling method:

In same position. The massagist places the 2nd, 3rd, 4th and 5th fingers of both hands on the back of shank near end of the patient, bends joints between palm and fingers and finger joints, places thumbs on the front and stretches upper limbs straight. Through the movement of stretching the waist backward, and with the joint force of five fingers, pull rear muscles of shank inward and forward. Repeat the manipulation 2-4 times (see Photo 73 and Fig. 52). Do one side, then the other.

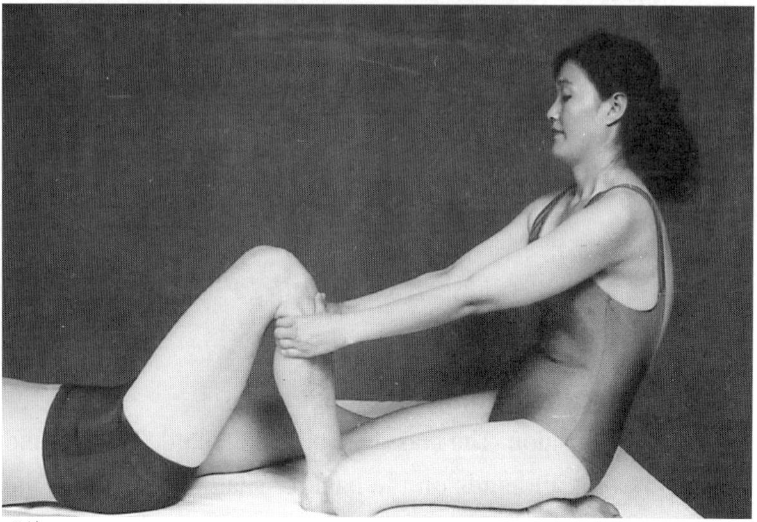
照片 (Photo) 73

圖示 (Fig.) 52
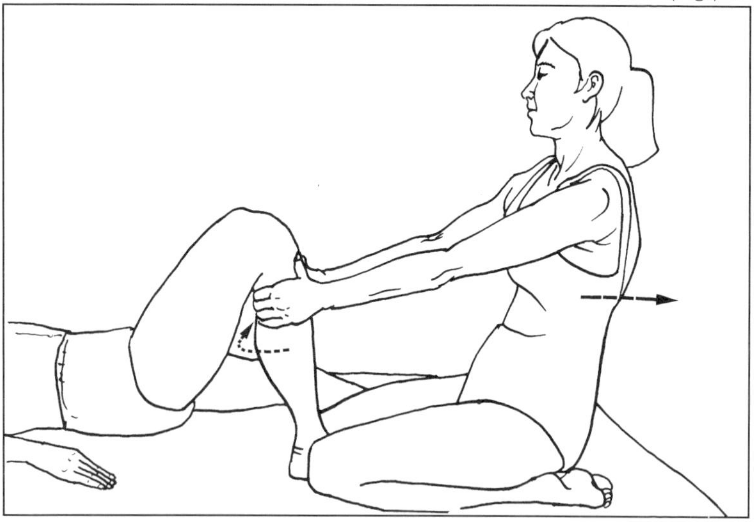

50 指揉小腿外側肌群：

體位同上。按摩者右手拇指置於被按摩者小腿近端的外側，其餘四指置於同水平內側，以拇指按揉之力，由小腿前外側近端向下按揉至踝關節上方（見照片74和圖示53），反復操作2－4次，左右手均可。一側完畢更換另一側。

Digital-rubbing outside muscles of shank:

In same position. The massagist places right thumb on the outside of near end shank of the patient and places the other four fingers on the inside at the same level. With the force of thumb pressing and rubbing, press and rub from the near end of front outside shank downward to the upper part of ankle joint (see Photo 74 and Fig. 53). Repeat the manipulation 2-4 times. Left and right hands can both do this. Do one side, then the other.

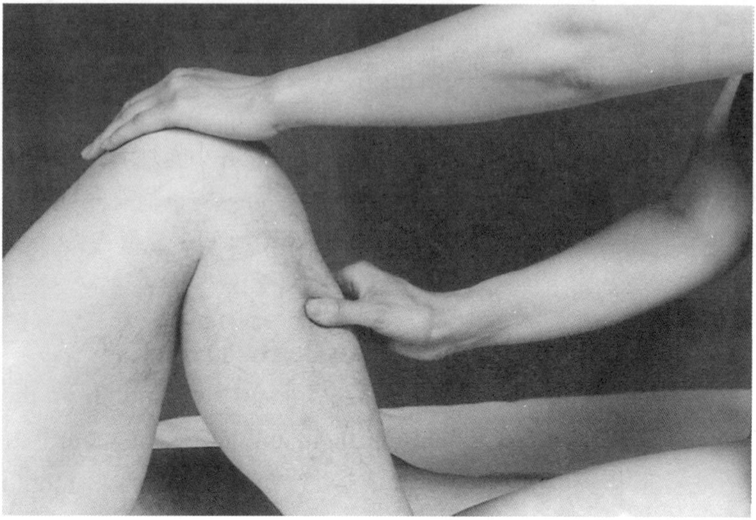
照片 (Photo) 74

圖示 (Fig.) 53
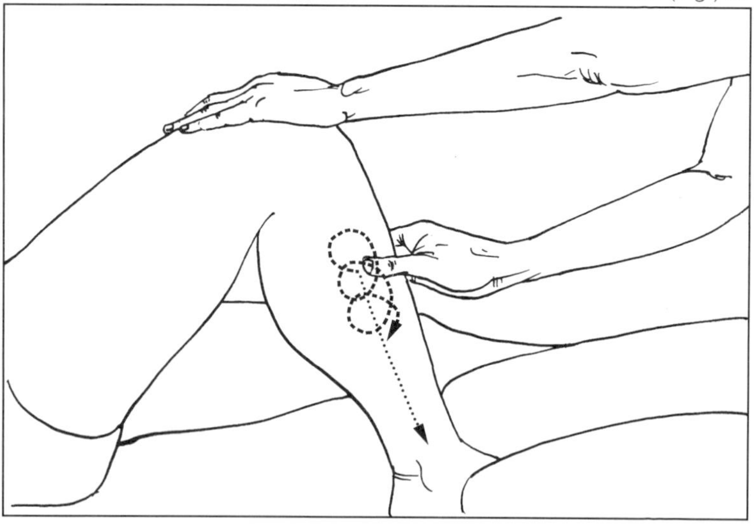

51 屈髖屈膝法：

被按摩者仰臥位，按摩者跪位於被按摩者足側，一手扶握被按摩者踝關節，一手按其膝關節向前推送，使其做被動屈髖屈膝動作，然後再牽伸下肢，反復操作2－4次（見照片75和圖示54）。一側完畢更換另一側。

Hip and knee bending method:

The patient lies flat on back. The massagist kneels at the side of patient's foot, holds the ankle joint with one hand and presses the knee joint with other hand pushes forward, making the patient bend hip and knee passively and then draws the lower limb. Repeat the manipulation 2-4 times (see Photo 75 and Fig. 54). Do one side, then the other.

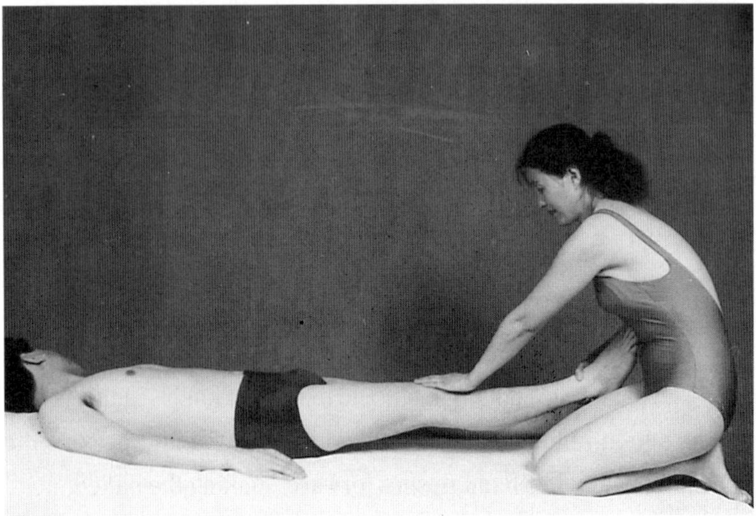

照片 (Photo) 75

圖示 (Fig.) 54

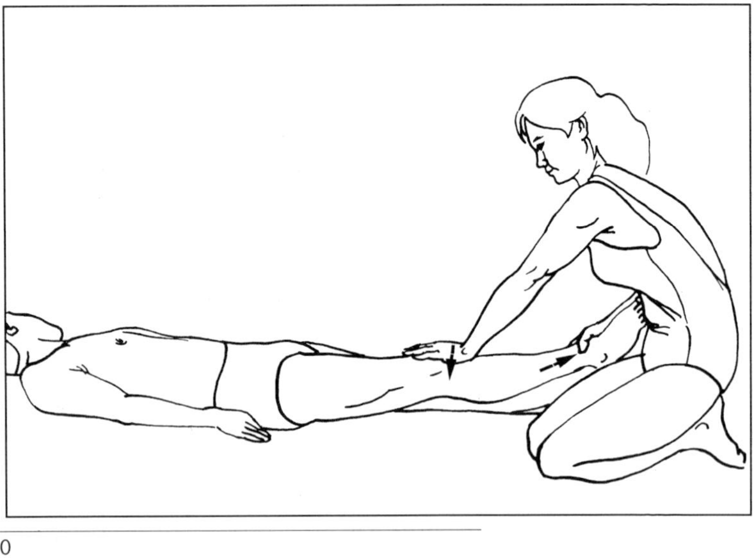

52 伸膝屈髖法：

體位同上，被按摩者下肢伸直，按摩者右手背伸腕關節，置於被按摩者膝關節前上方，向下壓，另一手握其足跟部，前臂置於足跖側，以軀幹右傾之力，使踝關節極度背伸，並向前推送足跟部，雙上肢伸直位，以下壓、內收之力，使其被動屈髖關節，幅度由小到大（見照片**76**和圖示**55**）。一側完畢更換另一側。

Knee stretching and hip bending method:

In same position. The patient stretches lower limbs straight. The massagist stretches the wrist joint of right hand backward and places it on the front upper side of patient's knee joint. Press downward. Hold the heel with other hand and place the forearm on the sole. With the force of inclining the trunk to right, make the ankle joint stretch backward to the utmost and push the heel forward. Stretch both upper limbs straight and with the force of pressing downward and pulling back, makes the patient bend hip joint passively from a small to big margin (see Photo 76 and Fig. 55). Do one side, then the other.

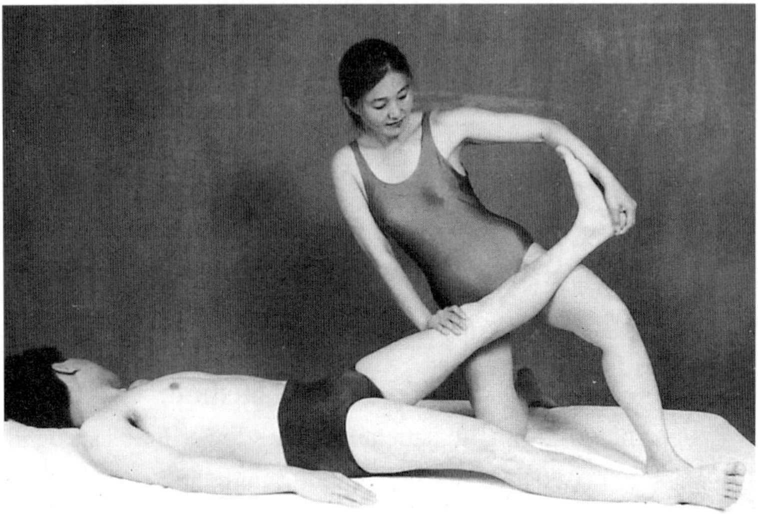

照片 (Photo) 76

圖示 (Fig.) 55

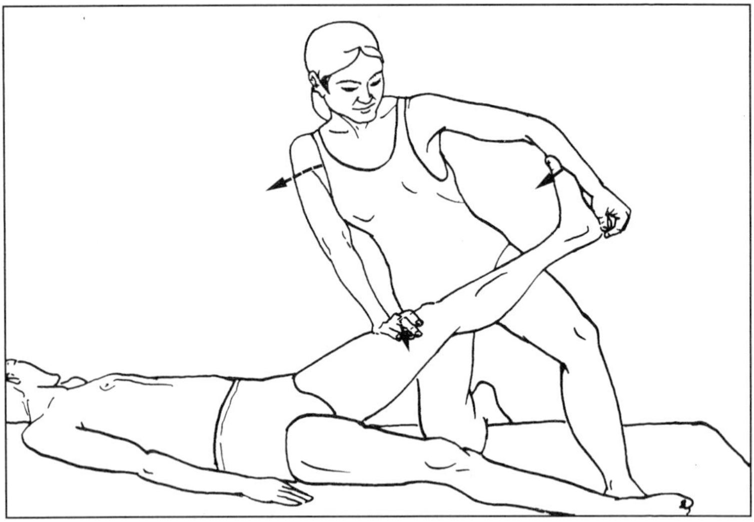

53 屈膝蹬壓法：

被按摩者仰臥位，按摩者坐於足側，右足向前蹬其左膝關節後上方，雙手緊握踝關節，向肢體遠心端牽拉，上下肢同時用力，邊蹬大腿後側肌群（見照片77和圖示56）邊向肢體近端挪移至臀溝處，握踝關節之手用力向遠心端牽拉（見照片78和圖示57）。一側完畢更換另一側。

Stamping and pressing bent knee method:

The patient lies flat on back. The massagist sits at the side of foot and stamps right foot forward on the rear upper part of left knee joint, grasps the ankle joint with both hands and draw toward the far center of limb. With the force of upper and lower limbs at the same time, stamp the rear muscles of thigh (see Photo 77 and Fig. 56) while moving to the buttock groove at the near end of limb, and draw to the far center with the force of both hands holding the ankle joint (see Photo 78 and Fig. 57). Do one side, then the other.

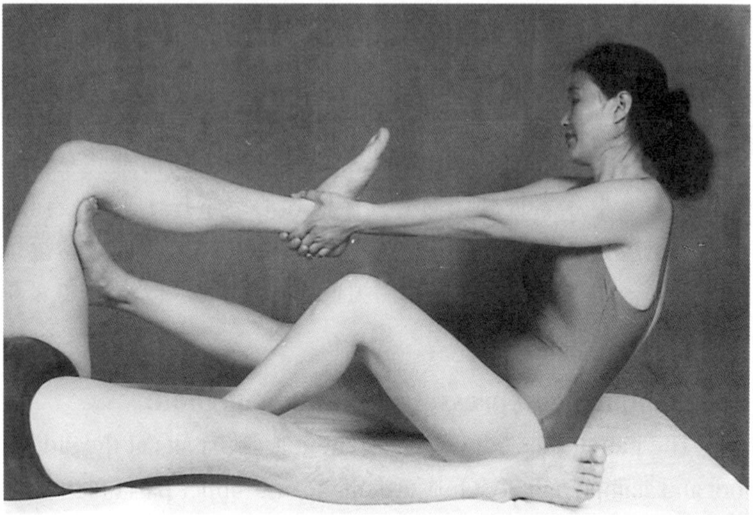

照片 (Photo) 77

圖示 (Fig.) 56

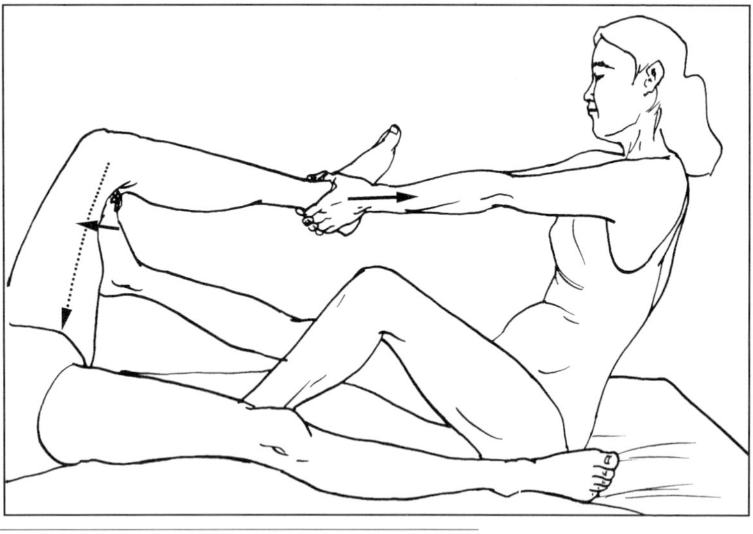

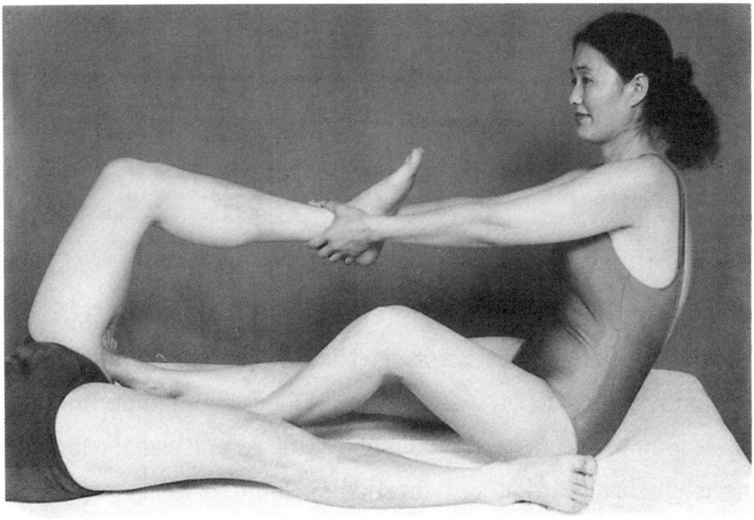

照片 (Photo) 78

圖示 (Fig.) 57

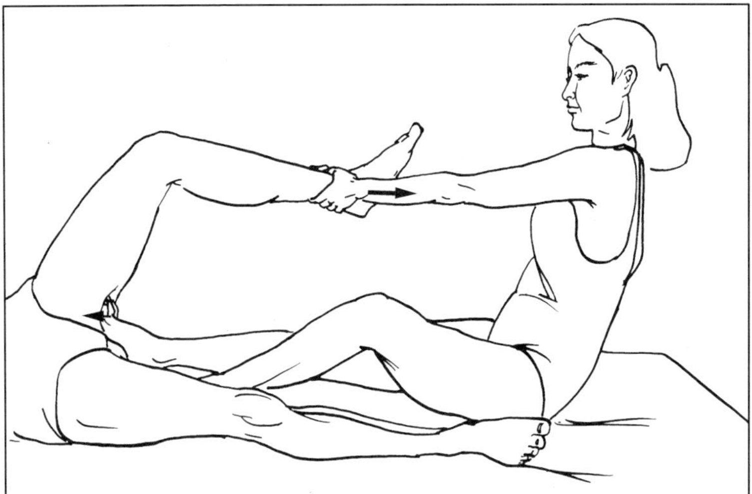

54 蹬拉法：

被按摩者仰臥位，按摩者坐於足側，左足向前蹬其坐骨結節處，雙手握踝關節，以後伸之力向遠端拉踝關節，反復操作**2－4**次（見照片**79**）。一側完畢更換另一側。

Stamping and pulling method:

The patient lies flat on back. The massagist sits at the side of foot and stamps the left foot forward on the ischium joint. Hold the ankle joint with both hands and pull it to the far end with the force of stretching backward. Repeat the manipulation 2-4 times (see Photo 79). Do one side, then the other.

照片 (Photo) 79

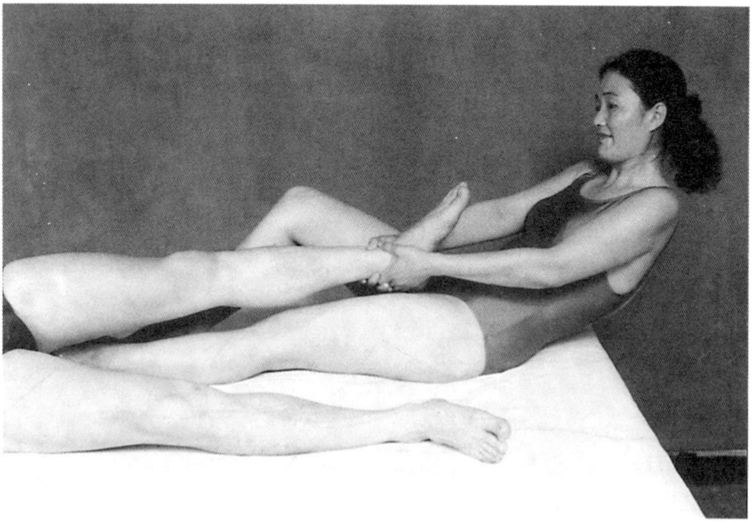

55 壓推小腿內側肌群：

被按摩者仰臥位，左下肢略屈髖屈膝，按摩者坐位於足背部，左足蹬推其坐骨結節處，雙手指置於膝關節後內下方，將小腿後內側肌群向前內方壓推至肢體遠端，反復操作**2－4**次（見照片**80**和圖示**58**）。一側完畢更換另一側。

Pressing and pushing inside muscles of shank:

The patient lies flat on back and slightly bends the hip and knee of the left lower limb. The massagist sits on the patient's dorsum of foot, stamps and pushes the left foot on the ischium joint and places both hands on the rear inside lower part of knee joint. Press and push the rear inside muscles of shank forward and inward to the far end of limb. Repeat the manipulation 2-4 times (see Photo 80 and Fig. 58). Do one side, then the other.

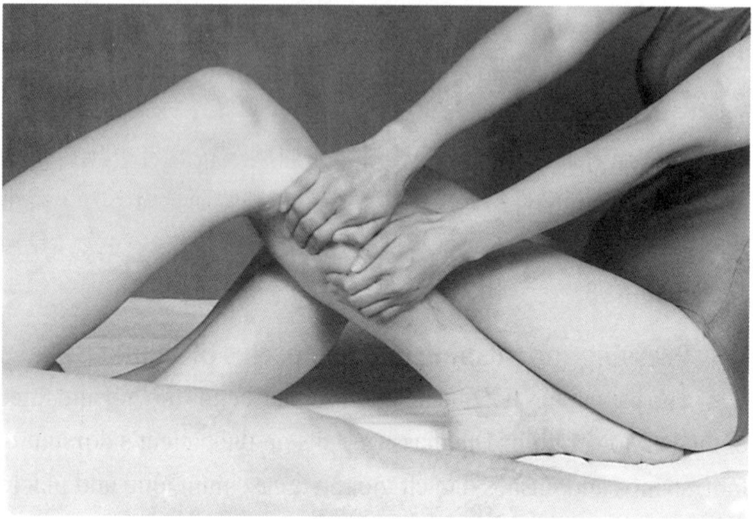

照片 (Photo) 80

圖示 (Fig.) 58

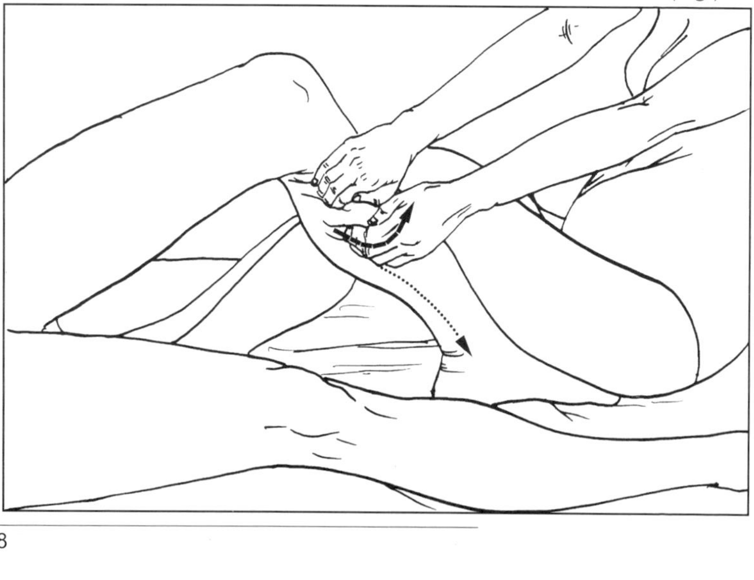

56 屈膝按壓法：

被按摩者仰臥位，右下肢外展屈膝小腿外旋位；按摩者跪其足側，右上肢伸直腕關節背伸，掌根部置於被按摩者膕窩內上方向下按壓，左手握其足外側（見照片**81**），邊屈膝關節邊按壓大腿後內側肌群，掌根向近端移動，反復操作**2－4**次（見照片**82**和圖示**59**）。一側完畢更換另一側。

Pressing bent knee method:

The patient lies flat on back, spreads the right lower limb outward, bends the knee and revolves the shank outward. The massagist kneels by the side of the foot of the patient, stretches the upper right limb straight, stretches the wrist joint backward and places the palm root on the upper inside part of hollow of knee and presses downward. Hold the outside of the foot with left the hand (see Photo 81), and bend the knee joint while pressing the rear inside muscles of the thigh and move the palm root to the near end. Repeat the manipulation 2-4 times (see Photo 82 and Fig. 59). Do one side, then the other.

照片 (Photo) 81

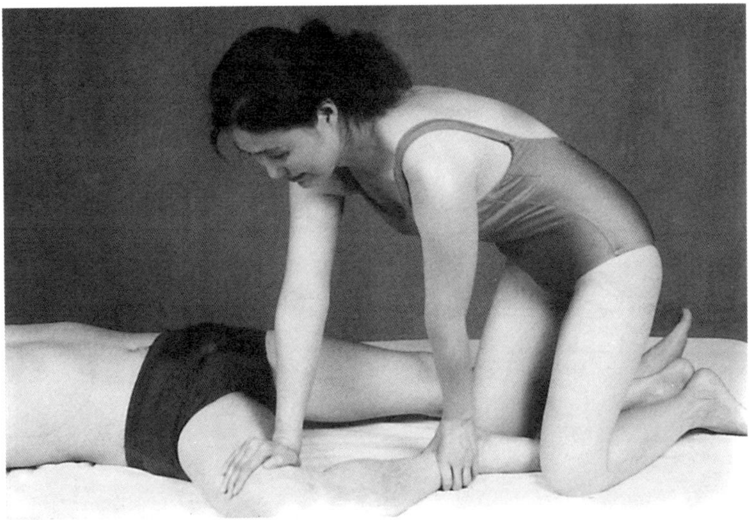

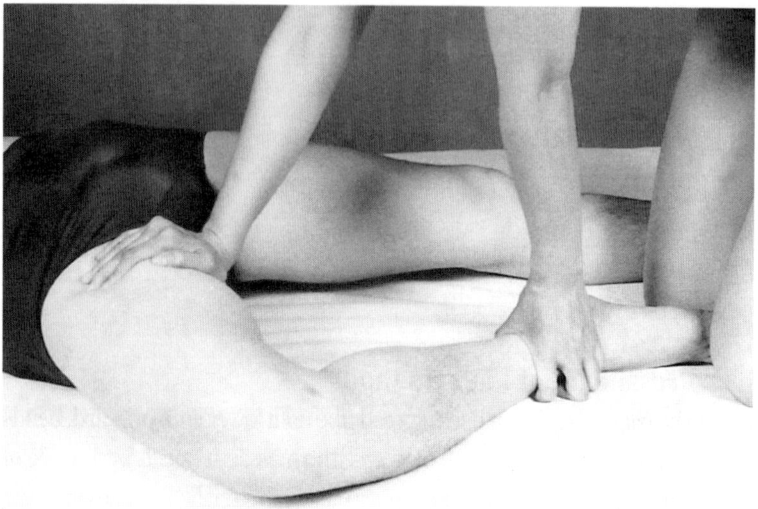

照片 (Photo) 82

圖示 (Fig.) 59

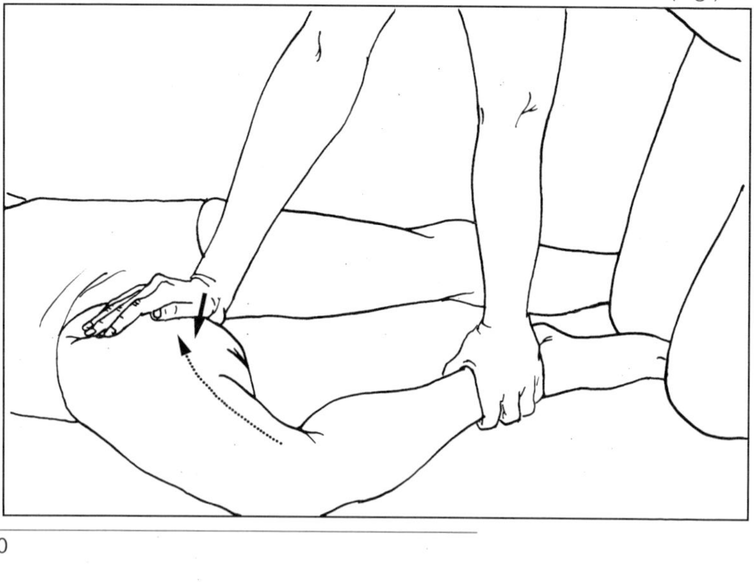

57 屈膝內旋法：

被按摩者體位同上。按摩者左下肢屈髖屈膝跪於床面之上，右下肢下蹲位，用膝關節內側按壓臥者膝關節外下方（見照片83），邊按壓邊增加被按摩者屈膝內旋的範圍，同時右手掌協同向下按壓（見照片84和圖示60），反復操作2－4次。一側完畢更換另一側。

Revolving bent knee inward method:

The patient in same position. The massagist bends the hip and knee of left lower limb and kneels on the bed. Squats down on the right lower limb and presses the lower outside of knee joint of the patient with the inside of knee joint (see Photo 83). Press while increasing the scope of revolving the patient's bent knee inward, and at the same time, press downward with help of right palm (see Photo 84 and Fig. 60). Repeat the manipulation 2-4 times. Do one side, then the other.

照片 (Photo) 83

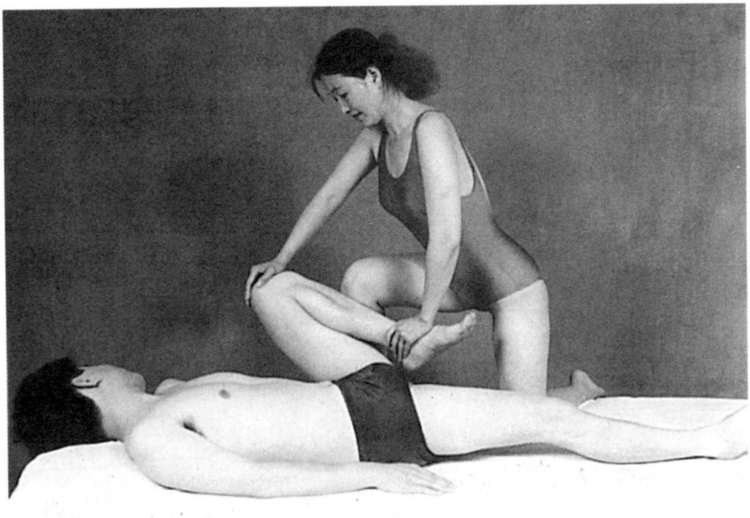

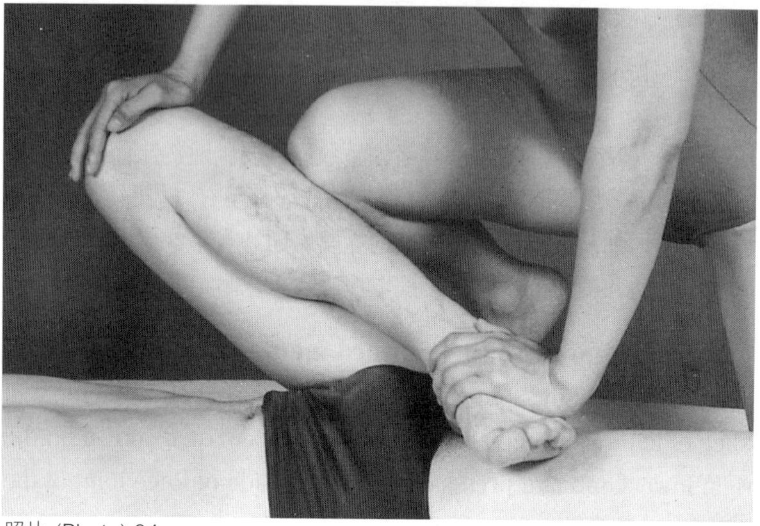

照片 (Photo) 84

圖示 (Fig.) 60

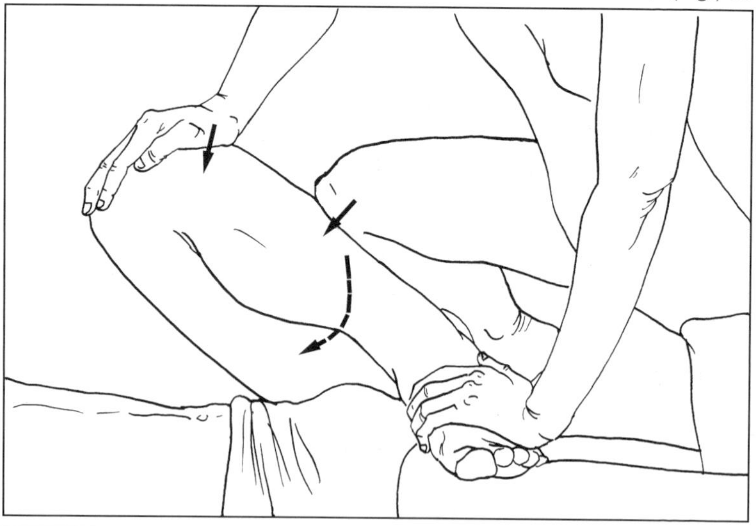

58 按壓下肢外側肌群：

被按摩者仰臥位，一側下肢內旋，屈膝關節，小腿外旋，按摩者跪位，雙上肢伸直，將手掌根置於大腿近端前外側，行向下按壓之力（見照片**85**），通過膝關節至踝關節處，按壓腿部外側肌群（見照片**86**和圖示**61**），反復操作**2－4**次。一側完畢更換另一側。

Pressing outside muscles of lower limb:

The patient lies flat on back, revolves a lower limb inward, bends knee joint and revolves the shank outward. The massagist kneels, stretches both upper limbs straight and places palm roots on the outside front of thigh near end. With force by pressing down (see Photo 85), presses the outside muscles of lower limb through the knee joint to the ankle joint (see Photo 86 and Fig. 61). Repeat the manipulation 2-4 times. Do one side, then the other.

照片 (Photo) 85

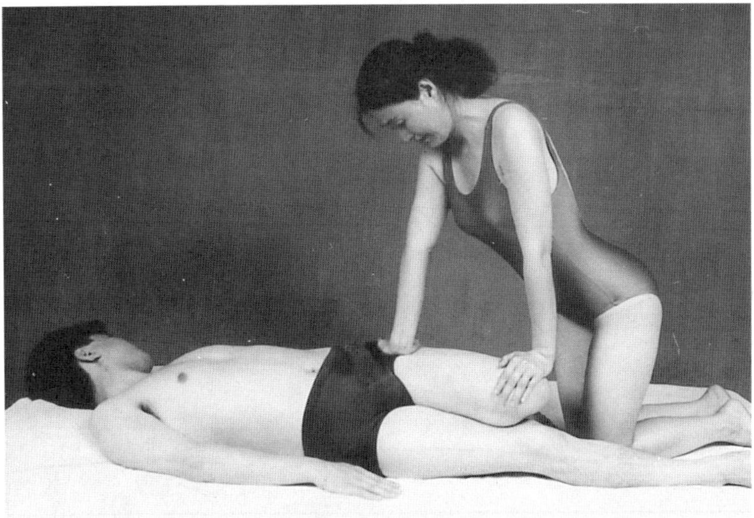

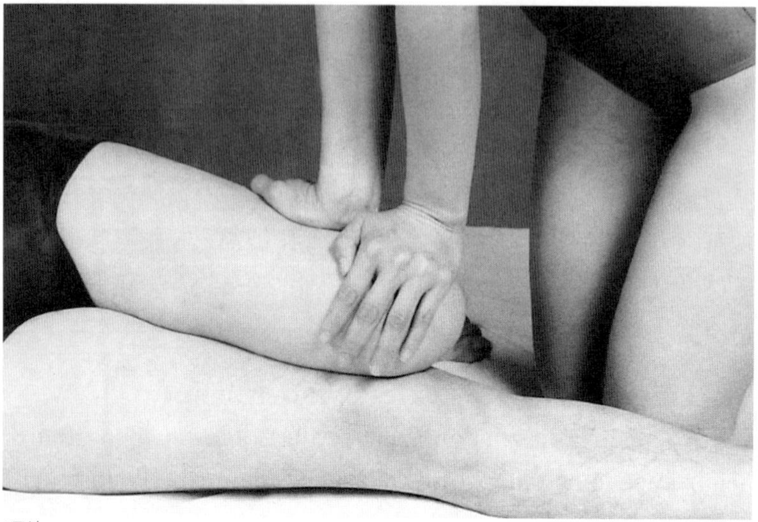

照片 (Photo) 86

圖示 (Fig.) 61

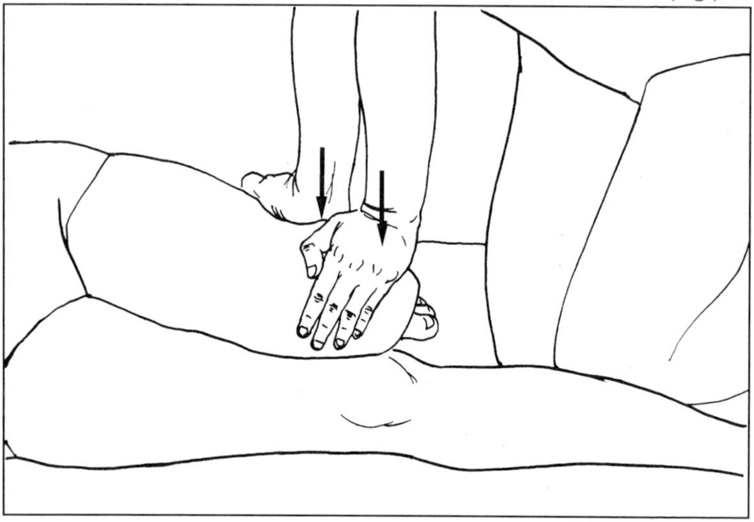

59 伸膝按壓法：

被按摩者仰臥位，右下肢伸直抬高約45度；按摩者左下肢屈髖屈膝，蹲於床面之上，右下肢跪位，右腕關節背伸，掌根着力被按摩者膝關節前上方，行向下按壓之力，至大腿近端前方肌群，同時左手置於足根部，以前臂遠端的掌側面按壓足部，使踝關節極度背伸，反復操作2－4次（見照片87和圖示62）。一側完畢更換另一側。

Pressing stretched knee method:

The patient lies flat on back, stretches the right lower limb straight, raised at about 45 degrees. The massagist bends the hip and knee of left lower limb and squats down on the bed; kneels down on right lower limb and stretches the right wrist joint backward. With force of palm root on the front upper part of knee joint of the patient, press down to front muscles at the near end of thigh. At the same time, place left hand on the heel and press the sole with the far end of front arm at the palm side, stretching the ankle joint backward to the utmost. Repeat the manipulation 2-4 times (see Photo 87 and Fig. 62). Do one side, then the other.

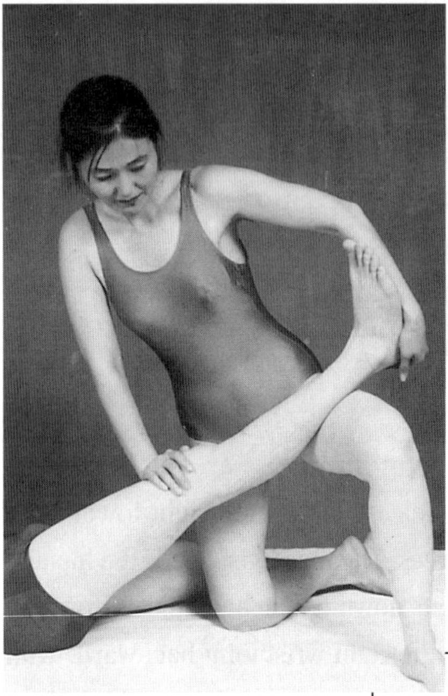

照片 (Photo) 87

圖示 (Fig.) 62

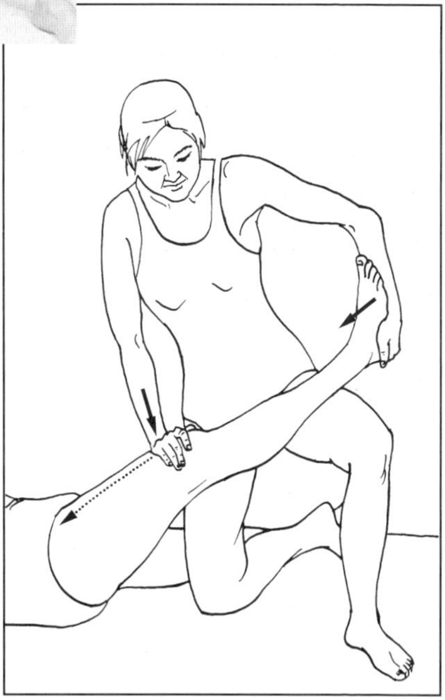

60 按壓小腿外側肌群：

被按摩者仰臥位，左側下肢內旋；按摩者屈膝關節跪位於同側，一手掌按壓左膝關節的前外方，一手按前足背側，用右膝關節的前下方按壓其小腿的前外側肌群，從膝關節至踝關節上方，反復操作2－4次（見照片88和圖示63）。一側完畢更換另一側。

Pressing outside muscles of shank:

The patient lies flat on back and revolves the left lower limb inward. The massagist bends knee joints and kneels on the same side. Press the outside front of left knee joint with one palm and press the dorsum of foot with the other hand. Press the outside front muscles of shank with the front lower part of right knee joint from knee joint to the upper part of ankle joint. Repeat the manipulation 2-4 times (see Photo 88 and Fig. 63). Do one side, then the other.

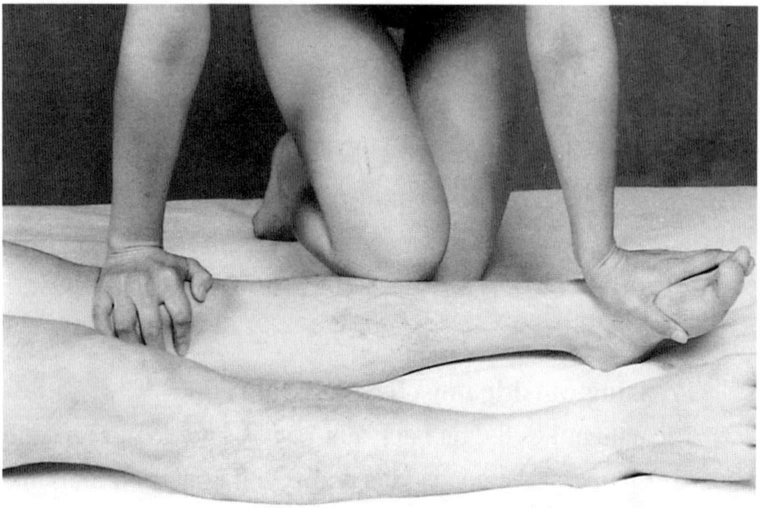

照片 (Photo) 88

圖示 (Fig.) 63

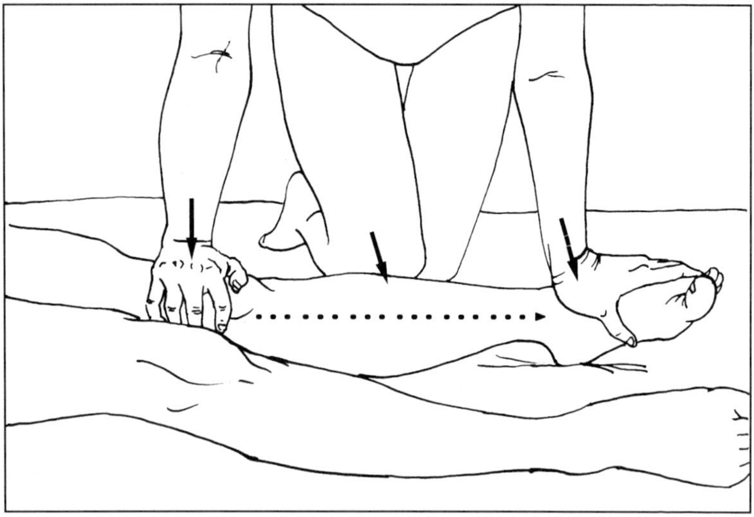

61 旋推大腿外側肌群：

體位同上。按摩者雙手拇指與其餘四指分開，置於被按摩者膝關節上方將其大腿前外側肌群向近心端旋推，反復操作2－4次（見照片89和圖示64）。一側完畢更換另一側。

Revolving and pushing outside muscles of thigh:

In same position. The massagist separates the thumbs with other four fingers of both hands and places them on the upper part of patient's knee joint. Revolve and push the outside front muscles of thigh to the near center. Repeat the manipulation 2-4 times (see Photo 89 and Fig. 64). Do one side, then the other.

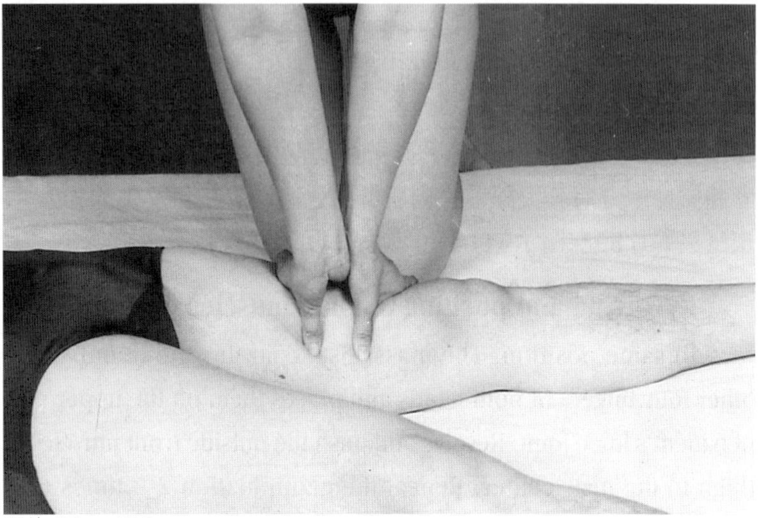

照片 (Photo)89

圖示 (Fig.) 64

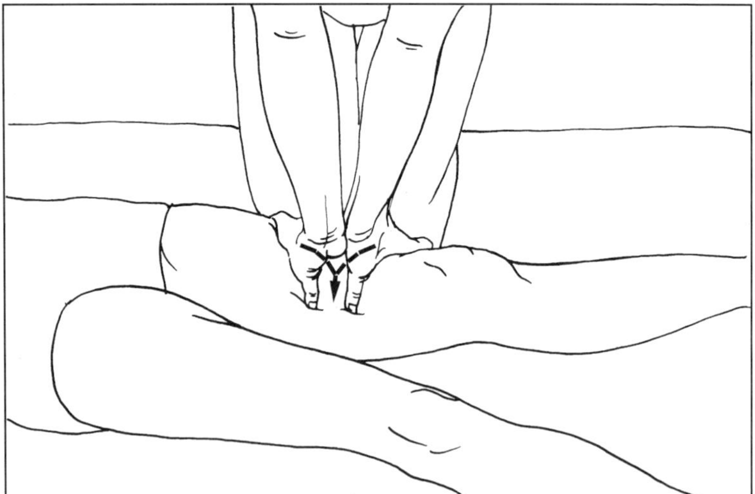

62 按壓大腿前方肌群：

被按摩者仰臥位，雙下肢中立位。按摩者跪位，雙膝關節夾住被按摩者右小腿，雙上肢伸直內旋，雙手五指交叉，置於被按摩者大腿正前方（見照片**90**），從腹股溝處向下按壓至膝關節處（見照片**91**和圖示**65**），反復操作**2－4**次。一側完畢更換另一側。

Pressing front muscles of thigh:

The patient lies flat on back with both legs straight. The massagist kneels and clamps the patient's right shank between both knee joints; stretches straight and revolves inward both upper limbs, crosses five fingers of both hands and places them on the front of thigh of the patient (see Photo 90) and then presses down from the groin to knee joint (see Photo 91 and Fig. 65). Repeat the manipulation 2-4 times. Do one side, then the other.

照片 (Photo) 90

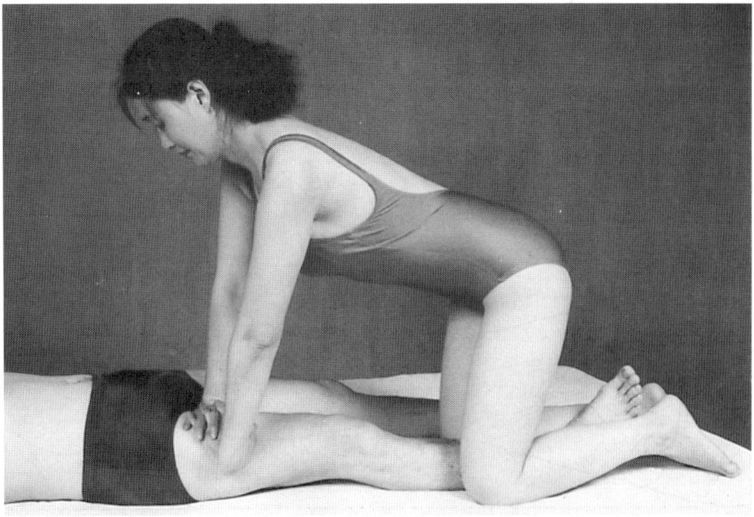

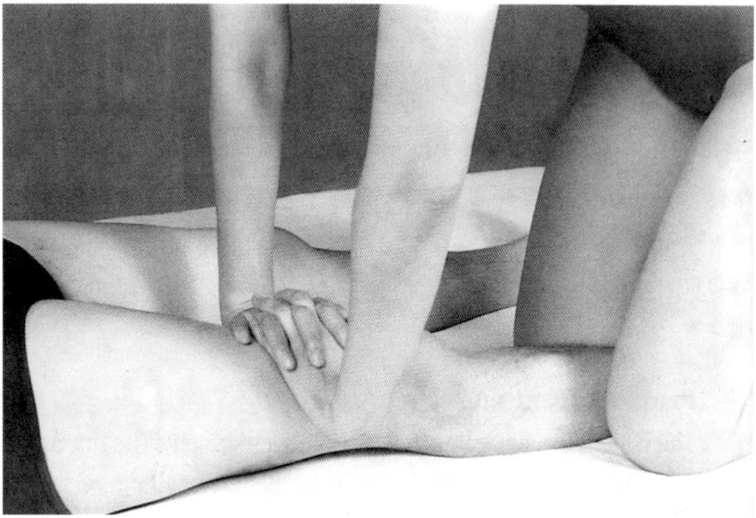

照片 (Photo) 91

圖示 (Fig.) 65

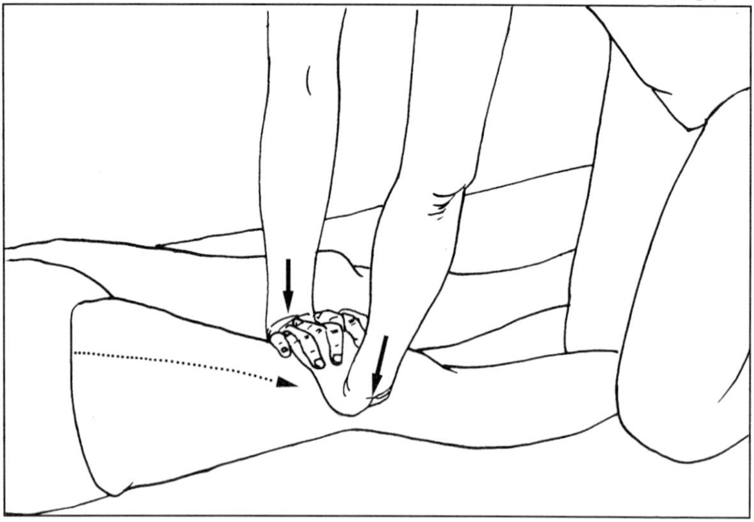

63 疊壓大腿前方肌群：

體位同上。按摩者上肢伸直內旋，雙手掌重疊置於被按摩者大腿正前方，從腹股溝處向下按壓至膝關節處，反復操作2－4次（見照片92和圖示66）。一側完畢更換另一側。

Overlapping hands to press front muscles of thigh:

In same position. The massagist stretches straight and revolves inside upper limbs and overlaps both palms on the front of the patient's thigh, and then presses downward from the groin to the knee joint. Repeat the manipulation 2-4 times (see Photo 92 and Fig. 66). Do one side, then the other.

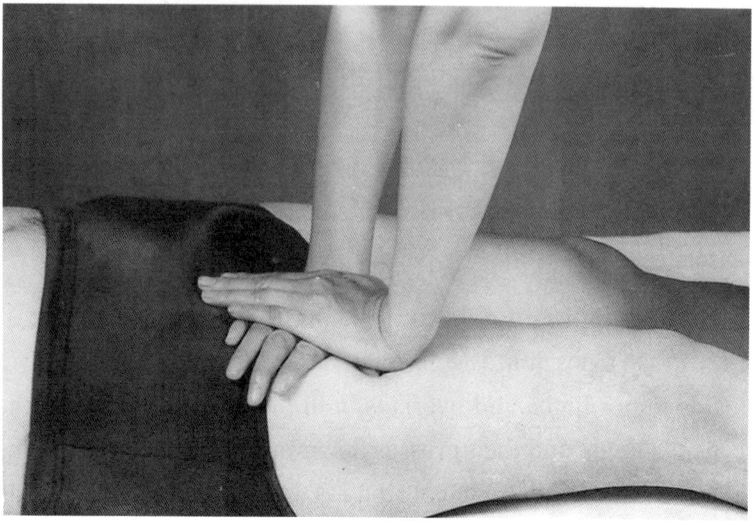

照片 (Photo) 92

圖示 (Fig.) 66

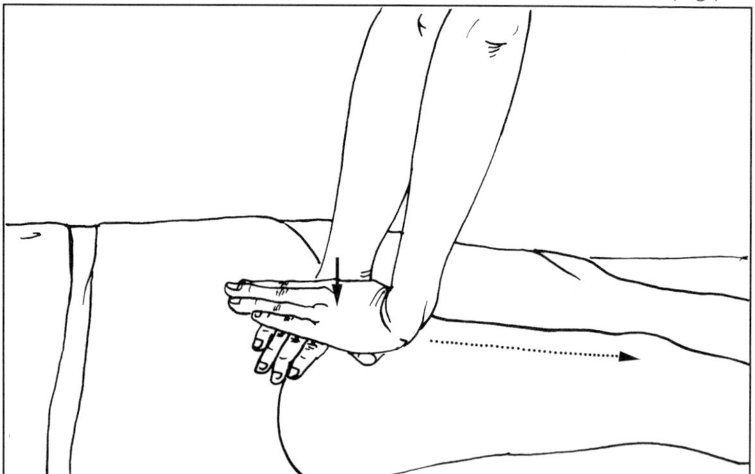

64 指叩法：

體位同上。按摩者跪坐於一側，雙手合十，五指分開，掌指及指間關節伸直位（見照片**93**），靠前臂旋前旋後動作，帶動腕關節，以小指尺側着力，叩擊被按摩者大腿前方肌群（見照片**94**和圖示**67**），從腹股溝處至膝關節，反復叩擊**2－4**次。一側完畢更換另一側。

Digital-tapping method:

In same position. The massagist kneels at one side with palms together, separates five fingers and stretches joints between palms and fingers and finger joints (see Photo 93); by the movement of inclining the wrist joint ulna and radius and with the force of little finger ulna, taps the front muscles of the patient's thigh (see Photo 94 and Fig. 67) from the groin to knee joint. Repeat the tapping 2-4 times. Do one side, then the other.

照片 (Photo) 93

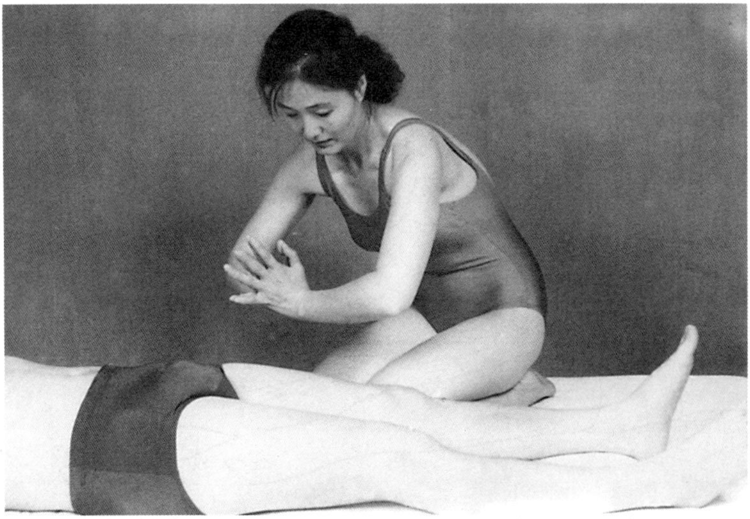

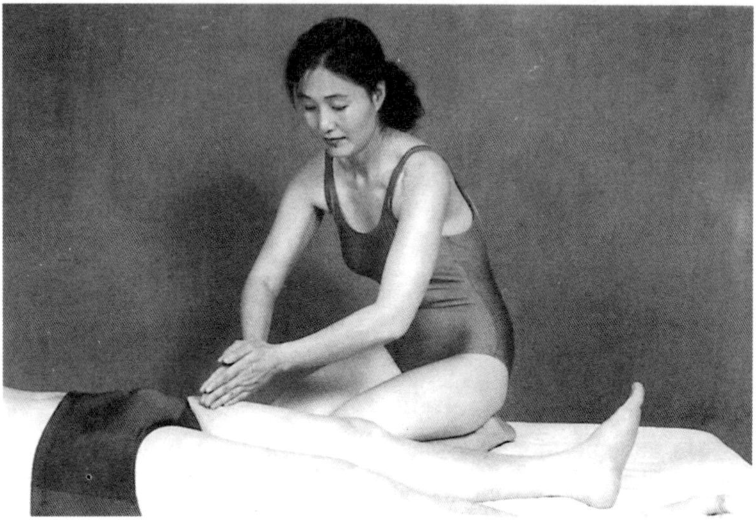

照片 (Photo) 94

圖示 (Fig.) 67

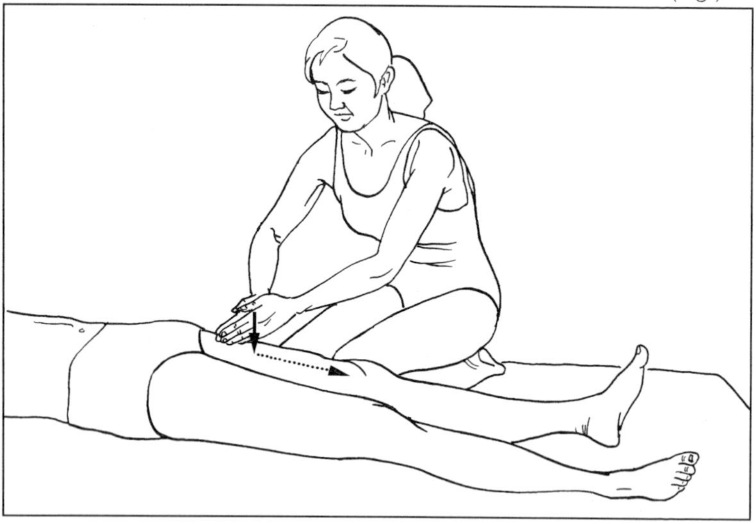

65 按壓肩關節：

被按摩者仰臥位，右上肢外展約90度。按摩者跪於同側，右上肢伸直，腕關節背伸，用掌根部按壓被按摩者肩關節前方，反復按壓2－4次（見照片95和圖示68）。一側完畢更換另一側。

Pressing shoulder joint:

The patient lies flat on back and stretches out the right upper limb at about 90 degrees. The massagist kneels on the same side, stretches the right upper limb straight and stretches wrist joint backward; then presses the front of the patient's shoulder joint with palm root. Repeat the pressing 2-4 times (see Photo 95 and Fig. 68). Do one side, then the other.

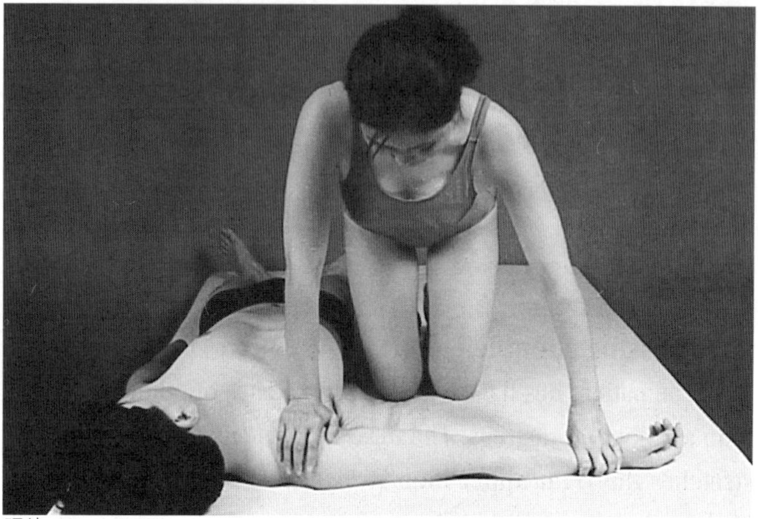
照片 (Photo) 95

圖示 (Fig.) 68

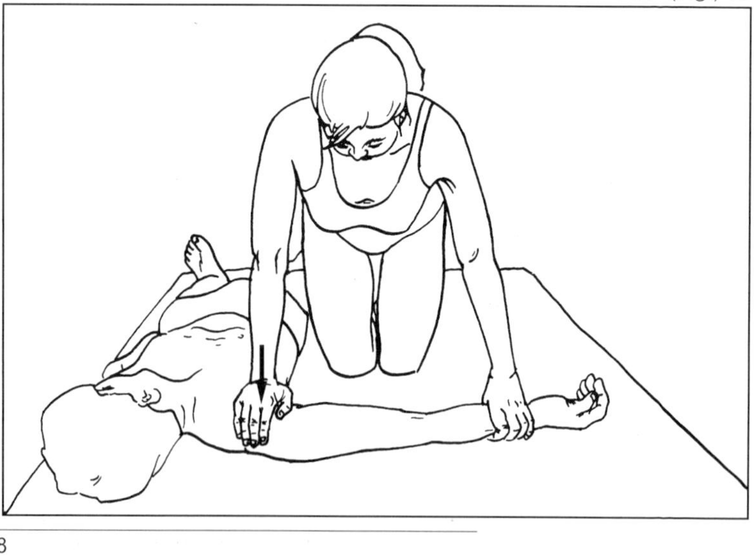

66 提拉肩部肌群

體位同上。按摩者雙手的2、3、4、5指置於被按摩者肩關節後方，以屈掌指及指間關節之力，將其頸肩部肌群向前方提拉，反復提拉4－6次（見照片96和圖示69）。一側完畢更換另一側。

Lifting and pulling shoulder muscles:

In same position. The massagist places the 2nd, 3rd, 4th and 5th fingers of both hands on the back of the patient's shoulder joint. With the force of bending joints between palm and fingers and finger joints, lift and pull the muscles of the patient's neck and shoulder and lift them forward. Repeat the lifting and pulling 4-6 times (see Photo 96 and Fig. 69). Do one side, then the other.

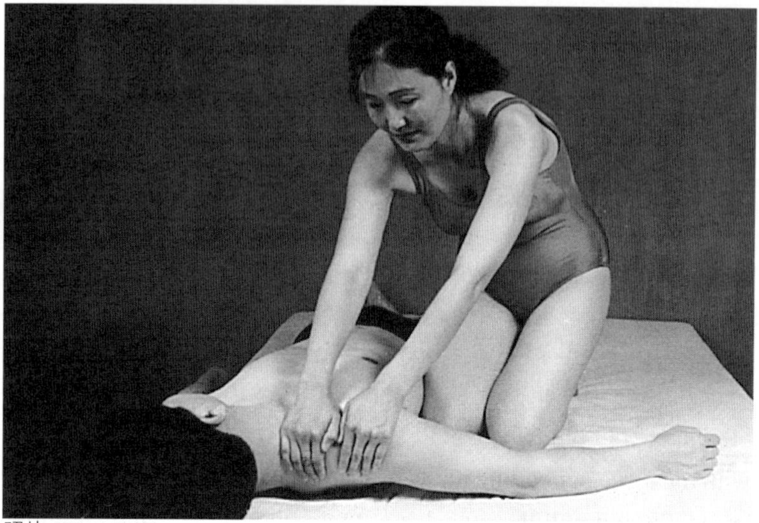

照片 (Photo) 96

圖示 (Fig.) 69

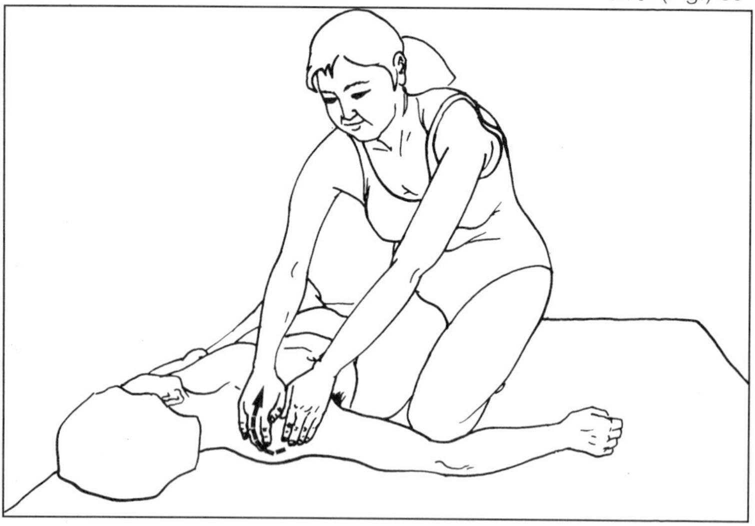

67 拇指按揉腋窩法：

體位同上。按摩者雙手上肢伸直，拇指伸直，以指腹為着力點，置於被按摩者腋窩處，分別行按法（見照片**97**和圖示**70**）和揉法（見圖示**71**），交替操作**2－4**次。一側完畢更換另一側。

Thumb-pressing and rubbing armpit method:

In same position. The massagist stretches both upper limbs straight as well as thumbs; with the force of finger insides, places them on the patient's armpit and carries out pressing (see Photo 97 and Fig. 70) and rubbing (see Fig. 71) methods respectively. Repeat the manipulation alternatively 2-4 times. Do one side, then the other.

照片 (Photo) 97

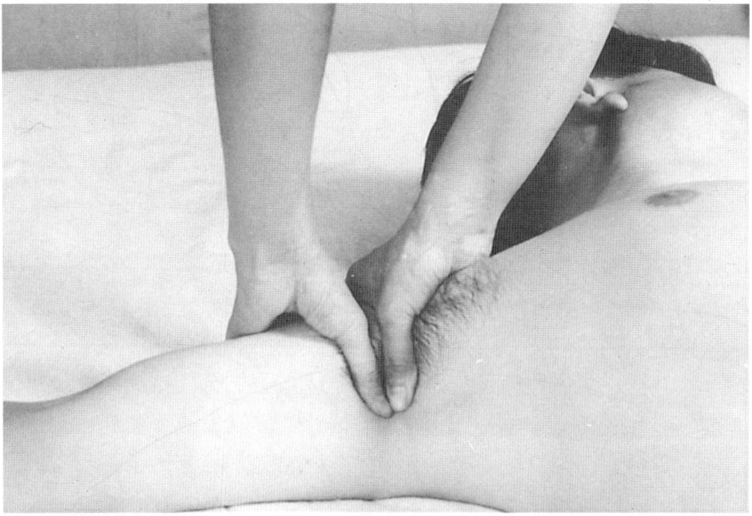

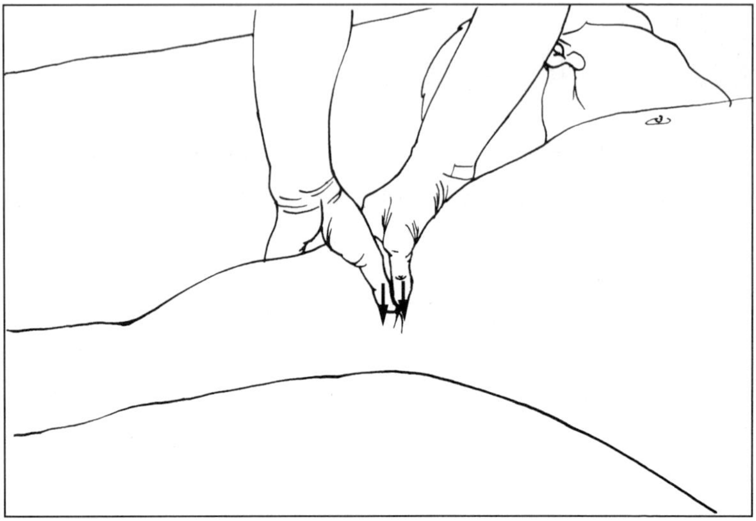

圖示 (Fig.) 70

圖示 (Fig.) 71

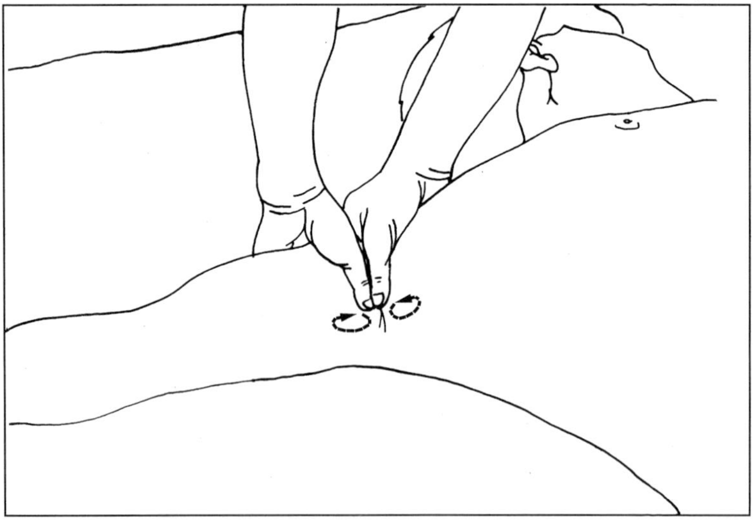

68 提拿上肢內側肌群：

被按摩者仰臥位，上肢外展90度，掌心向上。按摩者跪坐於同側，雙手拇指與其餘四指掌指及指間關節伸直（見照片98），以對指提拿之力，從按摩者腋窩處提拿上肢前內側肌群至腕關節（見照片99和圖示72），反復操作2－4次。一側完畢更換另一側。

Lifting inside muscles of upper limb:

The patient lies flat on back and stretches the right upper limb outward at an angle of 90 degrees with palm upward. The massagist kneels on the same side and stretches straight joints between palm and fingers and finger joints of the thumb and other four fingers of both hands (see Photo 98). With the force of finger lifting, lift the front inside muscles of the upper limb of the patient from the armpit to the wrist joint (see Photo 99 and Fig. 72). Repeat the manipulation 2-4 times. Do one side, then the other.

照片 (Photo) 98

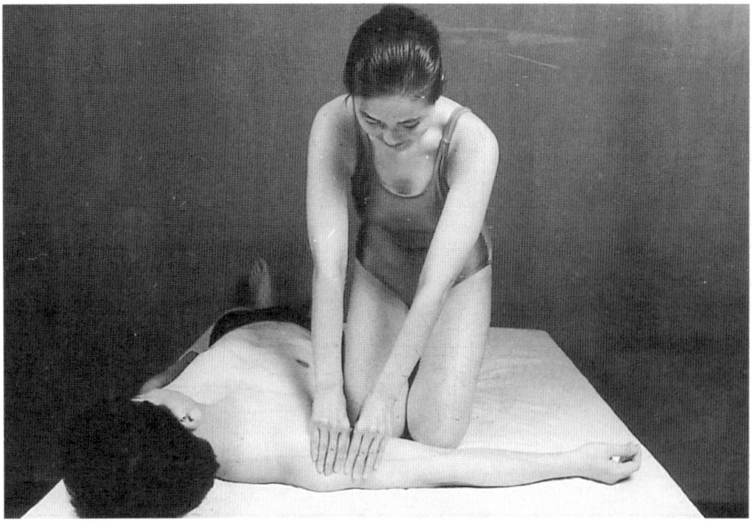

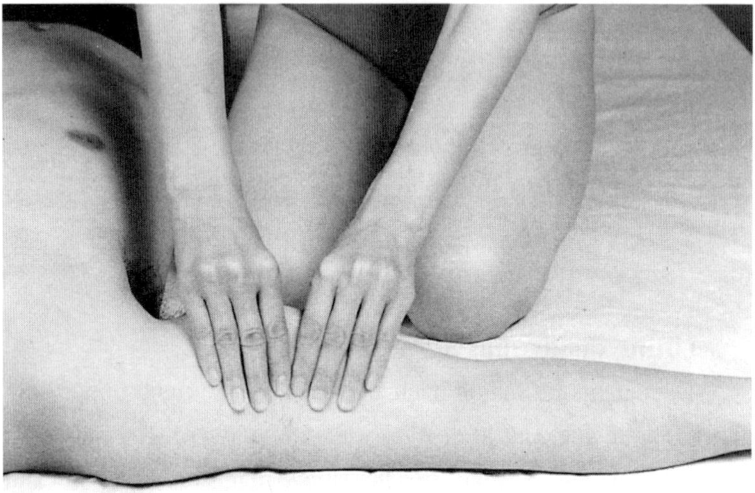

照片 (Photo) 99

圖示 (Fig.) 72

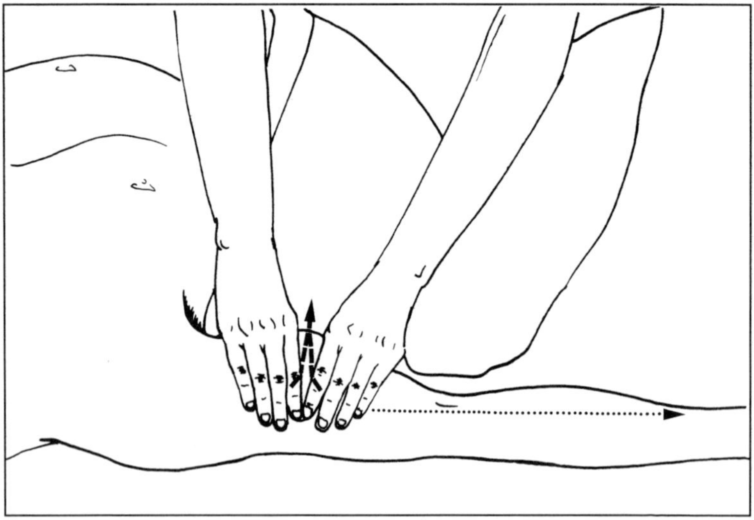

69 點揉捏拿法：

體位同上。按摩者先用拇指指端點揉被按摩者合谷穴（見照片**100**和圖示**73**），再依次捏拿拇指、食指、中指、無名指、小指的背側，從遠心端至掌指關節處（見照片**101**和圖示**74**），反復操作**2**次。一側完畢更換另一側。

Pointing, rubbing and kneading method:

In same position. The massagist first points and rubs the patient's Hegu acupoint with a thumb tip (see Photo 100 and Fig. 73) and then kneads the back of thumb, forefinger, middle finger, ring finger and little finger from far center to joints between palm and fingers (see Photo 101 and Fig. 74). Repeat the manipulation twice. Do one side, then the other.

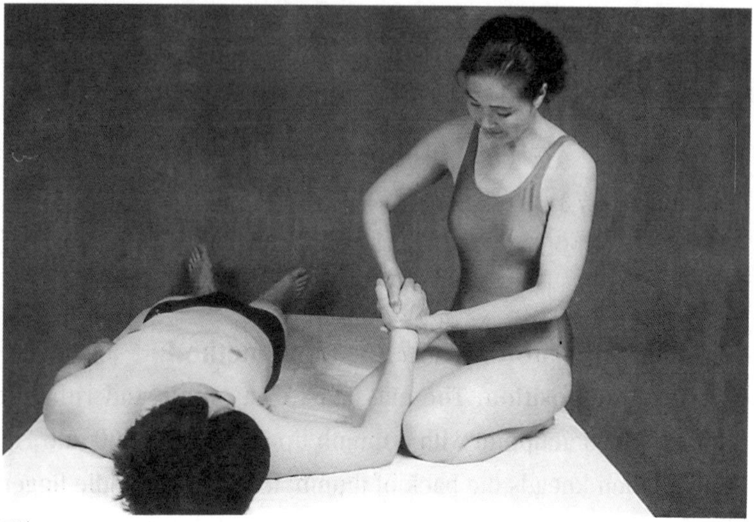
照片 (Photo) 100

圖示 (Fig.) 73
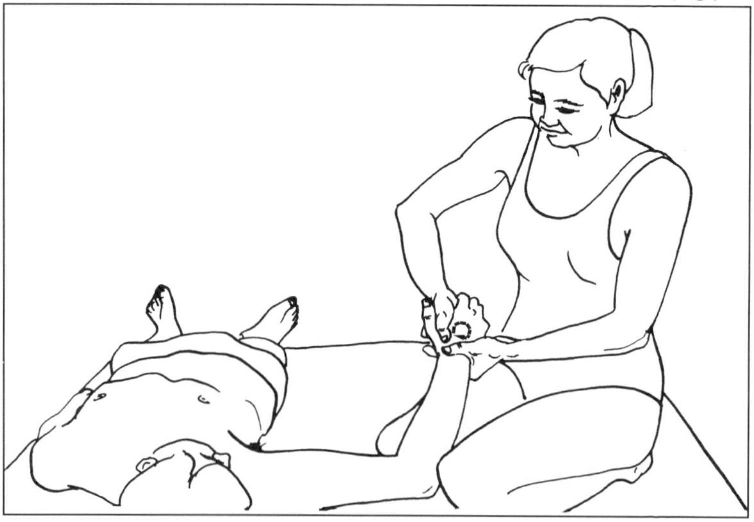

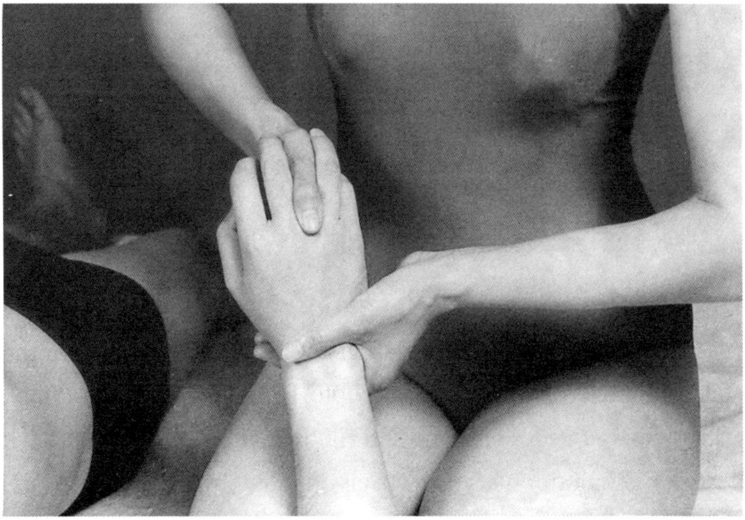

照片 (Photo) 101

圖示 (Fig.) 74

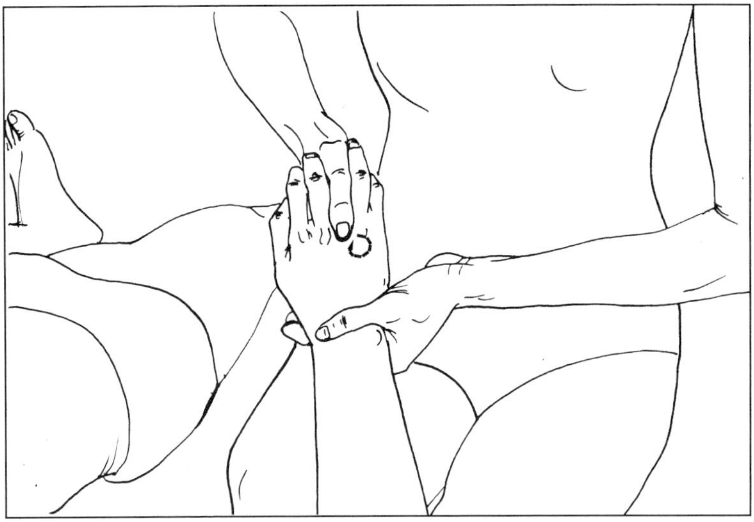

70 按揉法：

體位同上。按摩者雙手拇指置於被按摩者腕關節背側（見照片102和圖示75），以指腹按揉之力，依次按揉第1－5掌骨背側（見照片103），反復操作2次。一側完畢更換另一側。

Pressing and rubbing method:

In same position. The massagist places both thumbs on the back of patient's wrist joint (see Photo 102 and Fig. 75). With the force of finger insides pressing and rubbing, press and rub the back of Nos. 1-5 palm bones respectively (see Photo 103). Repeat the manipulation twice. Do one side, then the other.

照片 (Photo)102

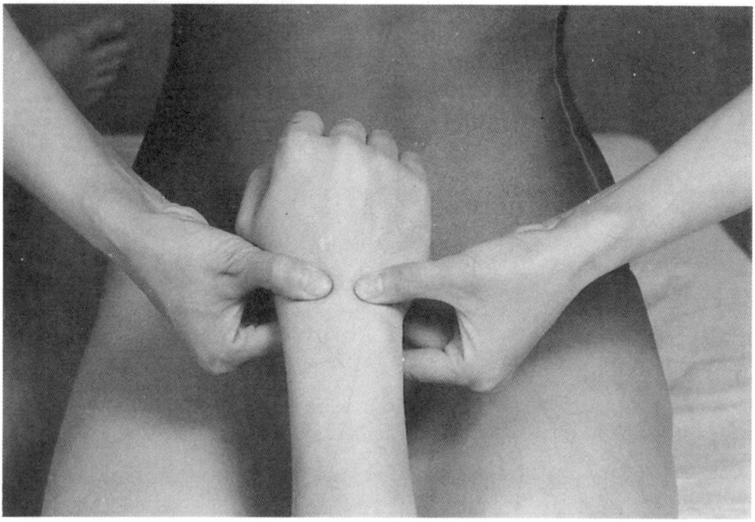

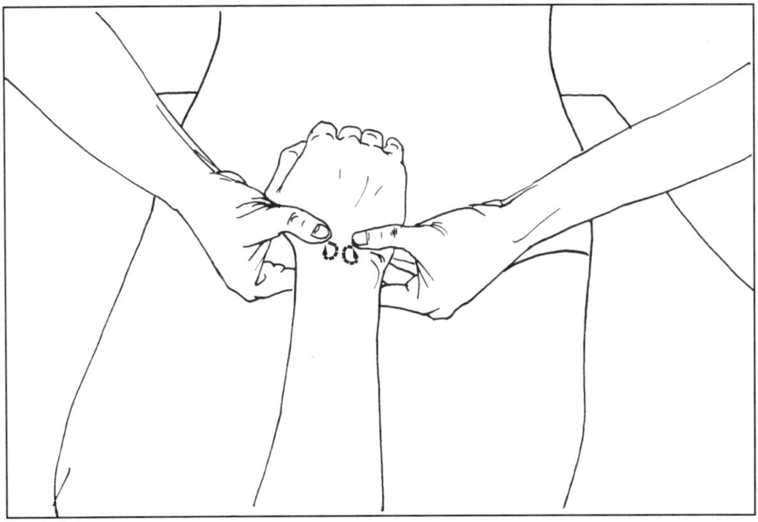

圖示 (Fig.) 75

照片 (Photo) 103

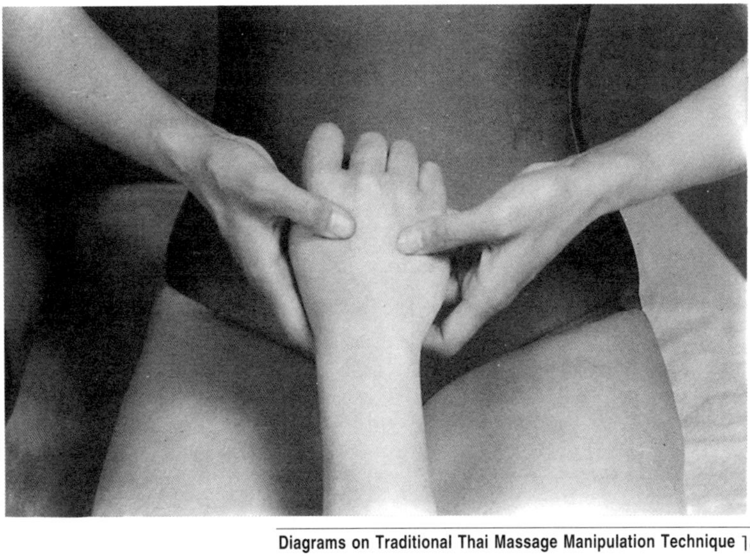

71 搖掌指關節法：

體位同上。按摩者一手扶握被按摩者腕關節，另一手的拇指和食指捏拿其拇指，做掌指關節的搖晃動作，依次從拇指至小指（見照片**104**和圖示**76**）。一側完畢更換另一側。

Shaking palm finger joints method:

In same position. The massagist holds the patient's wrist joint with one hand and kneads the thumb with the thumb and forefinger of other hand. Shake joints between palm and fingers from the thumb to little finger in an orderly way (see Photo 104 and Fig. 76). Do one side, then the other.

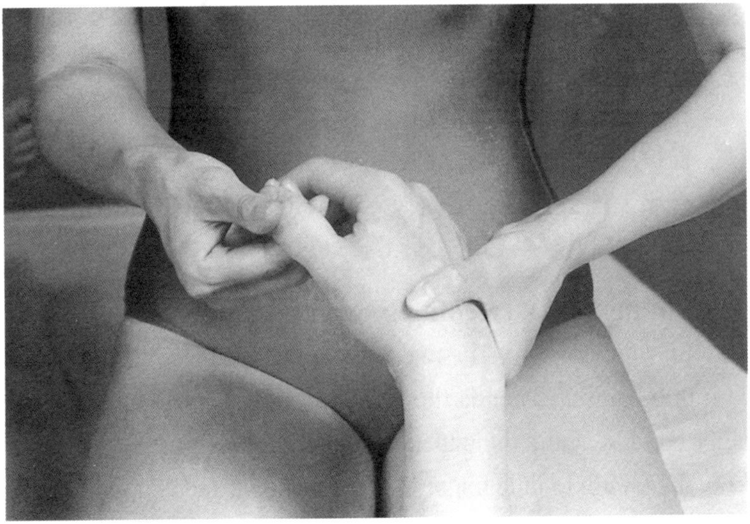
照片 (Photo) 104

圖示 (Fig.) 76

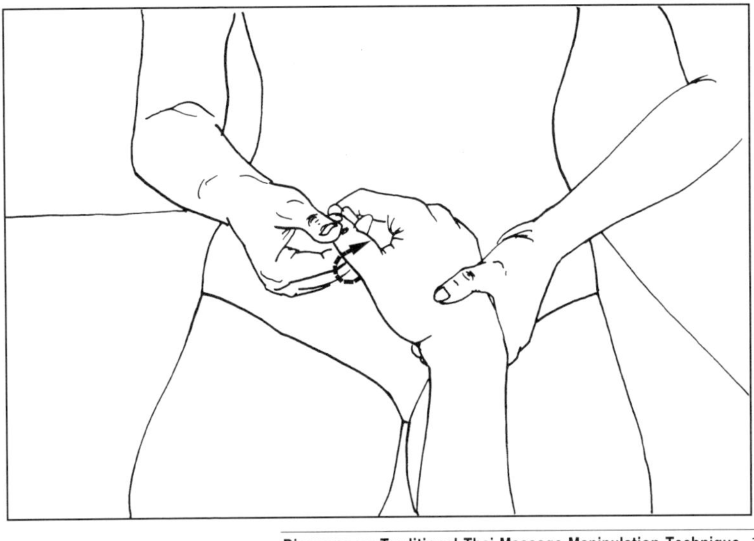

72 手指拔伸法：

體位同上。按摩者手扶握被按摩者腕關節，另一手的食、中指屈曲並夾住被按摩者手指向遠心端拔伸，依次從拇指至小指（見照片**105**和圖示**77**）。一側完畢更換另一側。

Pulling and stretching fingers method:

In same position. The massagist holds the patient's wrist joint with one hand and bends the forefinger and middle finger of the other hand to clamp the patient's finger and pull it to the far center from the thumb to little finger in an orderly way (see Photo 105 and Fig. 77). Do one side, then the other.

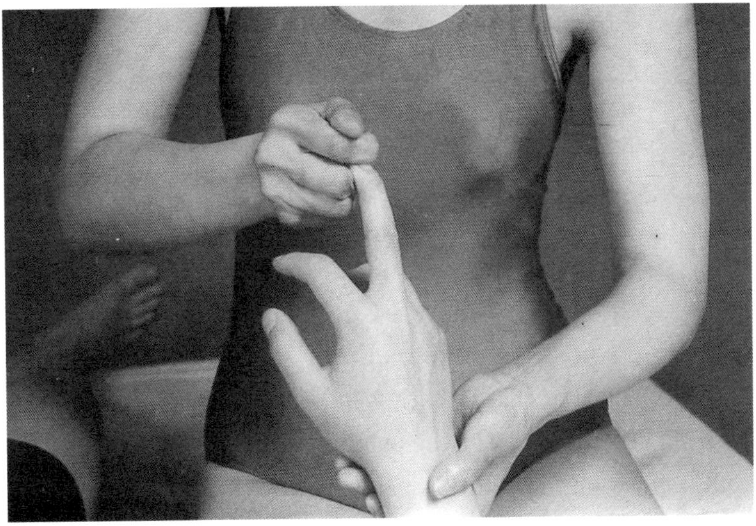

照片 (Photo) 105

圖示 (Fig.) 77

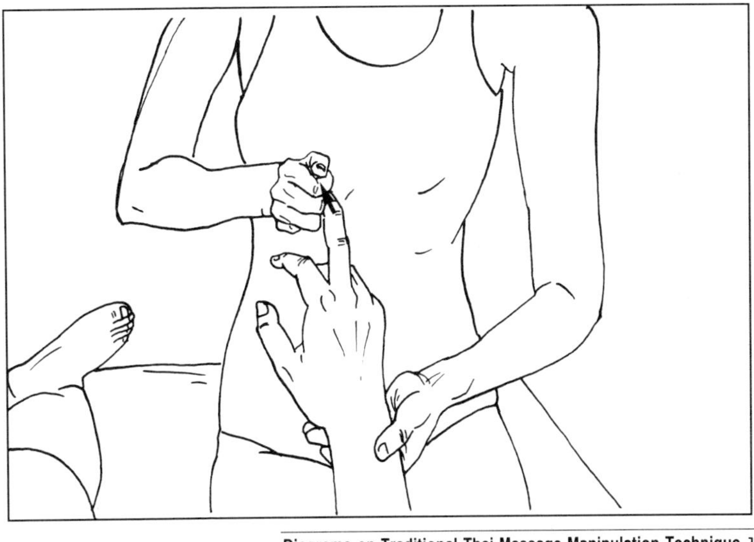

73 指推掌心法：

被按摩者仰臥位，屈肘關節，前臂旋前掌心向上。按摩者雙手拇指置於被按摩者掌根部以指腹着力，向其五指掌指關節處搓推（見照片**106**和圖示**78**），反復操作**2－4**次。一側完畢更換另一側。

Digital-pushing palm method:

The patient lies flat on back, bends an elbow joint and revolves the front arm forward with the palm upward. The massagist places both thumbs on the patient's palm root; with the force of thumb insides, kneads and pushes the joints between palm and five fingers (see Photo 106 and Fig. 78). Repeat the manipulation 2-4 times. Do one side, then the other.

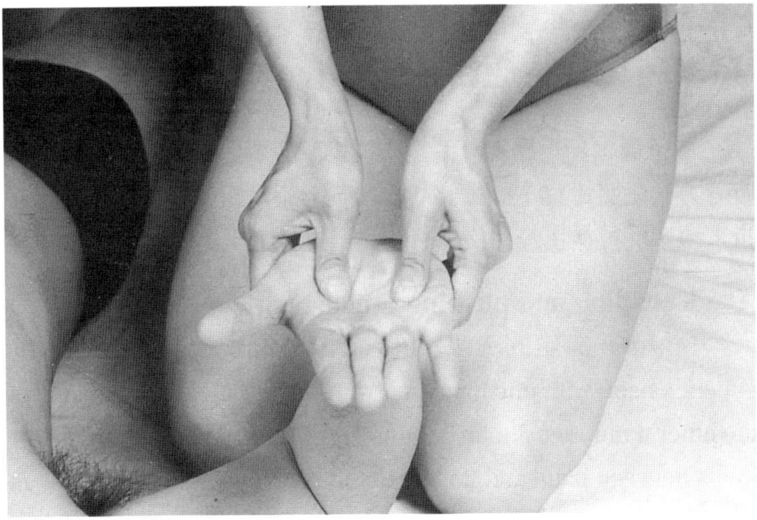
照片 (Photo) 106

圖示 (Fig.) 78

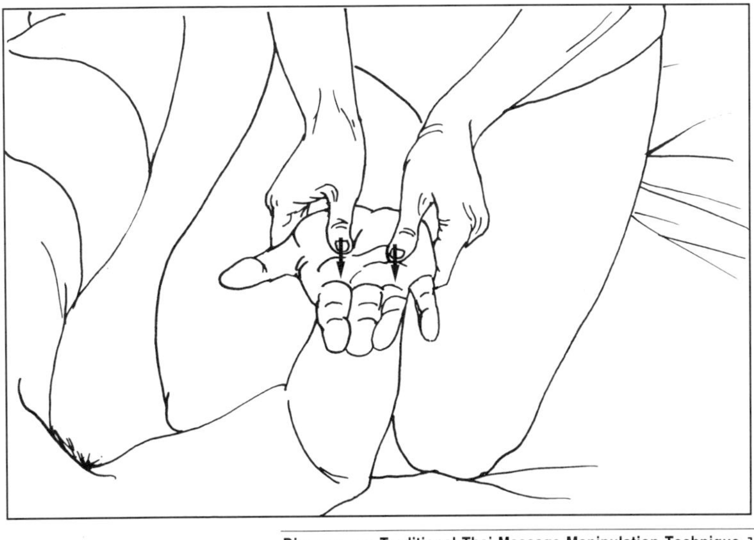

74 搓推指腹法：

體位同上。按摩者一手托扶被按摩者手背，另一手以拇指指腹着力（見照片**107**和圖示**79**），從五指掌指關節依次搓推至五指末節，反復操作**2－4**次。一側完畢更換另一側。

Kneading and pushing finger inside method:

In same position. The massagist holds the dorsum of the patient's hand with one hand and with the force of thumb inside of the other hand (see Photo 107 and Fig. 79), kneads and pushes the joints between palm and fingers to the last joint of five fingers in an orderly way. Repeat the manipulation 2-4 times. Do one side, then the other.

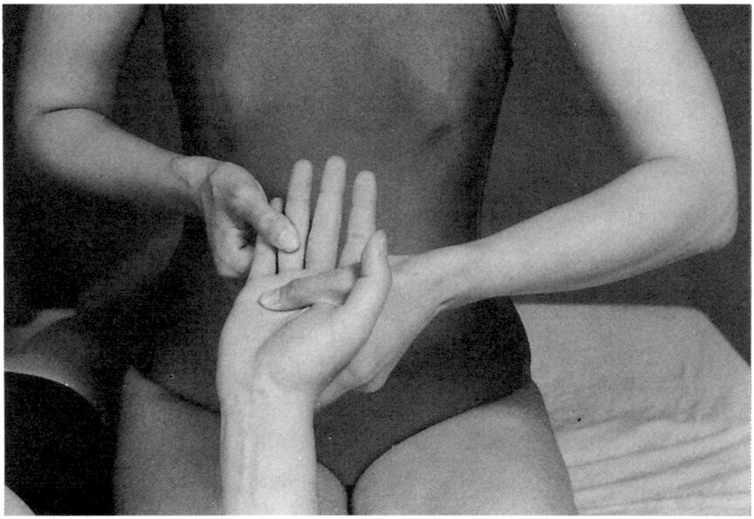

照片 (Photo) 107

圖示 (Fig.) 79

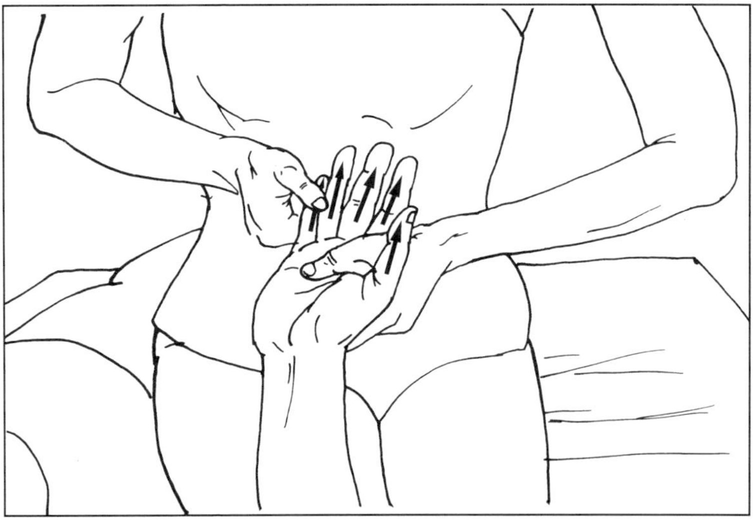

75 伸指間關節法：

體位同上。被按摩者前臂旋前，掌心向上；按摩者一手托扶其腕關節，另一手拇指伸直，向背側按壓其手指遠端，而食指屈曲向掌側按壓掌指關節處（見照片**108**和圖示**80**），依次從拇指至小指。注意按壓力不宜過重，避免造成掌指關節損傷。一側完畢更換另一側。

Stretching finger joints method:

In same position. The patient revolves a forearm forward with the palm upward. The massagist holds the patient's wrist joint with a hand and presses the far end of fingers backward with a stretched-straight thumb of the other hand and presses the joints between palm and fingers with a bent forefinger (see Photo 108 and Fig. 80) from the thumb to little finger in an orderly way. Note, do not use too heavy a force to avoid joints between palm and fingers getting injured. Do one side, then the other.

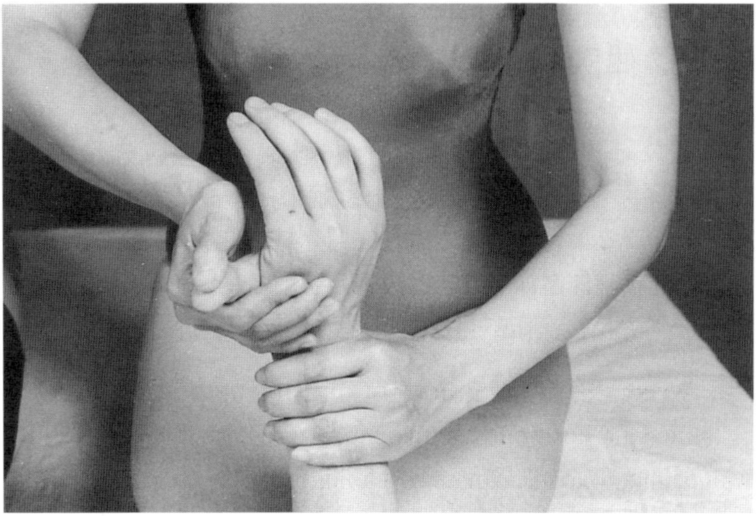

照片 (Photo) 108

圖示 (Fig.) 80

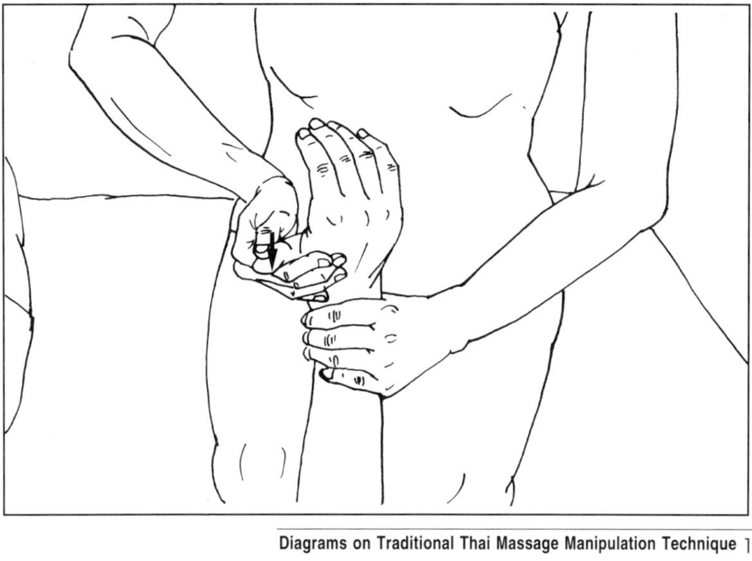

76 伸腕拔節法：

體位同上。被按摩者前臂旋前，掌心向上，按摩者一手扶握其腕關節，另一上肢屈肘，前臂旋前，掌心向下與其掌心相對，五指交叉，行向下壓之力（見照片**109**和圖示**81**），再借屈曲五指遠端指間關節之力向上拔提其腕關節（見照片**110** 和圖示**82**），如此反復操作**2－4**次。一側完畢更換另一側。

Wrist stretching and joint pulling method:

In same position. The patient revolves the forearm forward with palm upward. The massagist holds the patient's wrist joint with one hand and bends the elbow of the other upper limb and revolves the forearm forward with palm downward and opposite to the patient's palm and five fingers crossing to carry out the force of pressing down (see Photo 109 and Fig. 81). And, with the force of joints at the far end of five bent fingers, pull up the patient's wrist joint (see Photo 110 and Fig. 82). Repeat the manipulation 2-4 times. Do one side, then the other.

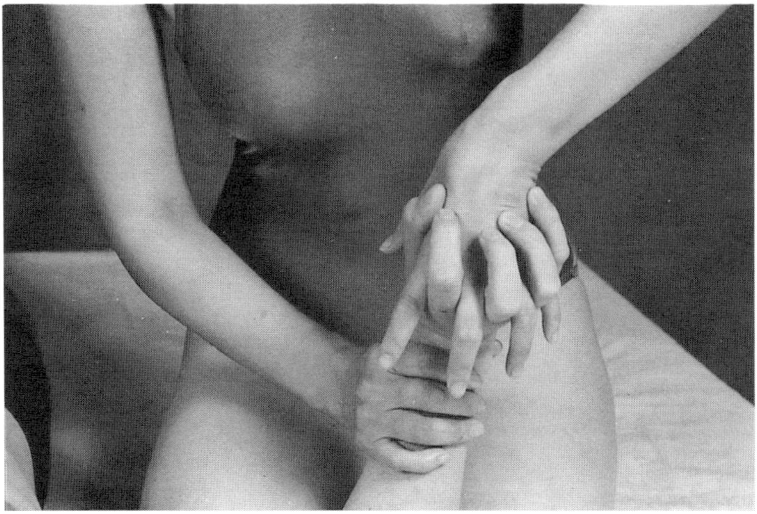
照片 (Photo) 109

圖示 (Fig.) 81

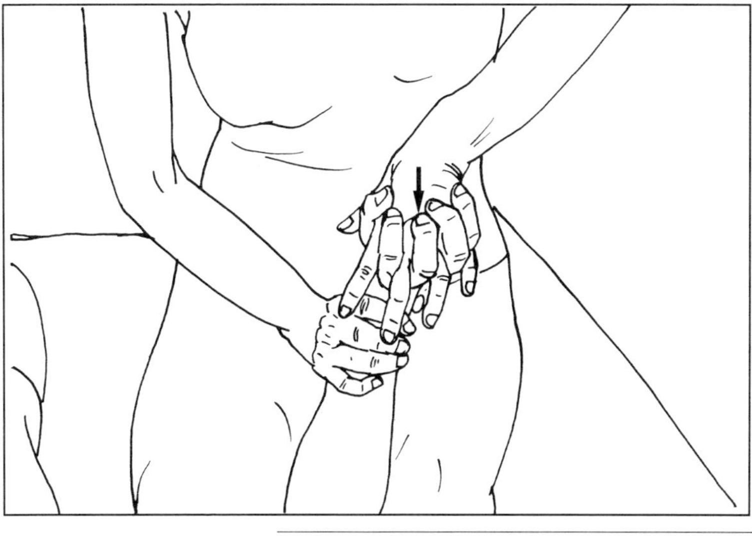

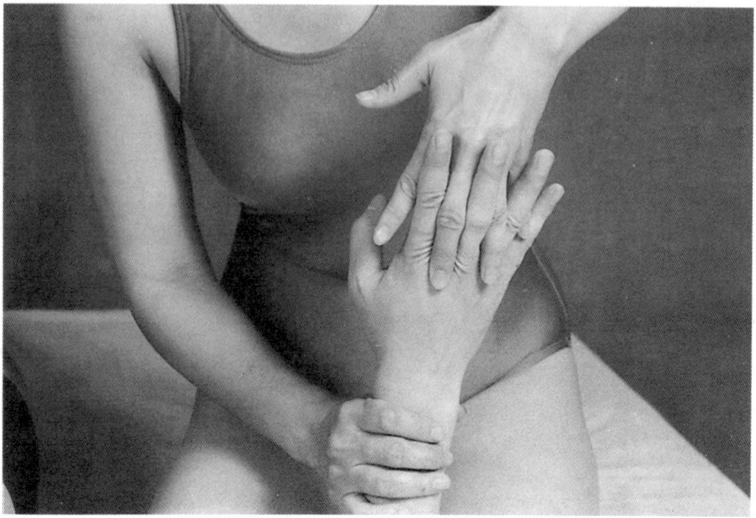

照片 (Photo) 110

圖示 (Fig.) 82

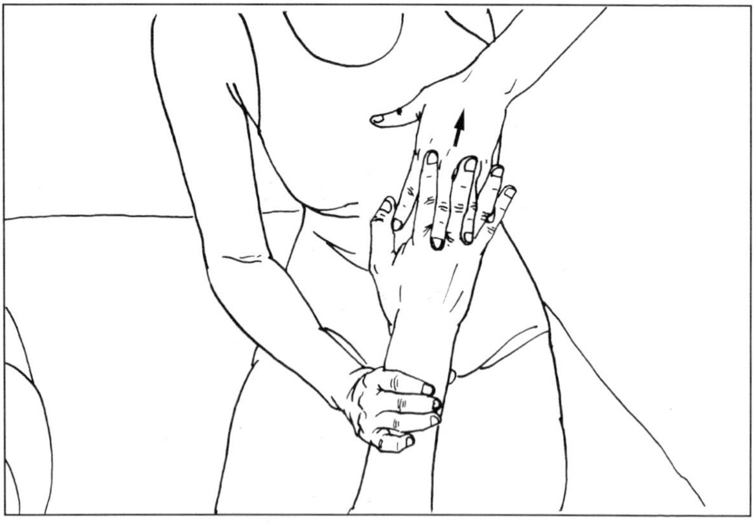

77 屈肘提拿法：

體位同上。被按摩者一側上肢上舉屈肘，前臂旋後，置於肩關節的後方（見照片**111**），按摩者一手向下按壓肘關節處，另一手拇指與其餘四指分開，以五指對合之力，將上肢近端後側肌群向內側提拿（見照片**112**和圖示**83**）。反復操作**2－4**次。一側完畢更換另一側。

Lifting bent-elbow method:

In same position. The patient raises an upper limb, bends the elbow, revolves the forearm backward and places it at the rear of shoulder joint (see Photo 111). The massagist presses the patient's elbow joint downward with one hand and separates the thumb from the other four fingers of the other hand; with the force of all five fingers, lifts up rear muscles of near end of the upper limb inward (see Photo 112 and Fig. 83). Repeat the manipulation 2-4 times. Do one side, then the other.

照片 (Photo) 111

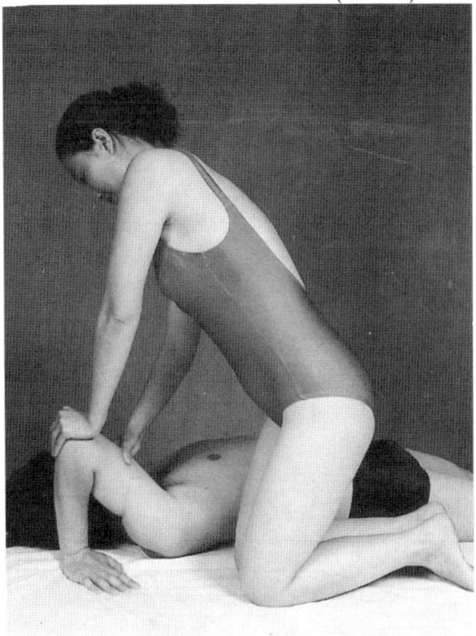

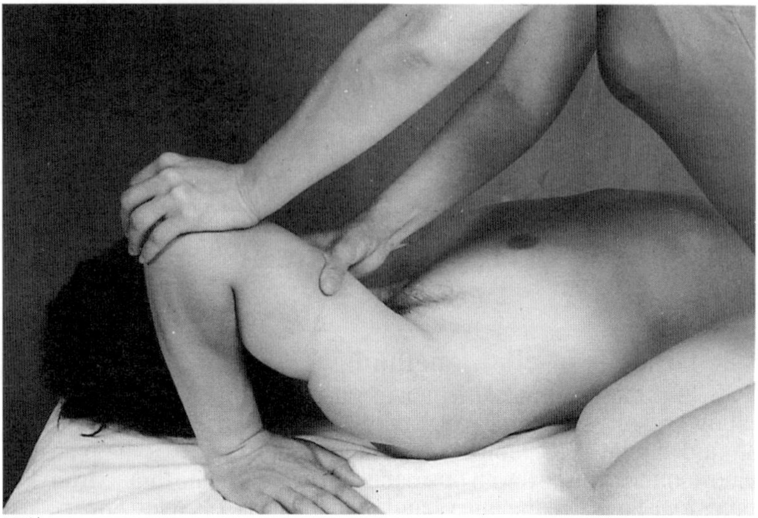
照片 (Photo) 112

圖示 (Fig.) 83
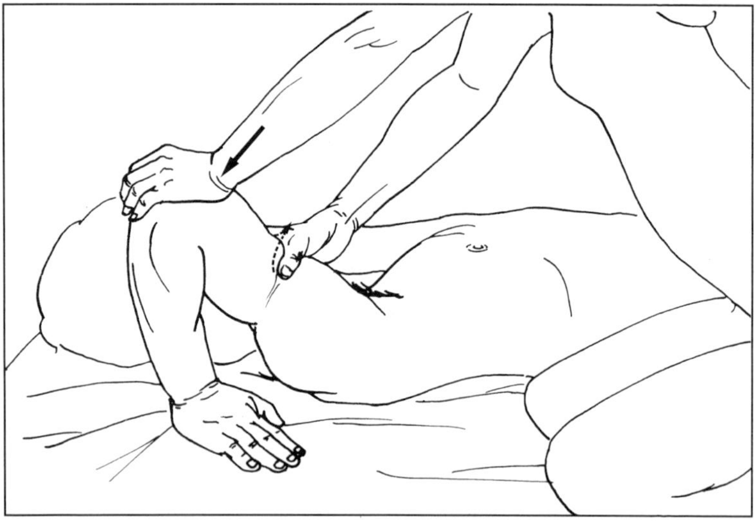

78 指叩上肢法：

被按摩者仰臥位，雙上肢置於軀幹兩側，按摩者跪坐於一側，雙手合十，五指分開，掌指關節及指間關節伸直（見照片**113**），以小指尺側着力，行扣擊法，從肩部扣擊至腕關節處（見照片**114**和圖示**84**）。一側完畢更換另一側。

Digital-tapping upper limb method:

The patient lies flat on back and places both upper limbs on both sides of the body. The massagist kneels at one side with the palms together, separates five fingers and stretches straight joints between palm and fingers and finger joints (see Photo 113); with the force of little finger ulna, taps from the shoulder to wrist joint (see Photo 114 and Fig. 84). Do one side, then the other.

照片 (Photo) 113

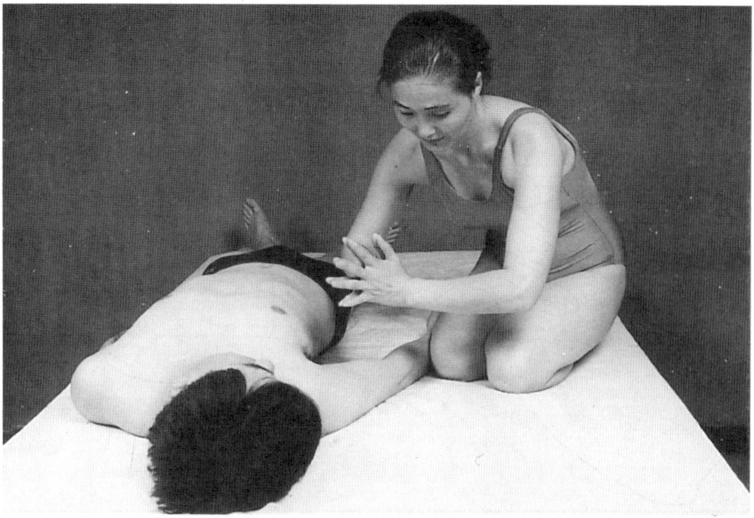

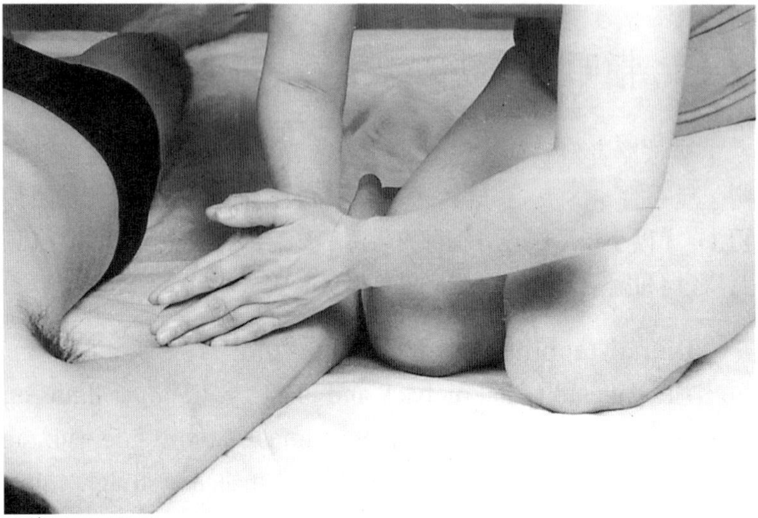
照片 (Photo) 114

圖示 (Fig.) 84

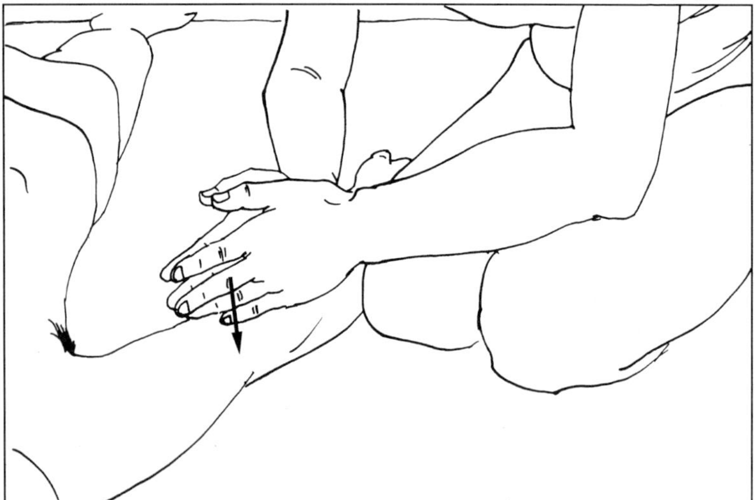

79 按壓夾脊穴：

被按摩者俯臥位，按摩者雙下肢略外展，屈膝跪於床上並將被按摩者的臀部夾住，兩手拇指掌指及指間關節伸直，以指腹為着力點，從腰部向頭側按揉夾脊穴（見照片**115**和圖示**85**），再從腰部向頭側按揉肩胛骨內緣垂線至頸部（見照片**116**和圖示**86**）反復操作**2－4**次。

Pressing Jiaji acupoint method:

The patient lies prone. The massagist slightly spreads both lower limbs outward, bends knees and kneels on bed and clamps the patient's buttocks and stretches joints between palm and fingers and finger joints of both thumbs straight; with the force of finger insides, presses and rubs the Jiaji acupoint from waist to head (see Photo 115 and Fig. 85) and then from waist to head presses and rubs the inside vertical line of the shoulder blade to the neck (see Photo 116 and Fig. 86). Repeat the manipulation 2-4 times.

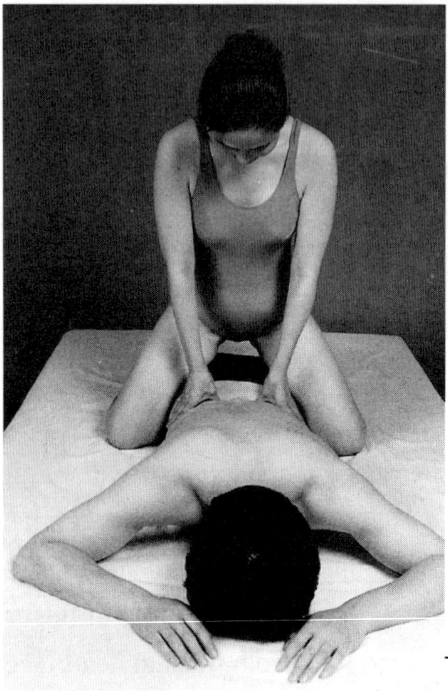

照片 (Photo) 115

圖示 (Fig.) 85

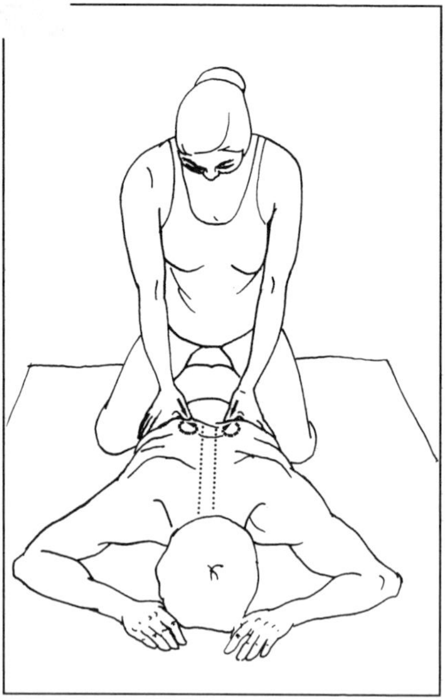

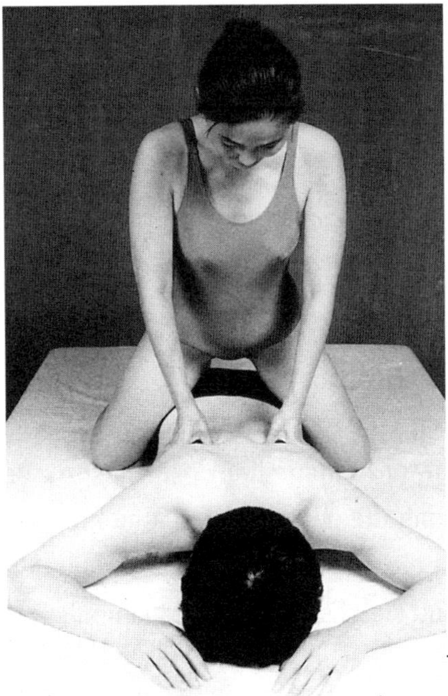

照片 (Photo) 116

圖示 (Fig.) 86

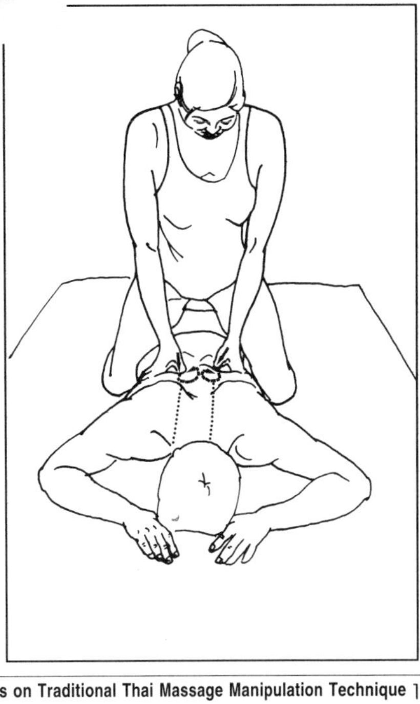

80 肘尖按揉法：

被按摩者體位同上。按摩者屈膝跪於被按摩者一側，一上肢屈肘，以肘尖為着力點，分別沿後正中線兩側旁開兩寸半的部位，依次從腰部按揉至頸肩部，再從頸肩部按揉至腰部（見照片117和圖示87）。反復操作2次。

Elbow-tip-pressing and rubbing method:

The patient in same position. The massagist kneels at the side of the patient and bends the elbow of an upper limb; with the force of elbow tip, presses and rubs along the parts two and a half inches apart from the central line from the waist to the neck and shoulder and vice versa (see Photo 117 and Fig. 87). Repeat the manipulation twice.

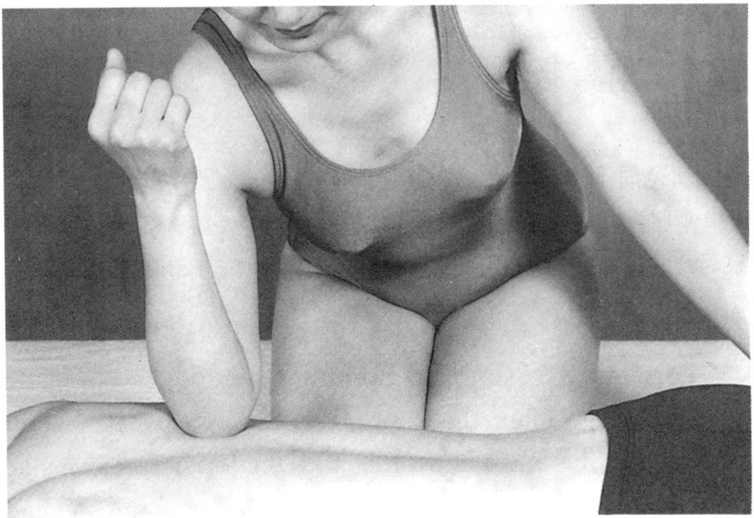

照片 (Photo) 117

圖示 (Fig.) 87

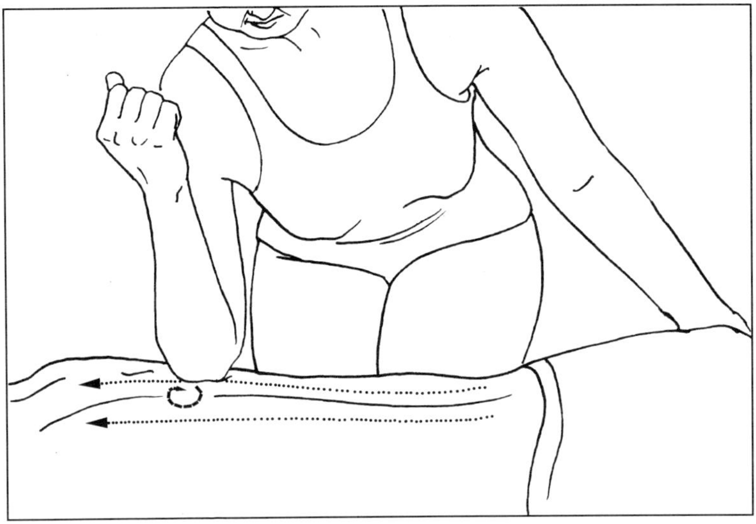

81 前臂按揉法：

體位同上。按摩者一上肢屈肘90度，前臂中立位，以前臂後內側肌群為着力點（見照片118和圖示88A），從被按摩者頸部，沿骶棘肌走行向腰部施按揉法（見照片119和圖示88B）。反復操作2次。

Forearm-pressing and rubbing method:

In same position. The massagist bends an upper limb at 90 degrees with the forearm neutral; with the force of rear inside muscles of the forearm (see Photo 118 and Fig. 88A), presses and rubs the patient's neck, along the musculus sacrospinalis to the waist (see Photo 119 and Fig. 88B). Repeat the manipulation twice.

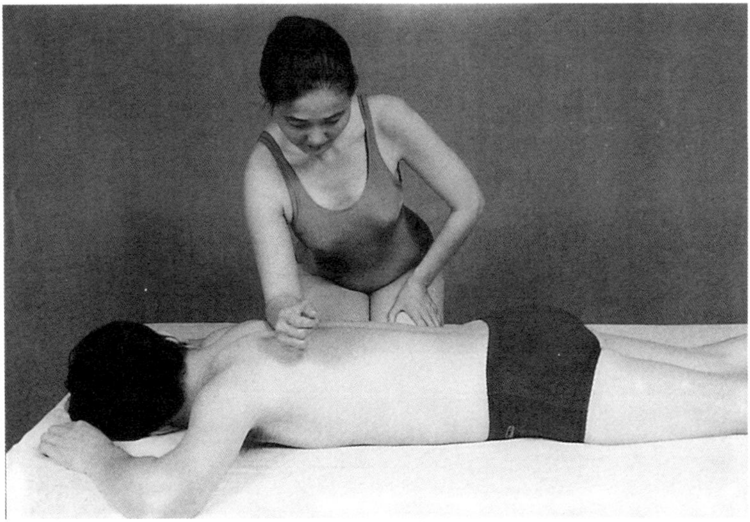
照片 (Photo) 118

圖示 (Fig.) 88A

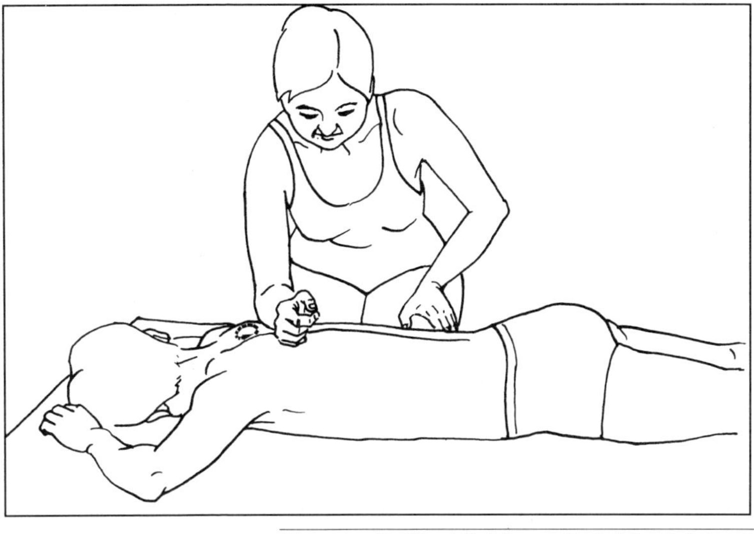

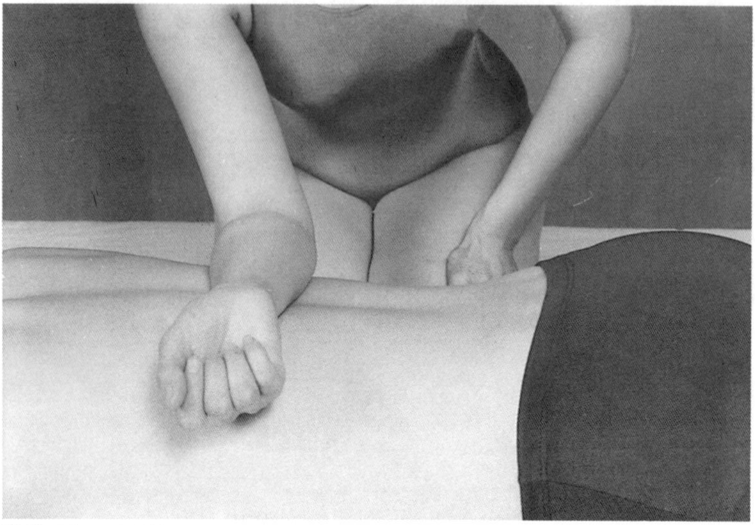
照片 (Photo) 119

圖示 (Fig.) 88B

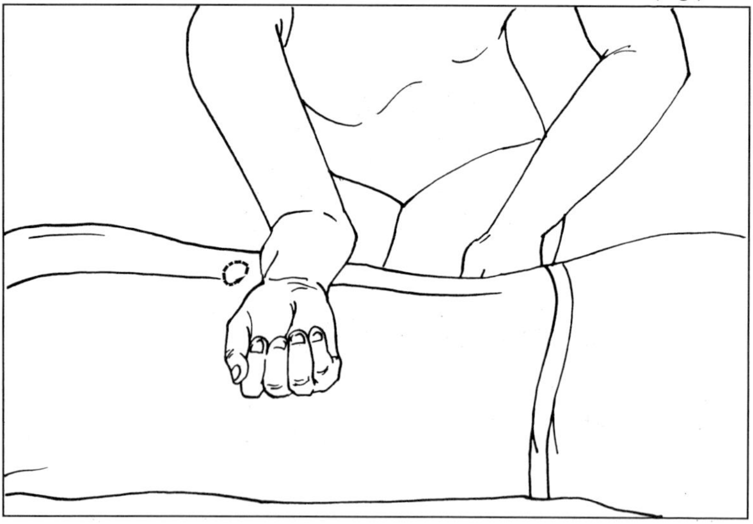

82 指叩後背法：

體位同上。按摩者雙手對合，五指分開，掌指關節及指間關節伸直（見照片120和圖示89A），以小指尺側為着力點，扣擊被按摩者從頸項後背到腰部（見照片121和圖示89B）。

Digital-tapping back method:

In same position. The massagist puts both hands together, separates five fingers and stretches joints between palm and fingers and finger joints straight (see Photo 120 and Fig. 89A); with the force of little finger ulna, taps from the back of the patient's neck to the waist (see Photo 121 and Fig. 89B).

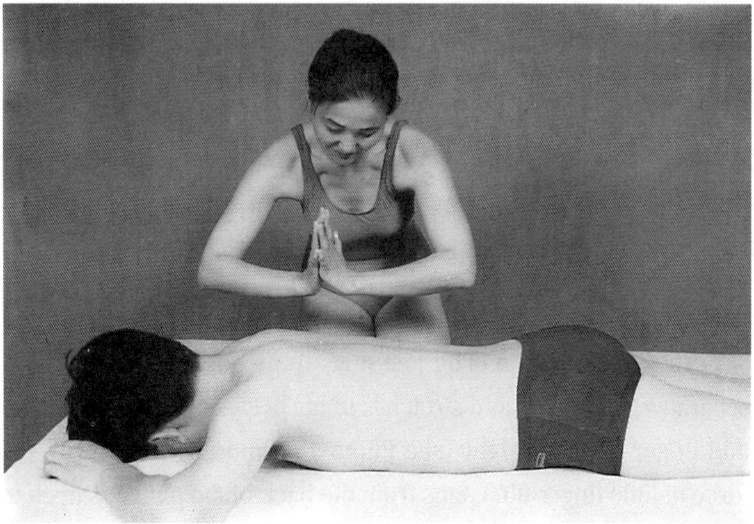

照片 (Photo) 120

圖示 (Fig.) 89A

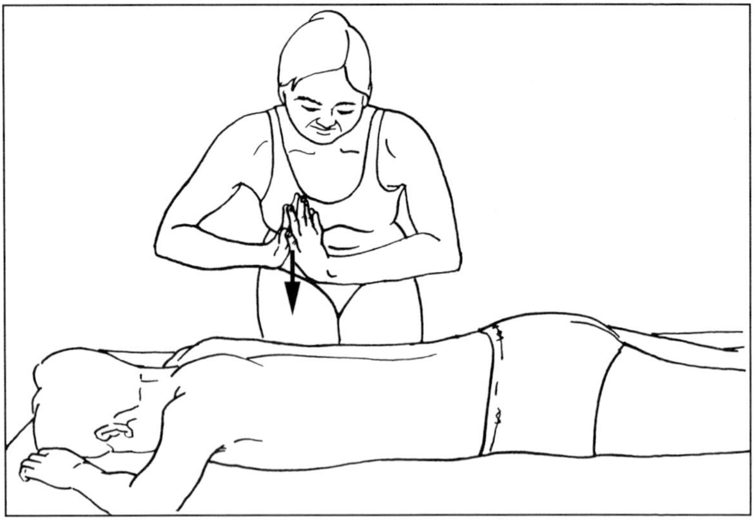

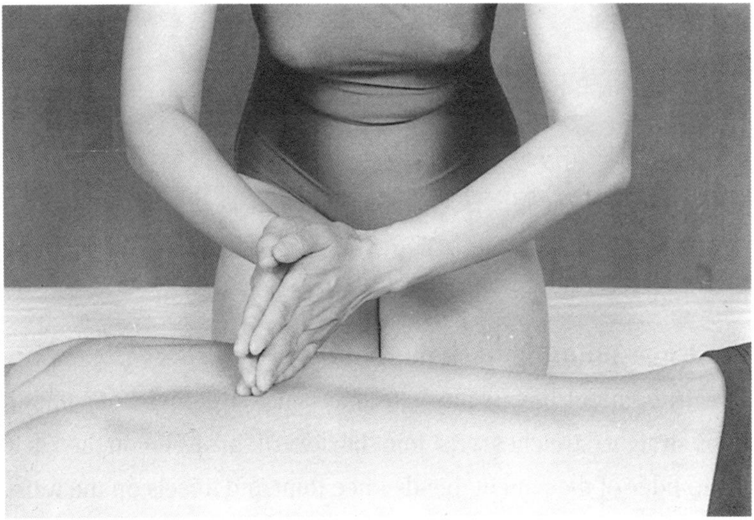

照片 (Photo) 121

圖示 (Γig.) 89B

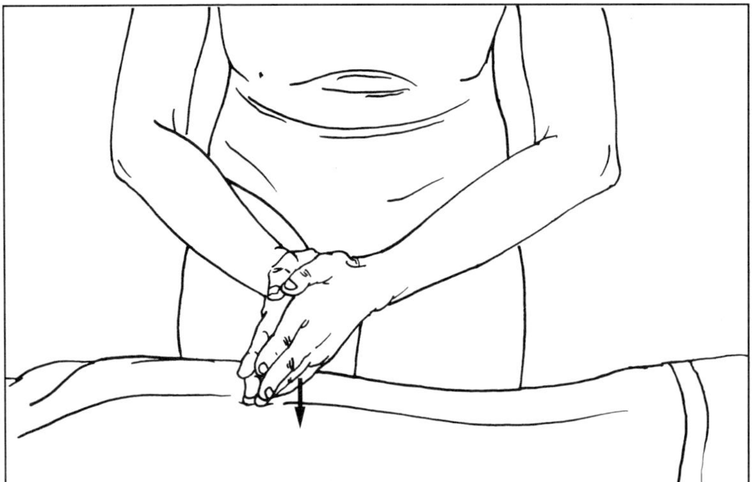

83 膝點後背法：

被按摩者俯臥位，按摩者雙上肢伸直，腕關節背伸，撐扶於被按摩者肩後方，膝關節屈曲跪於其腰部，以膝關節前方為着力點，點按雙側骶棘肌，從腰部至肩部，反復操作2次（見照片122和圖示90）。

Knee-pointing back method:

The patient lies prone. The massagist stretches both upper limbs straight, stretches wrist joint backward, props up on the back of shoulder of the patient, bends knee joint and kneels on the waist of the patient; with the force of the front of knee joint, points and presses musculus sacrospinalis at both sides from the waist to shoulder. Repeat the manipulation twice (see Photo 122 and Fig. 90).

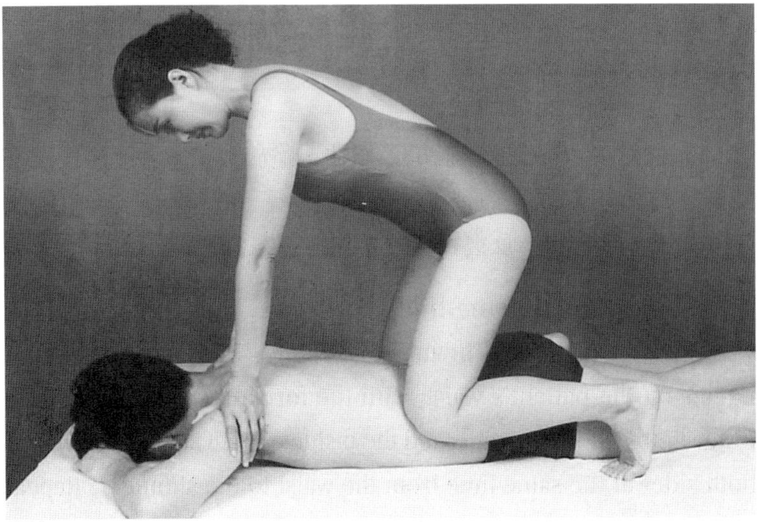

照片 (Photo) 122

圖示 (Fig.) 90

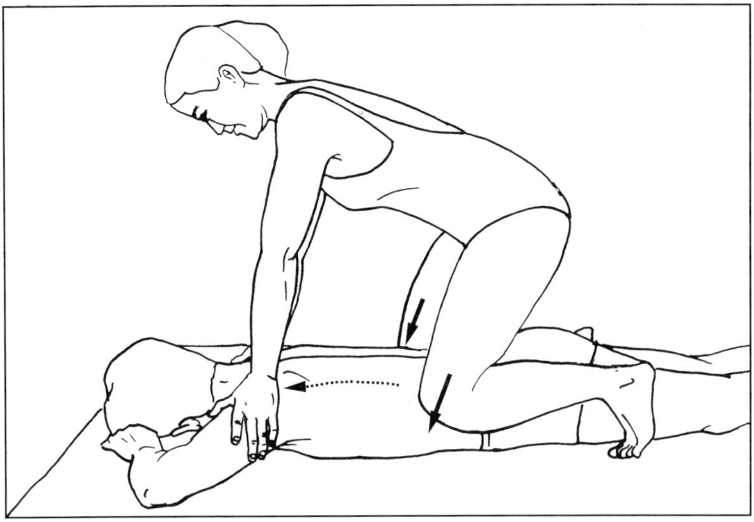

84 小腿分推法：

體位同上。按摩者雙膝關節屈曲，跪於被按摩者腰部，以下肢外展之力，以膝關節及雙小腿內側為着力點，同時向兩側分推，從腰部至肩部，反復操作2次（見照片123和圖示91）。

Shank-pushing method:

In same position. The massagist bends both knee joints and kneels on the patient's waist; with the force of spreading out the lower limbs, the knee joints and the inside of both shanks, pushes to both sides at the same time from the waist to the shoulder. Repeat the manipulation twice (see Photo 123 and Fig. 91).

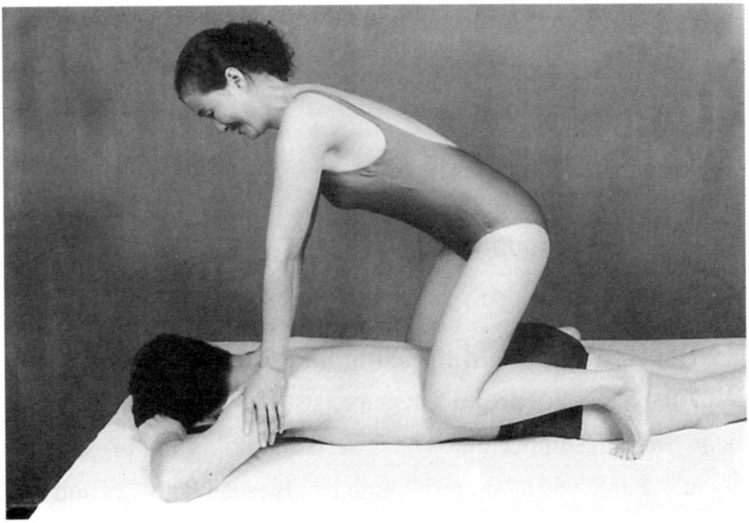
照片 (Photo) 123

圖示 (Fig.) 91

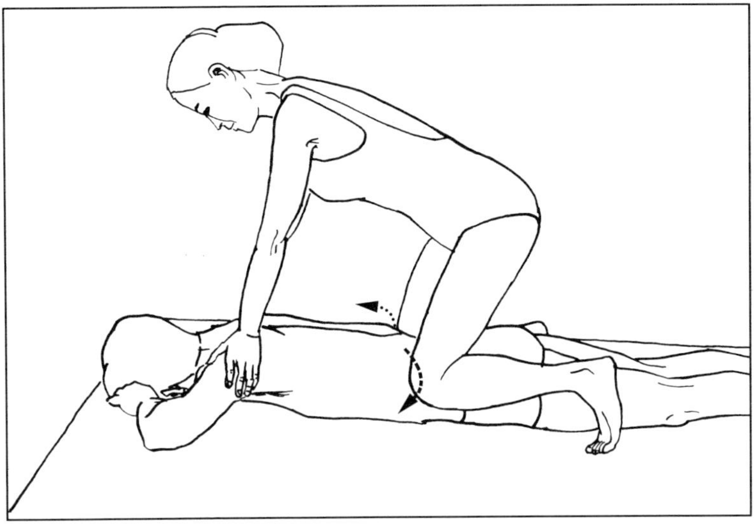

85 足跟點按法：

被按摩者俯臥位，按摩者坐於被按摩者大腿後方，上肢後伸，雙手扶按其小腿跟腱處（見照片124和圖示92A），以雙足跟為着力點，交替地點按腰3、4橫突部位（見照片125和圖示92B）。反復操作2－4次。

Heel-pointing and pressing method:

The patient lies prone. The massagist sits on the patient's back thighs, stretches upper limbs backward and holds and presses the patient's shank heel tendon with both hands (see Photo 124 and Fig. 92A); with the force of heels, presses Nos. 3 and 4 processus transversalis of waist alternately (see Photo 125 and Fig. 92B). Repeat the manipulation 2-4 times.

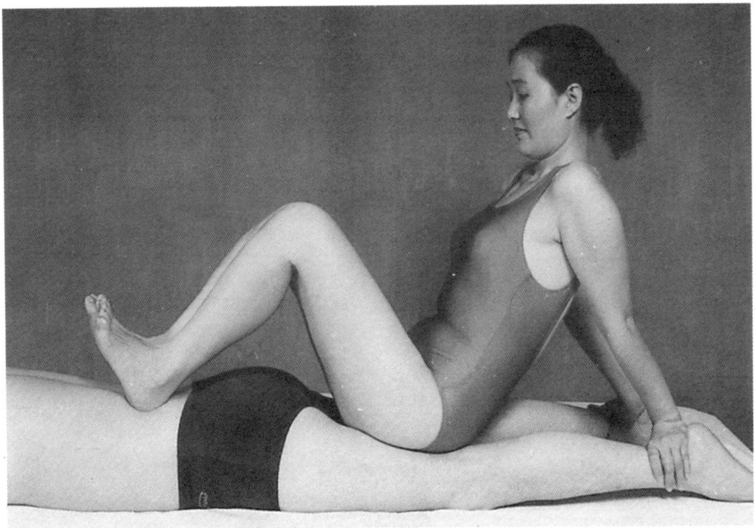

照片 (Photo) 124

圖示 (Fig.) 92A

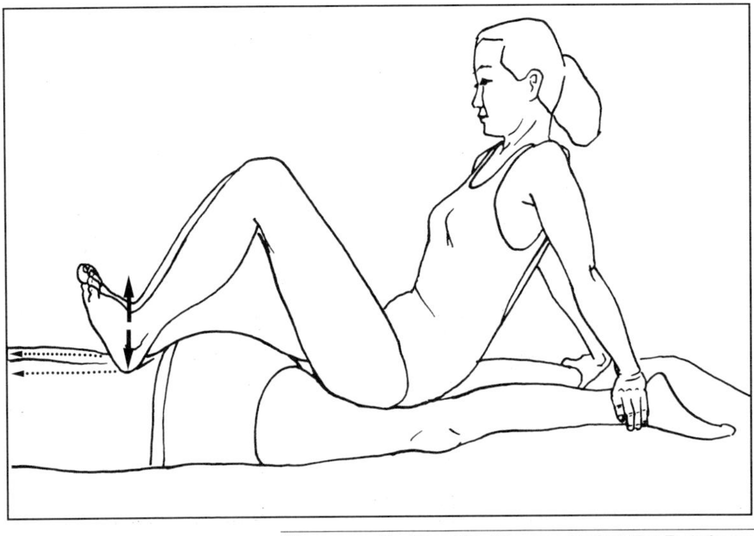

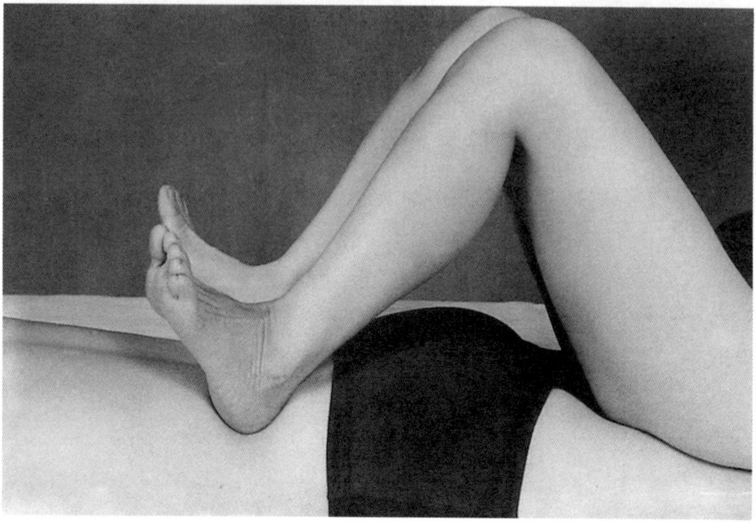

照片 (Photo) 125

圖示 (Fig.) 92B

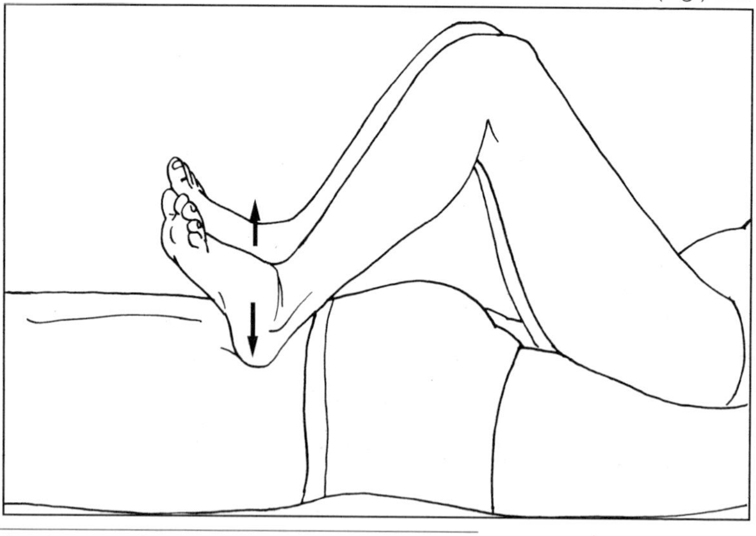

86 推踩後背法：

體位同上。按摩者以雙足跟為着力點，借膝關節屈伸動作，交替推踩被按摩者兩側骶棘肌，從腰部至頸肩部（見照片**126**、**127**和圖示**93A**、**93B**）。

Pushing and stamping back method:

In same position. With the force of both heels and the bending and stretching of knee joints, the massagist pushes and stamps on the patient's musculus sacrospinalis at both sides alternately from the waist to the neck and shoulder (see Photos 126, 127 and Figs. 93A , 93B).

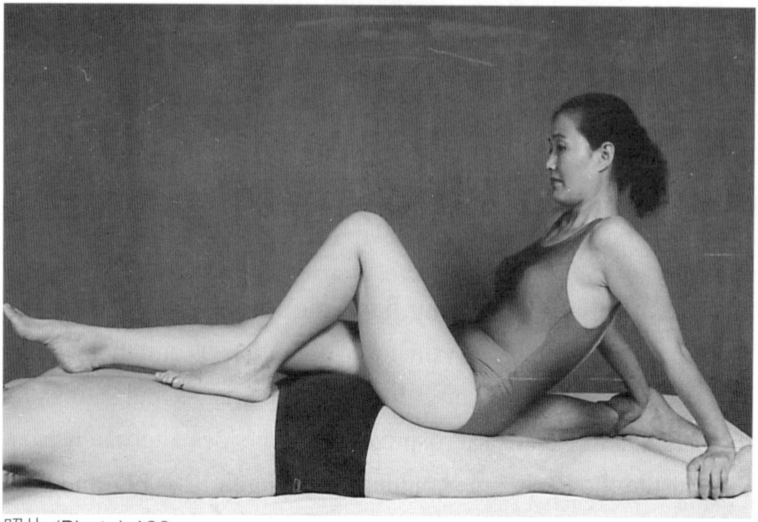

照片 (Photo) 126

圖示 (Fig.) 93A

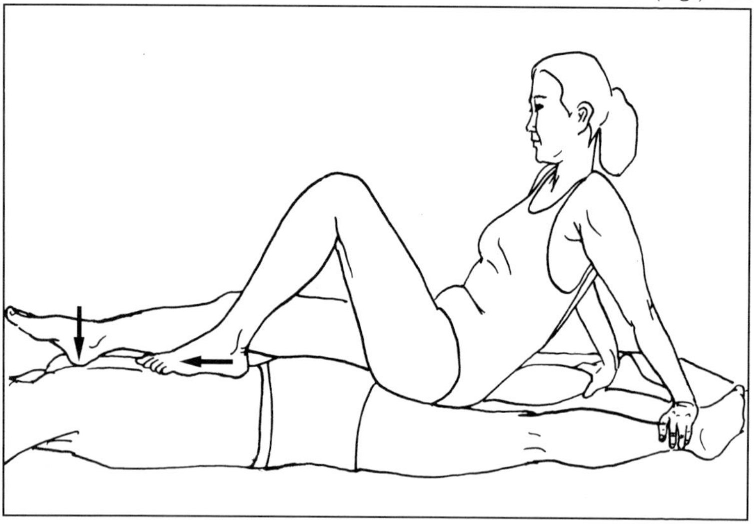

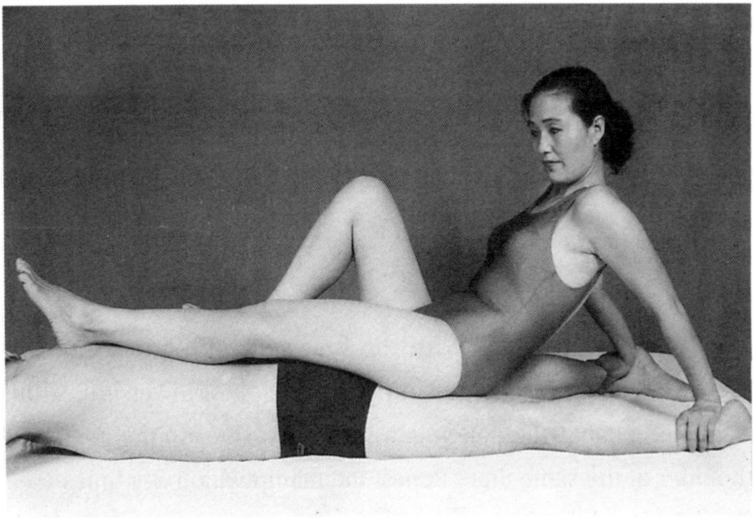

照片 (Photo) 127

圖示 (Fig.) 93B

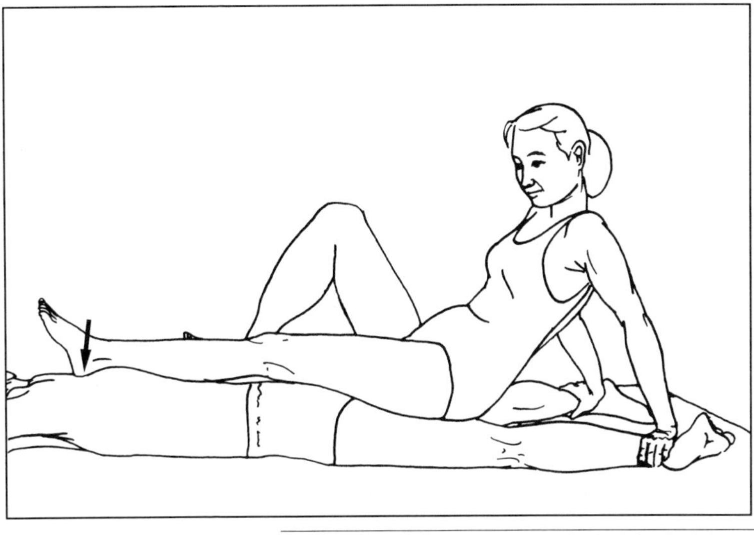

87 足底分推法：

體位同上。按摩者以雙足底為着力點，借下肢外展內收之動作，從被按摩者腰部同時向兩側分推至頸肩部，反復操作**2－4**次（見照片**128**和圖示**94**）。

Sole-pushing method:

In same position. With the force of both soles and the movement of spreading out and pulling back of lower limbs, the massagist pushes the patient's waist to two sides to the neck and shoulder at the same time. Repeat the manipulation 2-4 times (see Photo 128 and Fig. 94).

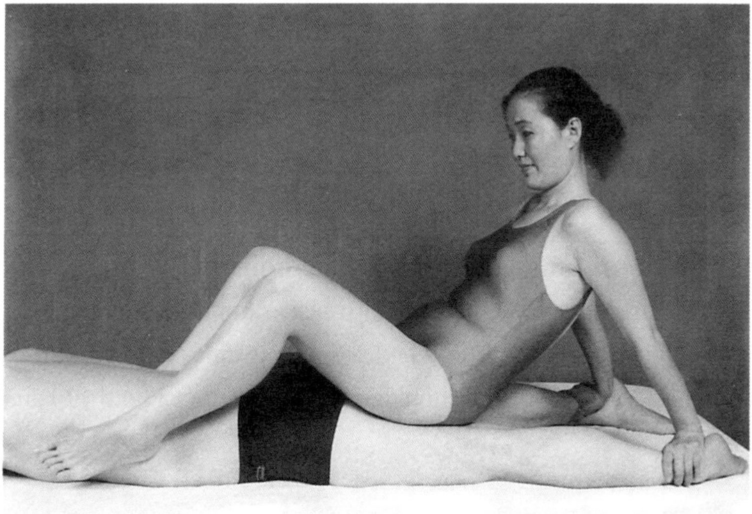

照片 (Photo) 128

圖示 (Fig.) 94

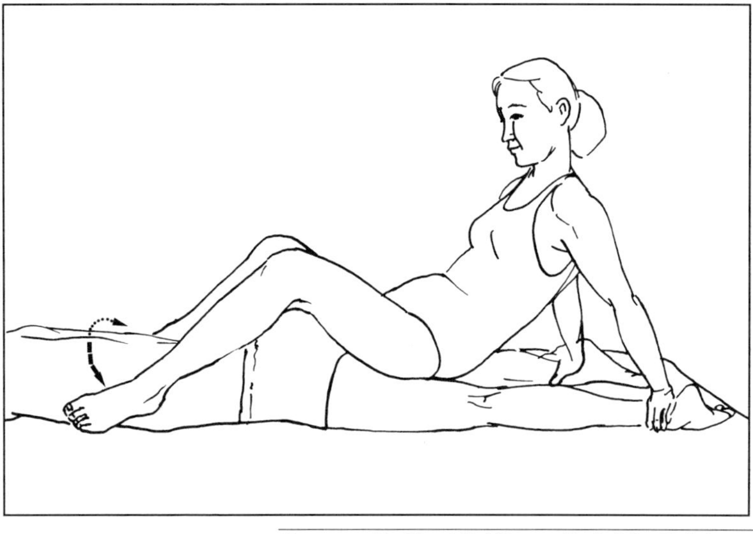

88 足底按揉法：

體位同上。按摩者雙足底跖側置於被按摩者肩關節後方，同時向下按揉肩後方肌群（見照片**129**和圖示**95**）。

Sole-pressing and rubbing method:

In same position. The massagist places both soles on the back of the patient's shoulder joints and at the same time presses and rubs the muscles at the back of shoulders downward (see Photo 129 and Fig. 95).

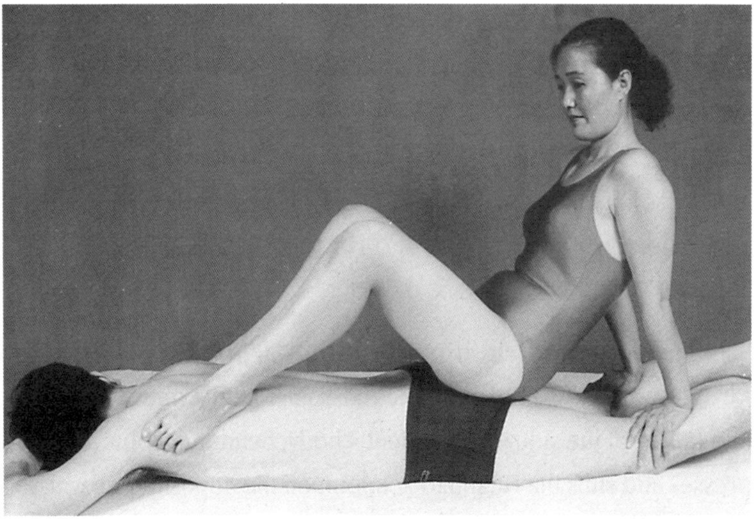
照片 (Photo) 129

圖示 (Fig.) 95

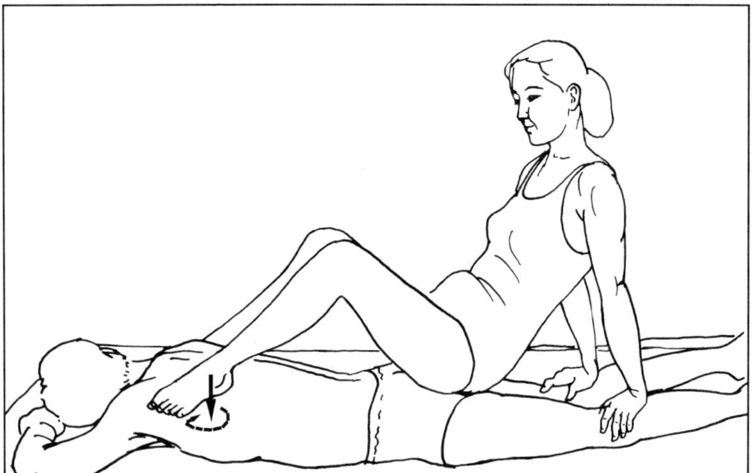

89 按揉環跳穴：

被按摩者俯臥位，按摩者雙膝關節屈曲跪於被按摩者軀幹部一側，肘關節屈曲，用尺骨鷹嘴部按揉對側的環跳穴（見照片**130**和圖示**96**）；然後再用前臂尺側按揉臀部肌群（見照片**131**和圖示**97**）。一側完畢更換另一側。

Pressing and rubbing Huantiao acupoint:

The patient lies prone. The massagist bends both knee joints and kneels at the side of the patient's body, bends an elbow joint and presses and rubs the Huantiao acupoint on the opposite side with the ulna hawk beak (see Photo 130 and Fig. 96) and then presses and rubs buttock muscles with the forearm ulna (see Photo 131 and Fig. 97). Do one side, then the other.

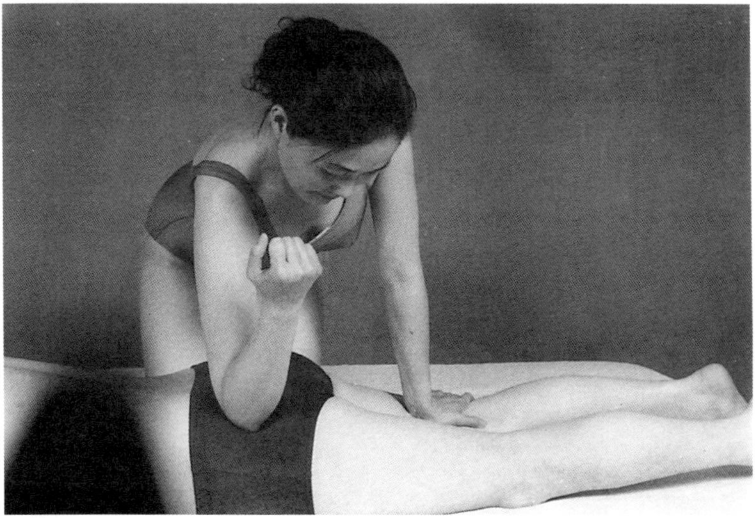
照片 (Photo) 130

圖示 (Fig.) 96

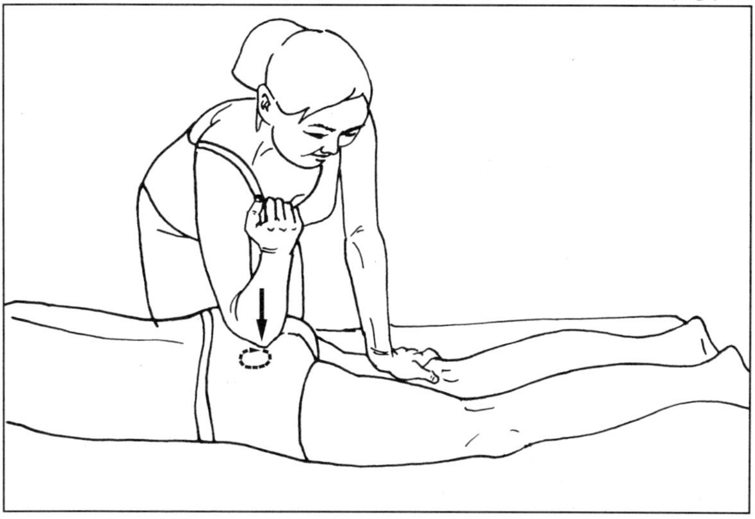

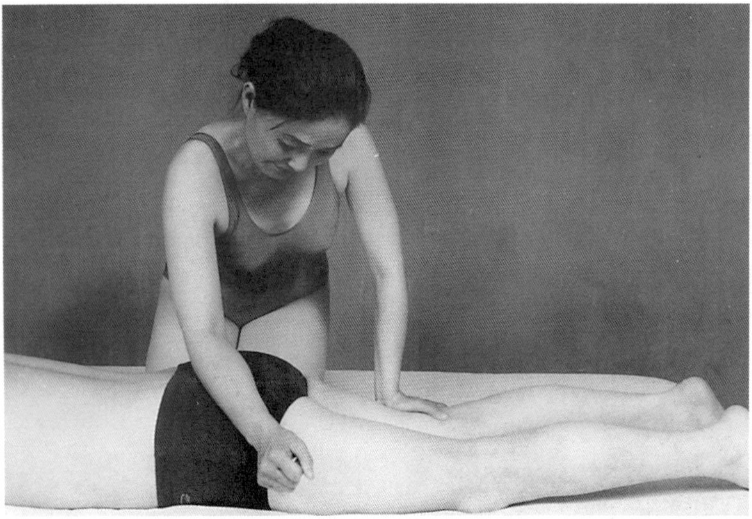

照片 (Photo) 131

圖示 (Fig.) 97

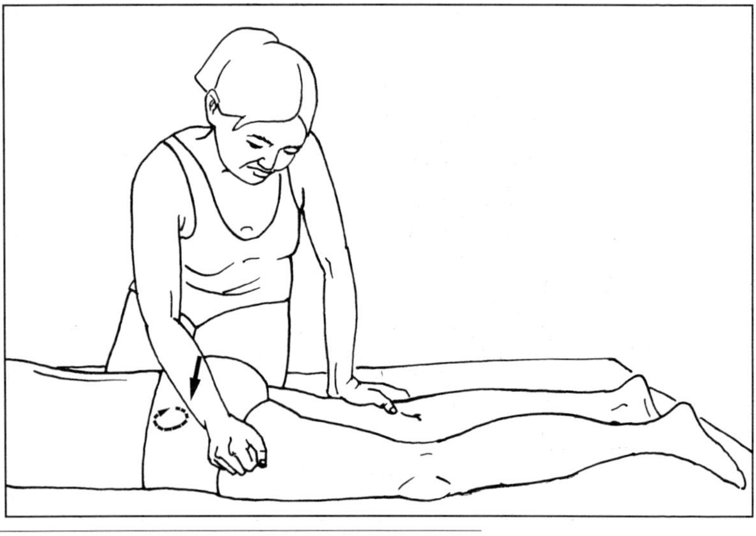

90 按揉臀部肌群：

被按摩者俯臥位，按摩者坐其腰背部，屈髖屈膝，小腿着床，雙腕關節背伸（見照片**132**和圖示**98A**），以掌根為着力點，按揉其臀部肌群（見照片**133**和圖示**98B**）。

Pressing and rubbing buttock muscles:

The patient lies prone. The massagist sits on the patient's waist back, bends hip and knees, places shanks on the bed and stretches both wrist joints backward (see Photo 132 and Fig. 98A); with the force of palm root, presses and rubs the patient's buttock muscles (see Photo 133 and Fig. 98B).

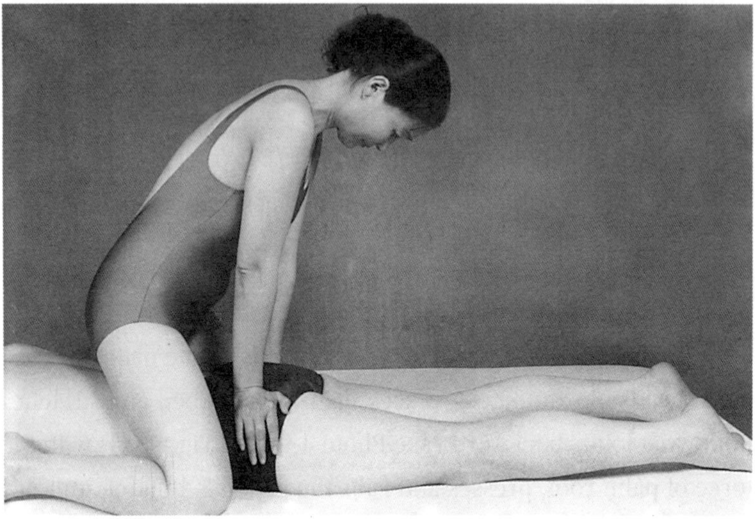

照片 (Photo) 132

圖示 (Fig.) 98A

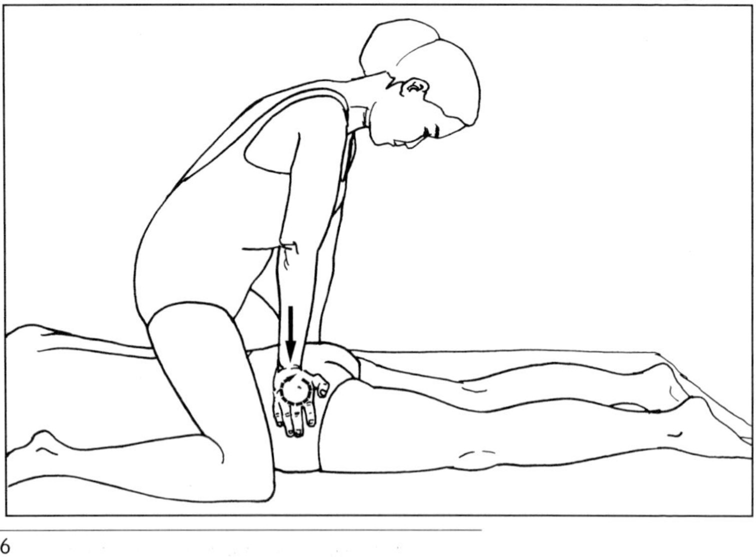

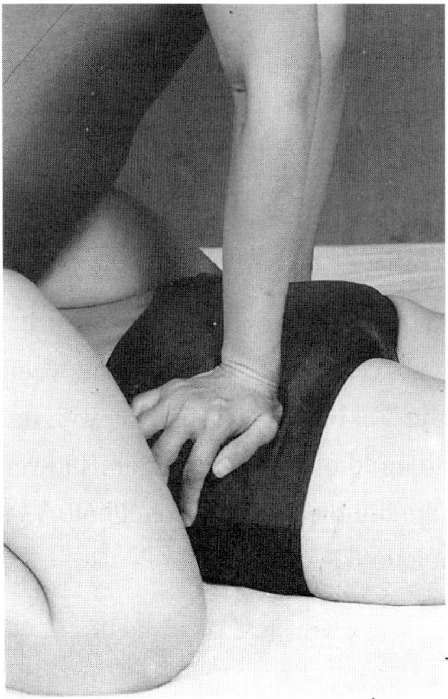

照片 (Photo) 133

圖示 (Fig.) 98B

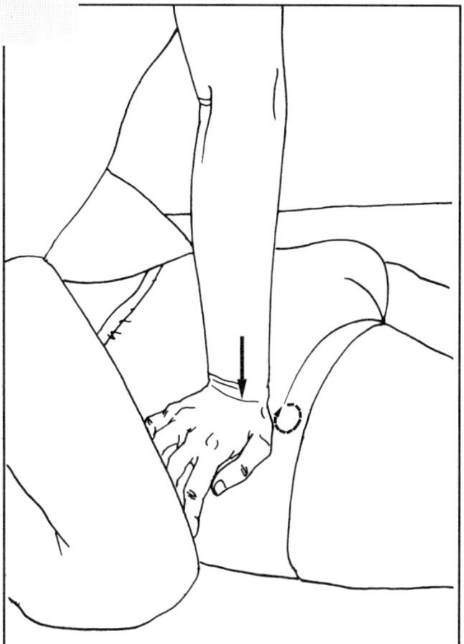

91 拇指循經按壓法：

體位同上。按摩者雙手拇指、掌指及指間關節伸直，以拇指指端着力，沿被按摩者下肢後正中線從近心端按壓至膕窩處（見照片134和圖示99），反復操作2－4次。

Thumb-pressing main channel (meridians) method:

In same position. The massagist stretches joints between thumb and fingers and finger joints of both hands straight; with the force of thumb tips, presses the middle line of the patient's lower rear limb from near center to the hollow of knees (see Photo 134 and Fig. 99). Repeat the manipulation 2-4 times.

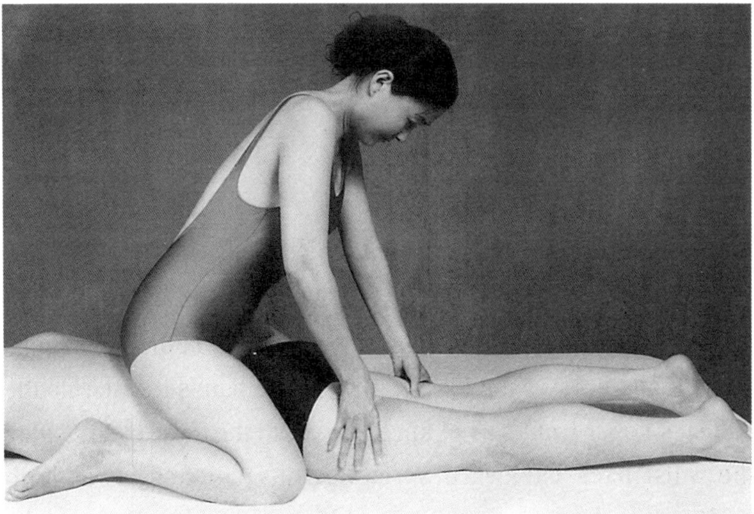

照片 (Photo) 134

圖示 (Fig.) 99

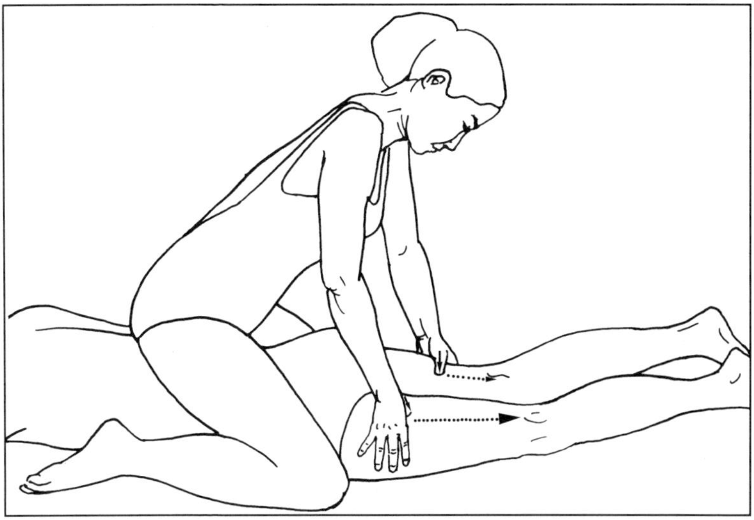

92 伸髖法：

體位同上。按摩者雙上肢伸直，雙手五指交叉環抱於被按摩者膝關節前上方，利用腰背部後伸之力，將其下肢極度後伸（見照片**135**和圖示**100**）。一側完畢更換另一側。

Hip stretching method:

In same position. The massagist stretches both upper limbs straight and crosses the five fingers of both hands to encircle the patient's upper front part of knee joint; with the force of stretching the waist back backward, stretches the patient's lower limb backward to the utmost (see Photo 135 and Fig. 100). Do one side, then the other.

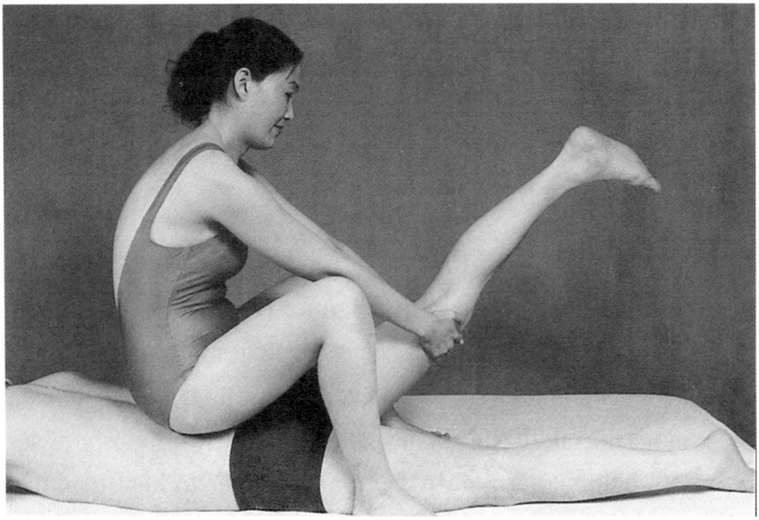

照片 (Photo) 135

圖示 (Fig.) 100

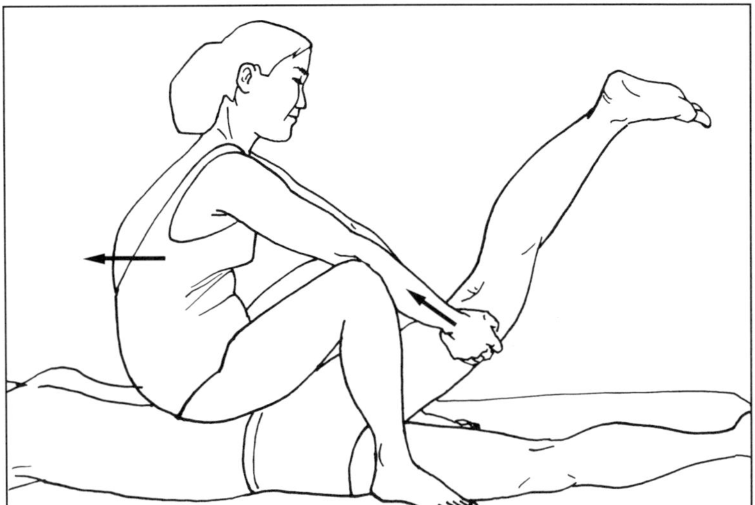

93 掌根循經按壓法：

體位同上。按摩者雙上肢伸直，腕關節背伸，以掌根為着力點，沿被按摩者下肢後正中線，雙手掌交替從近心端按壓至跟腱處，反復操作2－4次（見照片136和圖示101）。

Palm-root-pressing main channel (meridians) method:

In same position. The massagist stretches both upper limbs straight, and stretches wrist joints backward; with the force of palm roots, along the middle line of the patient's lower rear limbs, presses with both palms alternatively from near center to heel tendons. Repeat the manipulation 2-4 times (see Photo 136 and Fig. 101).

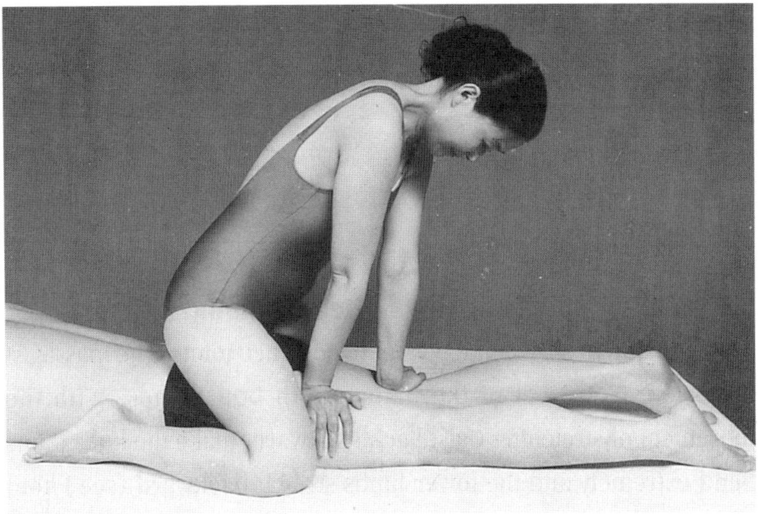

照片 (Photo) 136

圖示 (Fig.) 101

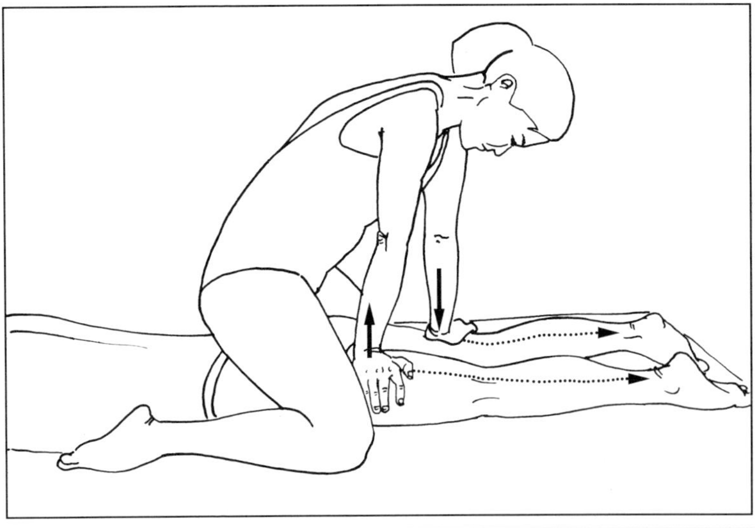

94 握足伸髖法：

體位同上。被按摩者膝關節屈曲，按摩者雙手握住其前足部，以腰背部的後伸動作，將其膝關節極度屈曲，並使其下肢後伸（見照片**137**和圖示**102**）。

Foot grasping and hip stretching method:

In same position. The patient bends knee joints. The massagist holds the front feet of the patient with both hands. With the movement of stretching waist back backward, make the knee joints bend extremely and the lower limbs stretch backward (see Photo 137 and Fig. 102).

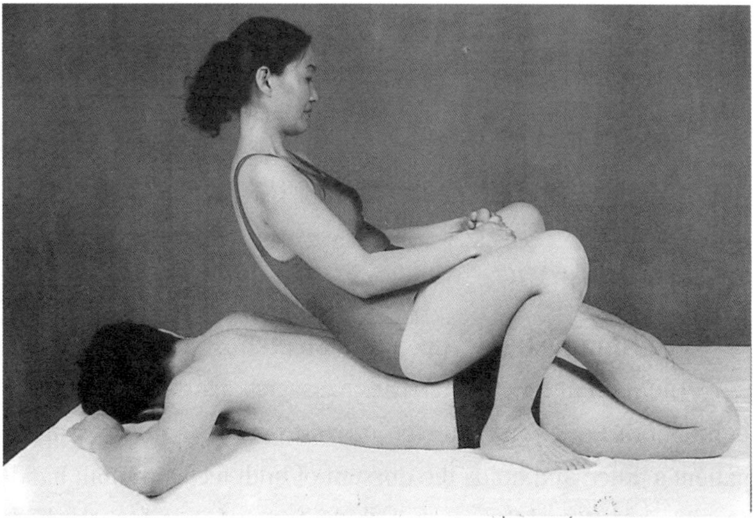
照片 (Photo) 137

圖示 (Fig.) 102

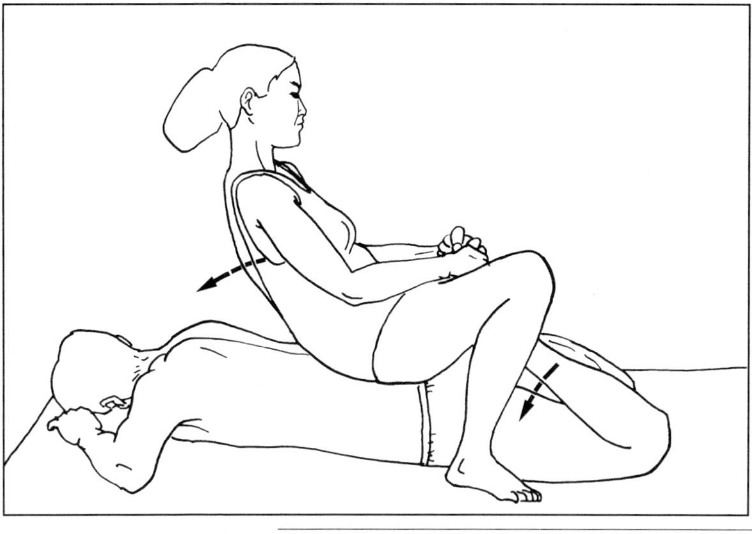

95 頂壓屈膝伸髖法：

被按摩者俯臥位，按摩者坐其臀部，雙膝關節屈曲，頂在被按摩者膕窩處，兩手握雙足的背側（見照片**138**和圖示**103**），利用軀幹後伸之力，使其行被動伸髖屈膝動作（見照片**139**、**140**和圖示**104A**、**104B**）。

Pressing by bent knees and stretching hips method:

The patient lies prone. The massagist sits on the buttocks, bends both knee joints to step on and press the hollows of the patient's knee and holds the dorsum of both feet with both hands (see Photo 138 and Fig. 103). With the force of stretching the body backward, make the patient stretch the hip and bend knees passively (see Photos 139, 140 and Figs. 104A, 104B).

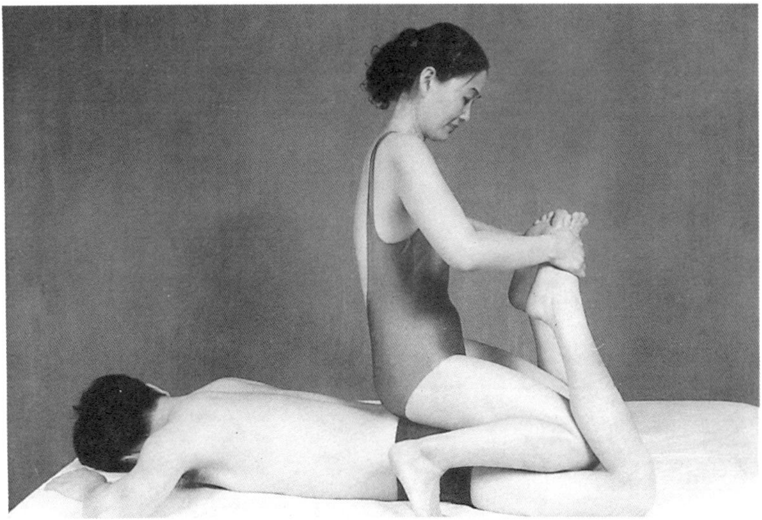
照片 (Photo) 138

圖示 (Fig.) 103

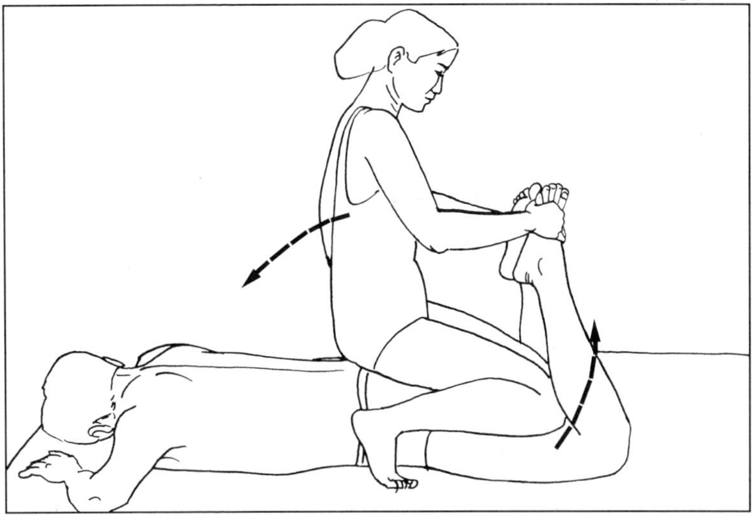

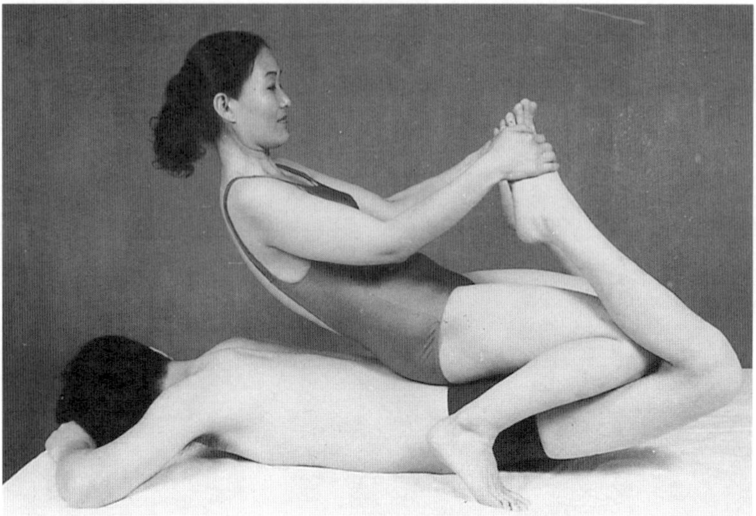

照片 (Photo) 139

圖示 (Fig.) 104A

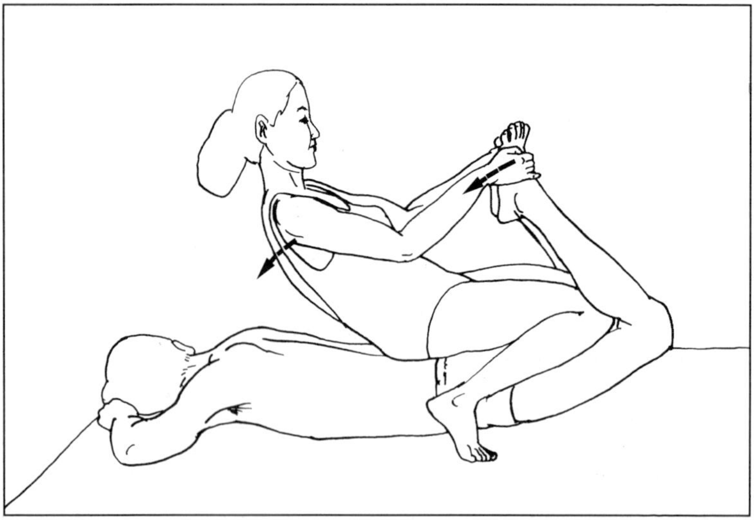

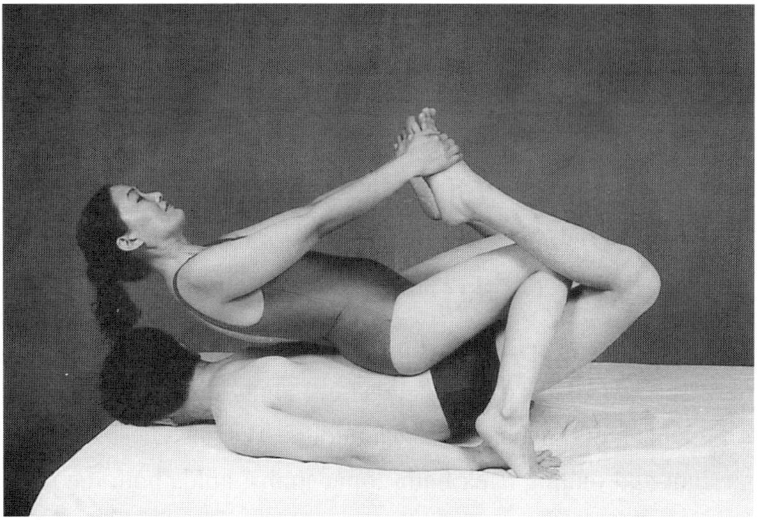

照片 (Photo) 140

圖示 (Fig.) 104B

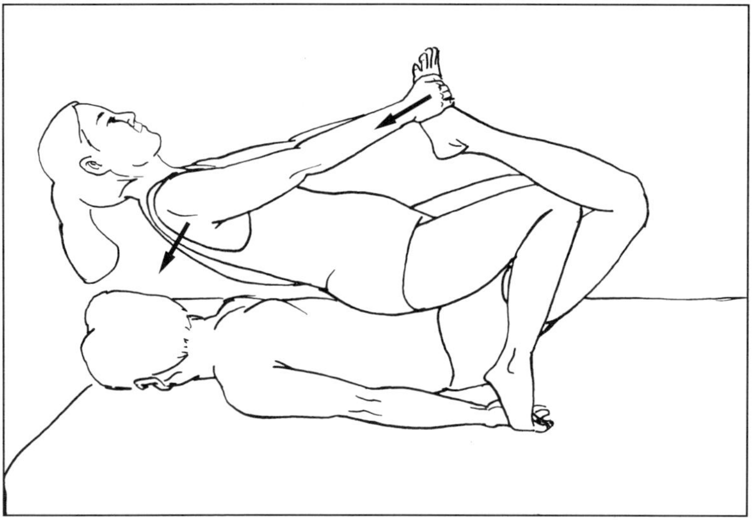

96 扶膝伸髖法：

被按摩者俯臥位，膝關節屈曲，雙足分別置於按摩者兩肩後方；按摩者雙上肢伸直內收，兩手扶握被按摩者雙膝關節前方（見照片**141**和圖示**105A**），借軀幹後伸之力，將被按摩者雙髖關節被動後伸（見照片**142**和圖示**105B**），反復操作**2－4**次。

Knee supporting and hip stretching method:

The patient lies prone, bends knee joints and places both feet on the back of the massagist's shoulders. The massagist stretches straight and pulling back both upper limbs, holds both the front knee joints of the patient with both hands (see Photo 141 and Fig. 105A); with the force of stretching body backward, makes the patient stretch both hip joints backward passively (see Photo 142 and Fig. 105B). Repeat the manipulation 2-4 times.

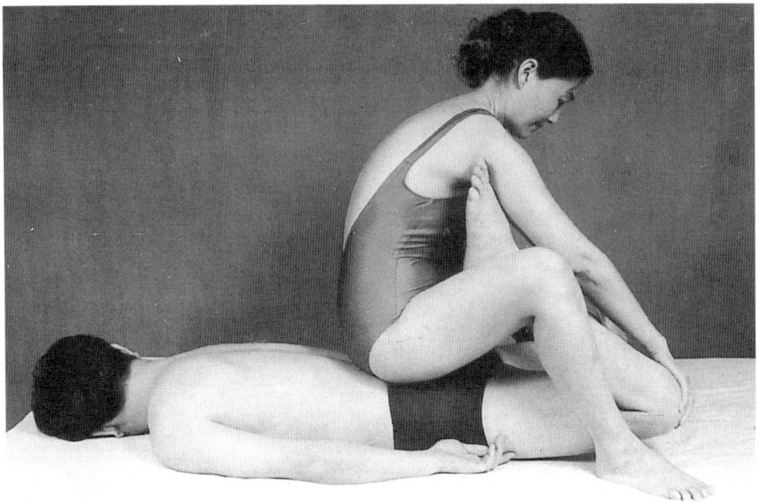

照片 (Photo) 141

圖示 (Fig.) 105A

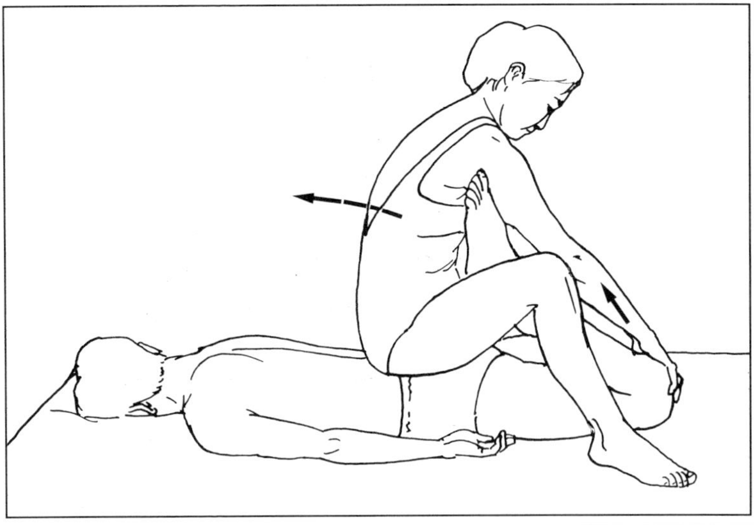

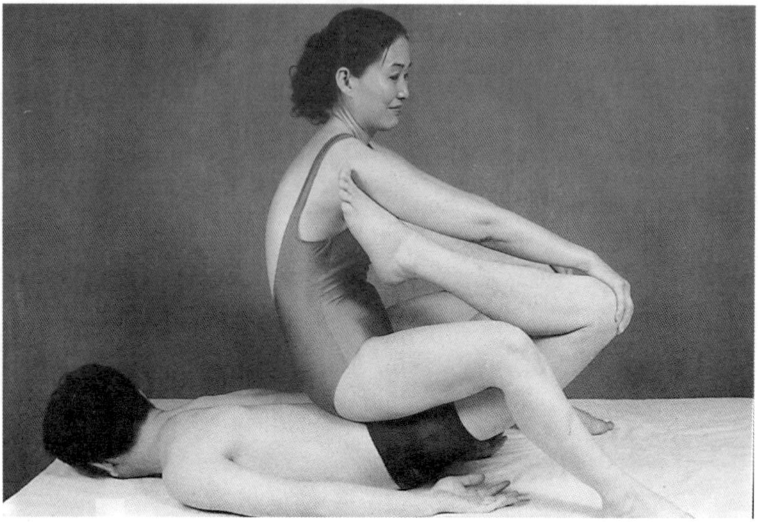
照片 (Photo) 142

圖示 (Fig.) 105B

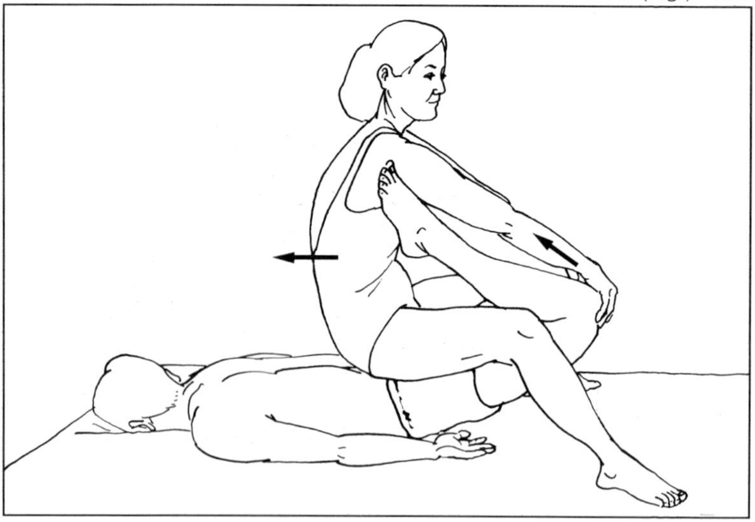

97 指壓涌泉穴：

被按摩者俯臥位，雙膝關節屈曲**9 0**度，踝關節背伸；按摩者跪或立於被按摩者足側，兩手拇指伸直，以指端為着力點，按壓其涌泉穴處，掌根按壓前足跖側，反復操作**2－4**次（見照片**143**和圖示**106**）。

Digital-pressing Yongquan acupoint:

The patient lies prone, bends both knee joints at 90 degrees and stretches ankle joints backward. The massagist kneels or stands at the side of the patient's feet and stretches both thumbs straight; with the force of thumb tips, presses the Yongquan acupoint and presses the front soles with palm roots. Repeat the manipulation 2-4 times (see Photo 143 and Fig. 106).

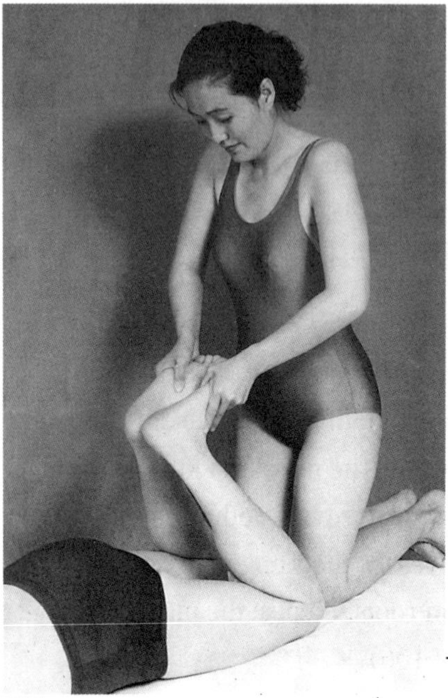

照片 (Photo) 143

圖示 (Fig.) 106

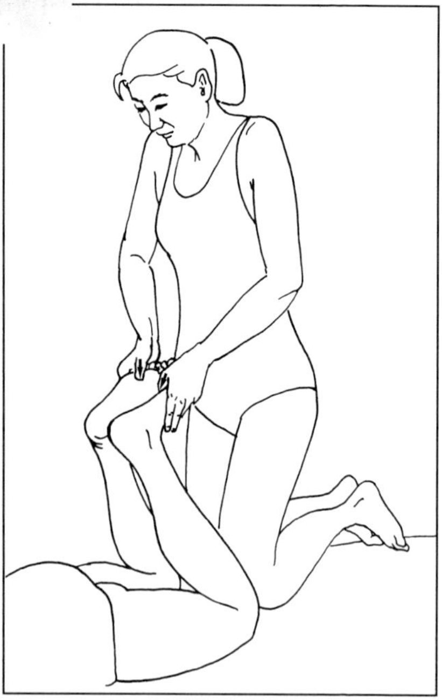

98 跟臀屈膝法：

體位同上。按摩者兩手握其雙足，向下按壓，使被按摩者膝關節屈曲到最大幅度，儘量以足跟貼近臀部為宜，反復操作**2－4**次（見照片**144**和圖示**107**）。

Heels-to-buttocks knee bending method:

In same position. The massagist holds both feet of the patient with both hands and presses downward so that the patient's knee joints bend to the utmost, best place the heels close to buttocks as much as possible. Repeat the manipulation 2-4 times (see Photo 144 and Fig. 107).

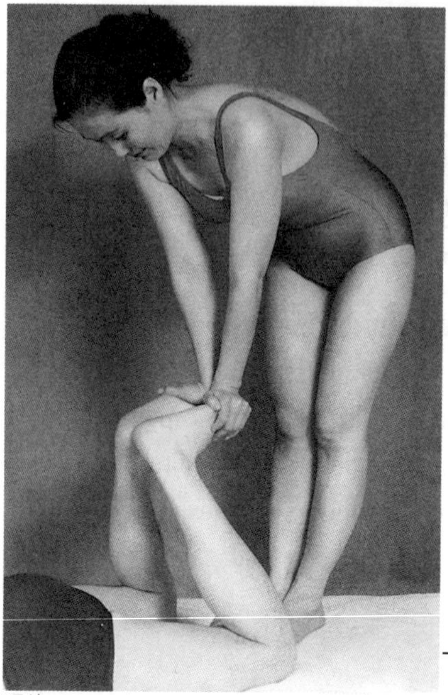

照片 (Photo) 144

圖示 (Fig.) 107

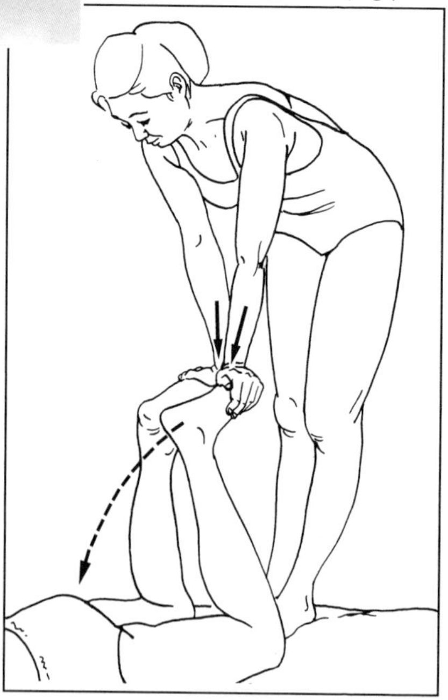

99 按壓小腿前外側肌群：

體位同上。按摩者雙膝關節屈曲，以膝關節前下方，按壓被按摩者小腿前外方肌群，從踝關節（見照片**145**和圖示**108A**）至膝關節處（見照片**146**和圖示**108B**），反復操作**2**次。

Pressing front outside muscles of shank:

In same position. The massagist bends both knee joints and presses the patient's front outside muscles of shanks with the lower front part of knee joints from ankle joints (see Photo 145 and Fig. 108A) to knee joints (see Photo 146 and Fig. 108B). Repeat the manipulation twice.

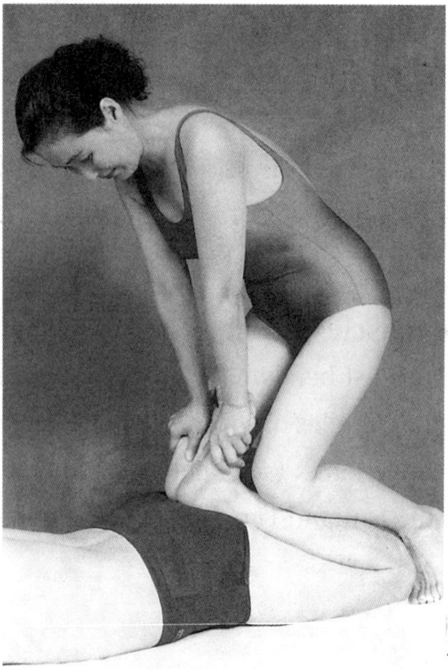

照片 (Photo) 145

圖示 (Fig.) 108A

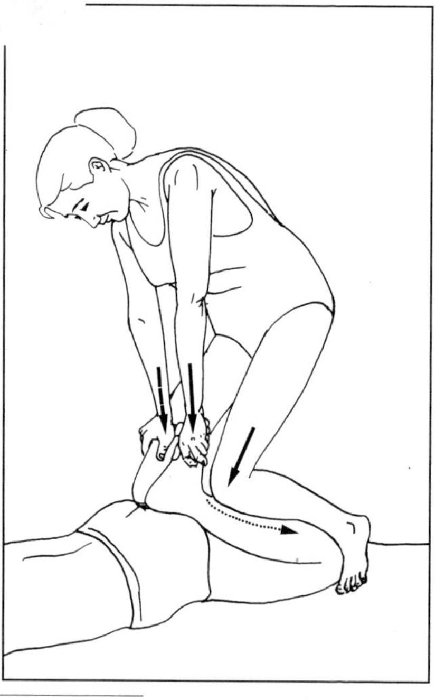

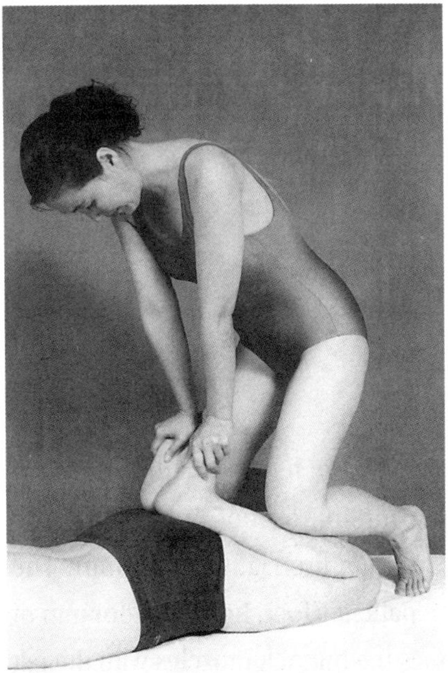

照片 (Photo) 146

圖示 (Fig.) 108B

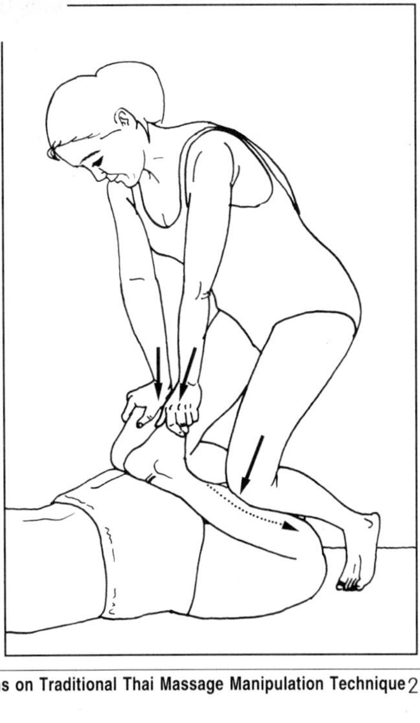

100 按壓大腿後側肌群：

被按摩者俯臥位，左下肢內旋，膝關節屈曲，足背置於對側膕窩處，右下肢屈膝。按摩者跪於被按摩者足側，右手握足背部，左手由近心端（見照片**147**和圖示**109A**）向遠心端自上而下按壓臀部肌群至膕窩處（見照片**148**和圖示**109B**）。一側完畢更換另一側。反復操作**2－4**次。

Pressing rear muscles of thigh:

The patient lies prone, revolves the left lower limb inward, bends the knee joint, places the dorsum of foot on the opposite hollow of knee and bends the knee of the right lower limb. The massagist kneels at the side of the patient's foot, holds the dorsum of foot with the right hand and presses the buttock muscles with the left hand from near center (see Photo 147 and Fig. 109A) to far center, from up to down, to the hollow of knee (see Photo 148 and Fig. 109B). Do one side, then the other. Repeat the manipulation 2-4 times.

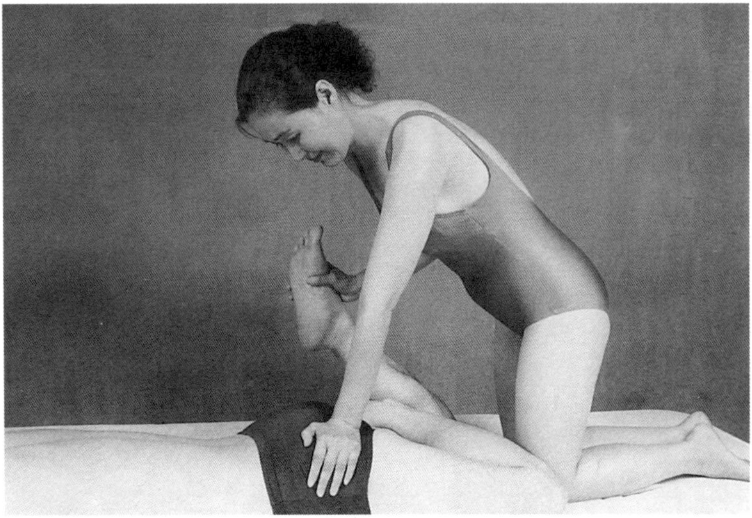
照片 (Photo) 147

圖示 (Fig.) 109A

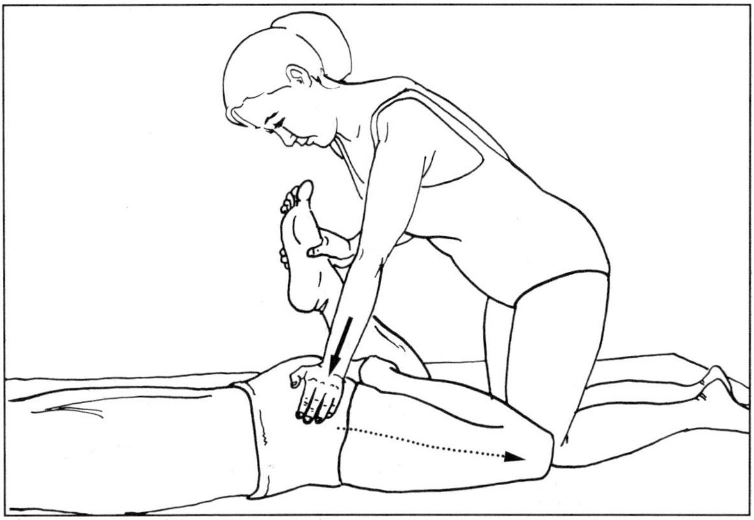

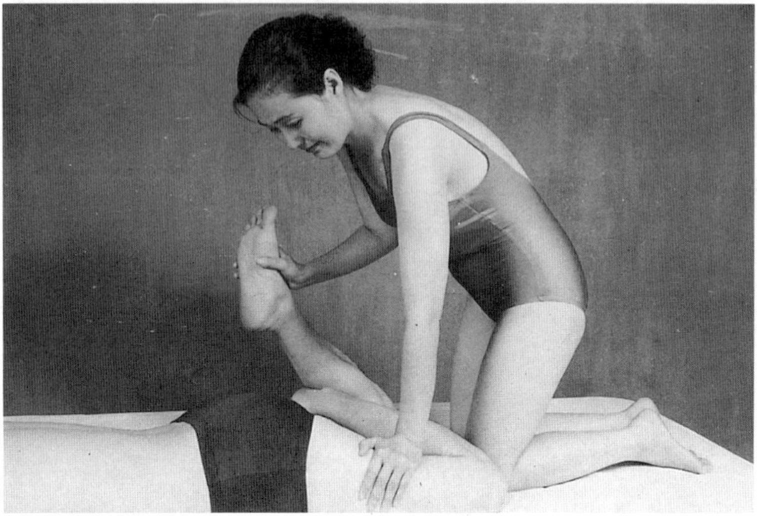
照片 (Photo) 148

圖示 (Fig.) 109B
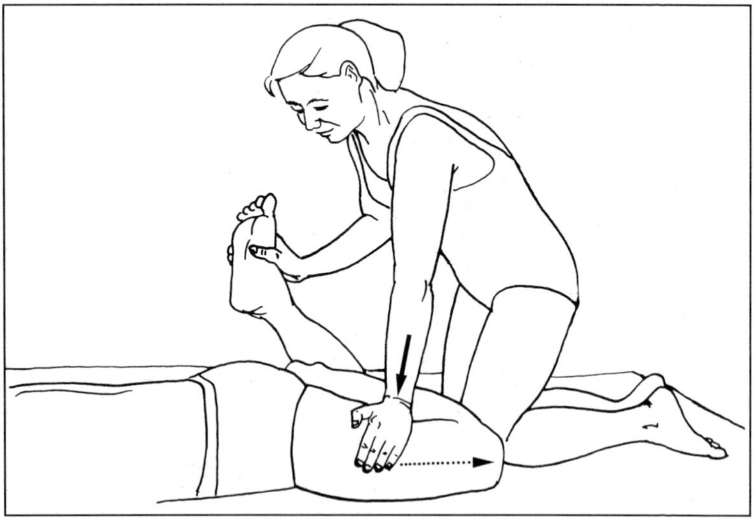

101 拉搬法：

體位同上。按摩者一手扶握被按摩者足背部，另一手扶握同側膝關節前上方（見照片**149**和圖示**110**），做向後拉搬動作，使髖關節被動後伸（見照片**150**），反復操作**2－4**次。一側完畢更換另一側。

Pulling and moving method:

In same position. The massagist holds the patient's dorsum of foot with one hand and holds the upper front part of knee joint at the same side with the other hand (see Photo 149 and Fig. 110). Do pulling back movement to make hip joints stretch backward passively (see Photo 150). Repeat the manipulation 2-4 times. Do one side, then the other.

照片 (Photo) 149

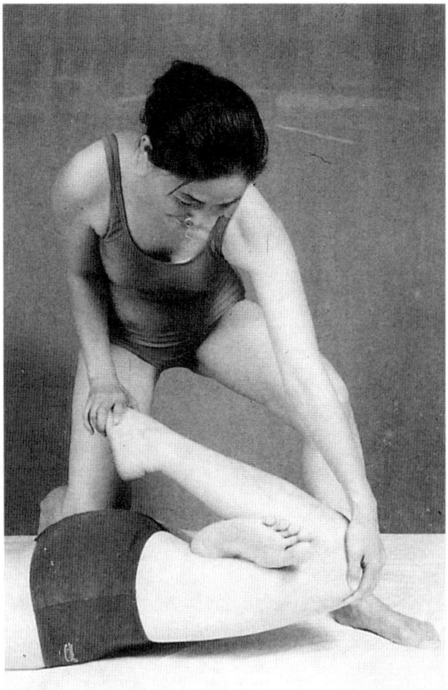

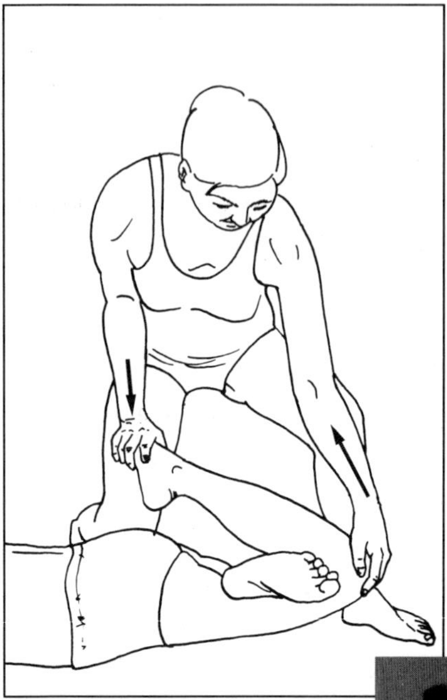

圖示 (Fig.) 110

照片 (Photo) 150

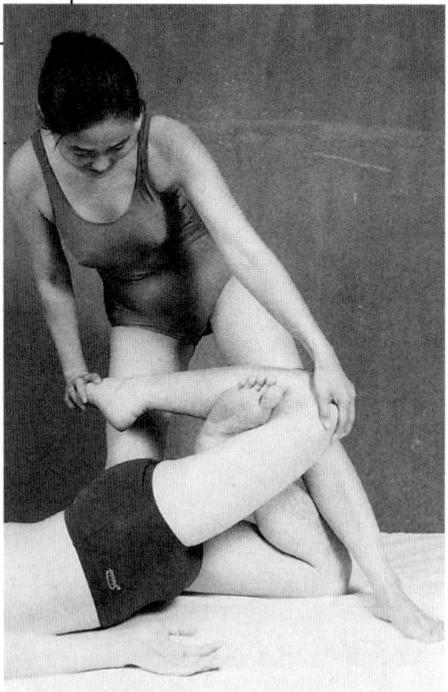

102 踩提法：

被按摩者俯臥位，雙膝關節屈曲；按摩者站立位，用足跖側從被按摩者臀部踩壓至膕窩處，同時雙手扶握被按摩者雙踝關節前方並向上提足（見照片**151**和圖示**111**）。一側完畢更換另一側。反復操作**2－4**次。

Stamping and lifting method:

The patient lies prone and bends both knee joints. The massagist stands and stamps the patient from the buttocks to the hollow of knee with the sole and at the same time holds the front ankle joints and lifts both feet up with both hands (see Photo 151 and Fig. 111). Do one side, then the other. Repeat the manipulation 2-4 times.

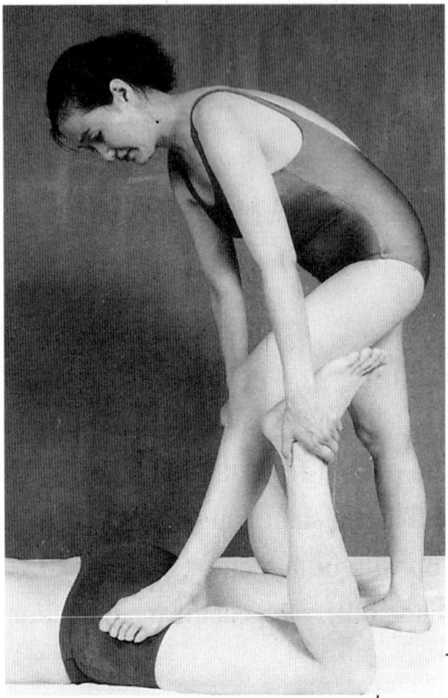

照片 (Photo) 151

圖示 (Fig.) 111

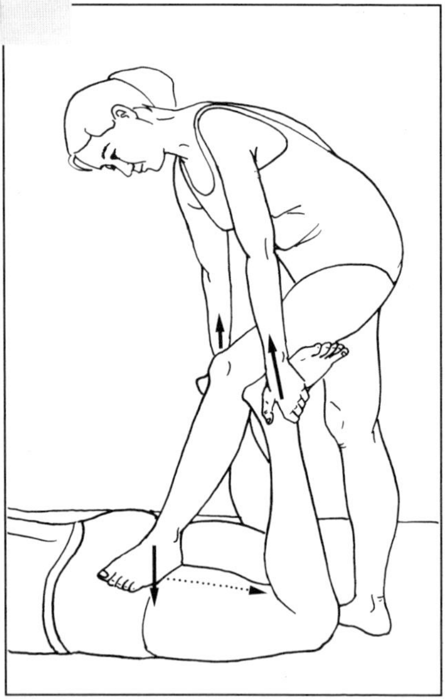

103 伸腰法：

被按摩者俯臥位，雙手五指交叉環抱於後頭部，屈膝約9 0度；按摩者坐被按摩者足跖側，兩手扶握其雙肘（見照片152A和圖示112A），反復向後牽拉三次，使其極度背伸腰部（見照片152 B和圖示112B）。

Waist stretching method:

The patient lies prone, encircles back of head with five fingers of both hands crossed and bends knees at about 90 degrees. The massagist sits on the patient's soles, holds both elbows with both hands (see Photo 152A and Fig. 112A) and repeatedly pulls them backward thrice so that the waist stretches backward to the utmost (see Photo 152B and Fig. 112B).

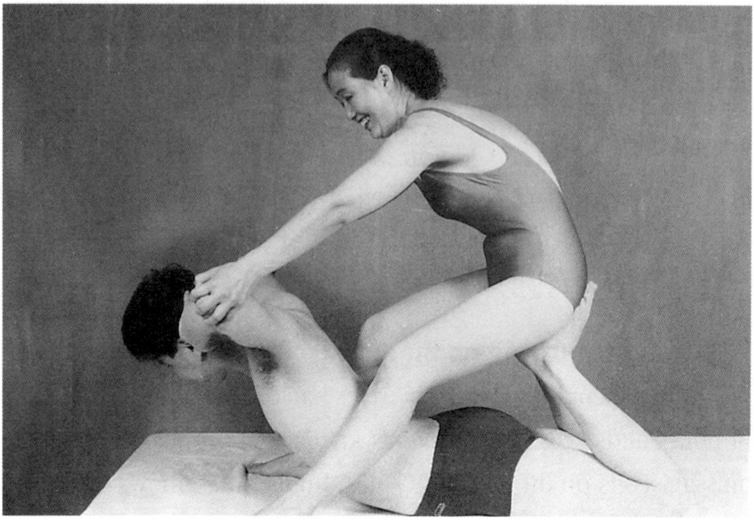

照片 (Photo) 152A

圖示 (Fig.) 112A

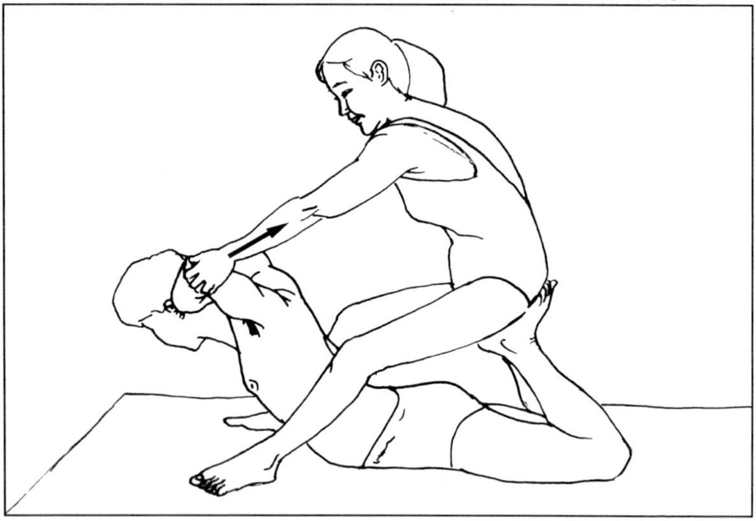

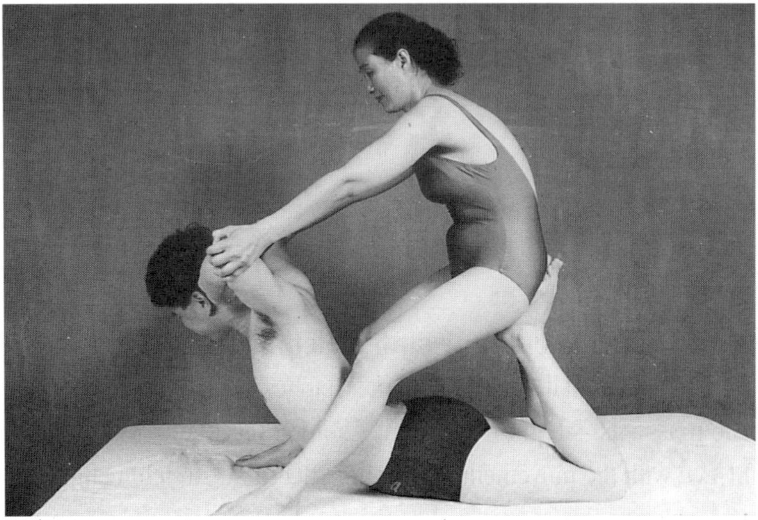

照片 (Photo) 152B

圖示 (Fig.) 112B

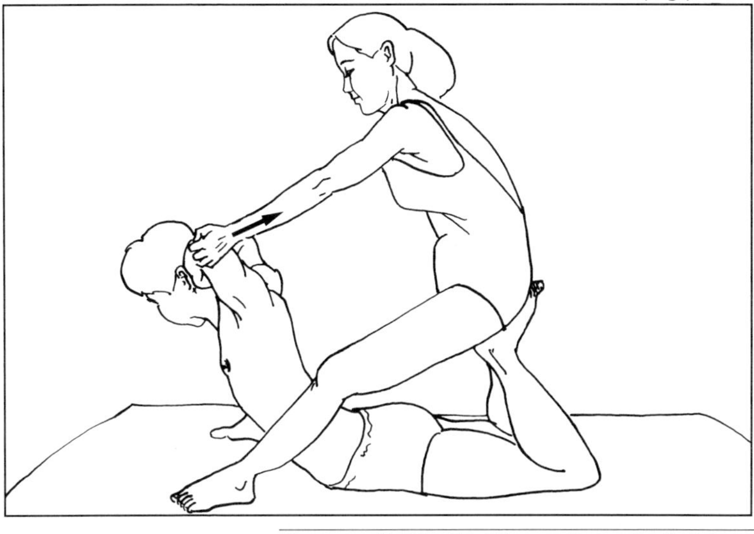

104 坐位屈膝法：

體位同上。被按摩者踝關節背伸，按摩者坐其足跖側（見照片153和圖示113A），借屈膝伸髖，向下坐壓足底，使被按摩者足跟儘量靠近臀部（見照片154和圖示113B）。反復操作2－4次。

Bending knee while sitting method:

In same position. The patient stretches ankle joints backward. The massagist sits on the patient's soles (see Photo 153 and Fig. 113A); with the movement of bending knees and stretching hips, sits and presses the soles so that the patient's heels approach the buttocks as much as possible (see Photo 154 and Fig. 113B). Repeat the manipulation 2-4 times.

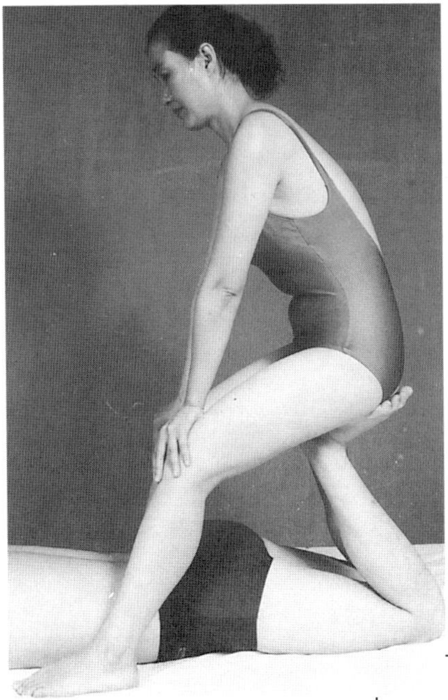
照片 (Photo) 153

圖示 (Fig.) 113A
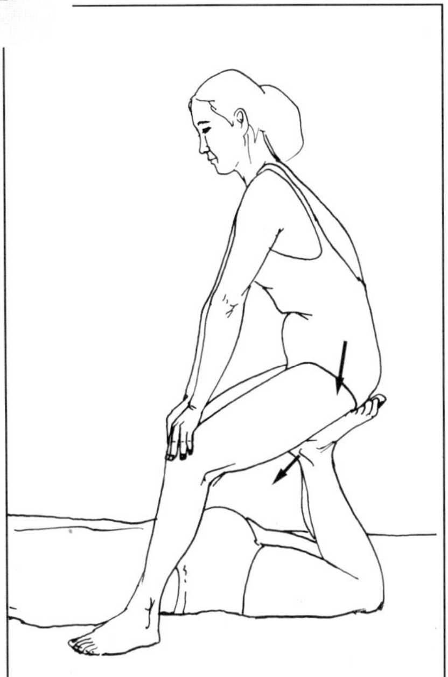

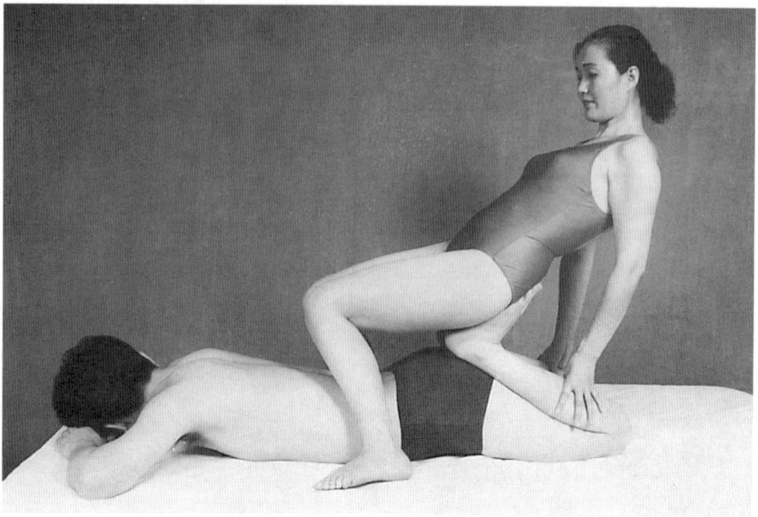

照片 (Photo) 154

圖示 (Fig.) 113B

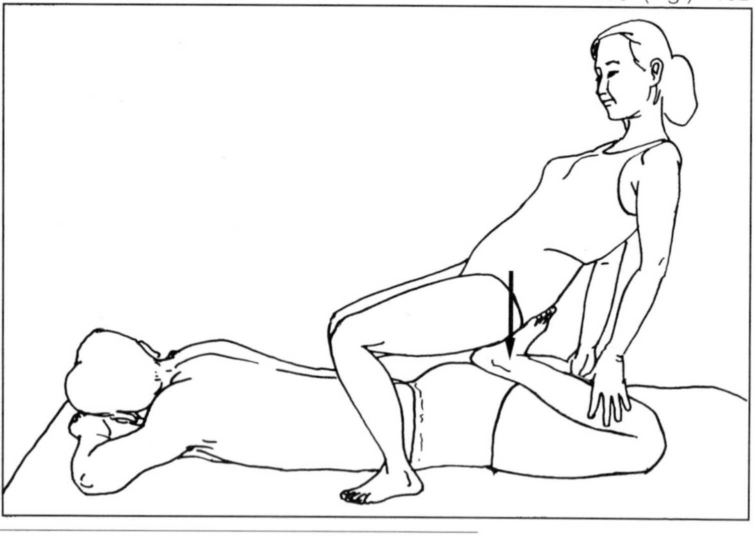

105 提腕伸腰法：

被按摩者俯臥位，雙上肢伸直並後伸；按摩者站立其臀溝處，雙上肢伸直握住被按摩者兩腕關節（見照片**155**和圖示**114A**），借軀幹後伸動作，牽拉其上肢，反復操作**2－4**次。（見照片**156**和圖示**114B**）。注意用力應適中，避免造成肩關節的損傷。

Wrist lifting and waist stretching method:

The patient lies prone and stretches both upper limbs straight and backward. The massagist stands on the buttock groove, stretches both upper limbs straight and holds the two wrist joints of patient with both hands (see Photo 155 and Fig. 114A); with the movement of stretching the body backward, lifts the upper arms. Repeat the manipulation 2-4 times (see Photo 156 and Fig. 114B). Note, use moderate force to avoid shoulder joint injury.

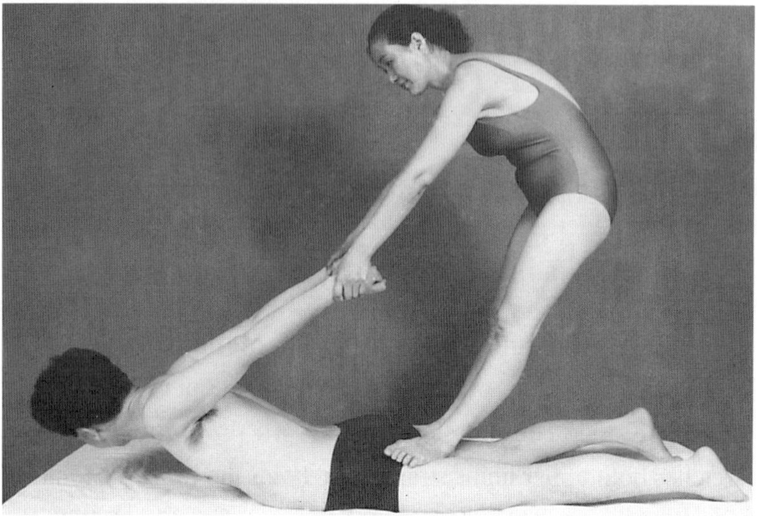
照片 (Photo) 155

圖示 (Fig.) 114A
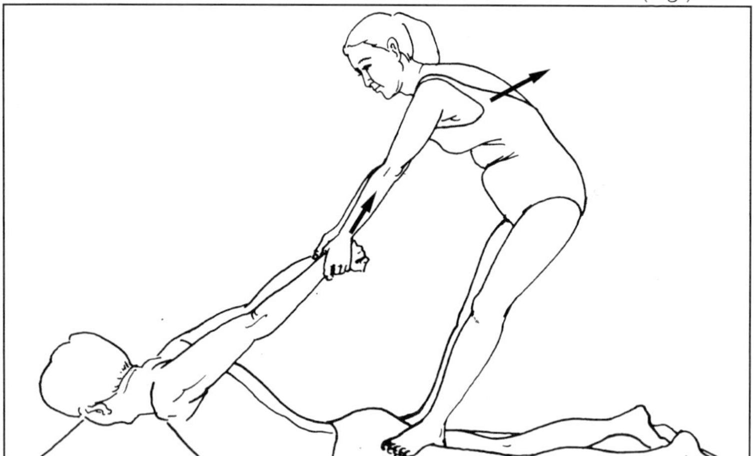

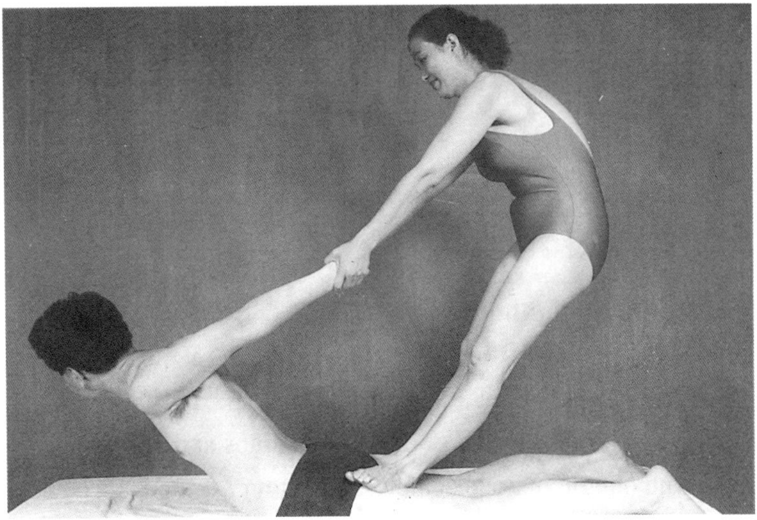

照片 (Photo) 156

圖示 (Fig.) 114B

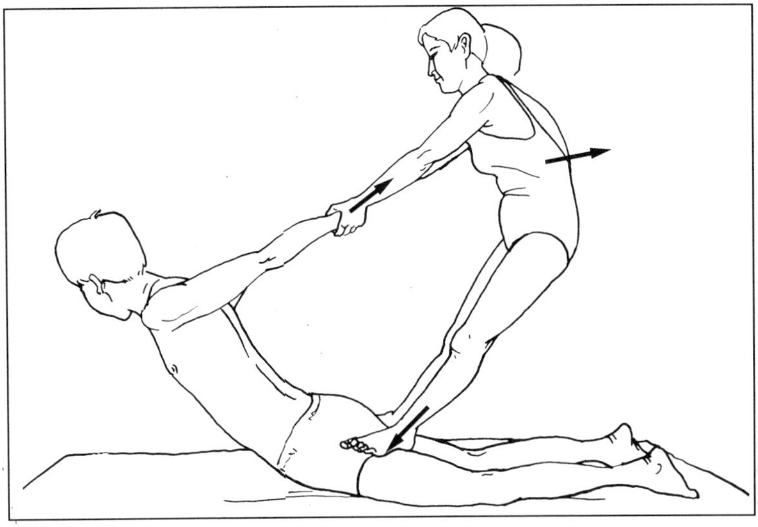

106 踩踏法：

被按摩者俯臥位，按摩者站於足側，雙手緊握踝關節前方，一腳置於雙下肢近端之間，另一腳踩踏脊柱，反復操作**2－4**次（見照片**157**和圖示**115**）。

Stamping method:

The patient lies prone. The massagist stands at the side of foot, grasps the patient's front ankle joints with both hands and places a foot between the near end of both lower limbs and stamps on the spine with other foot. Repeat the manipulation 2-4 times (see Photo 157 and Fig. 115).

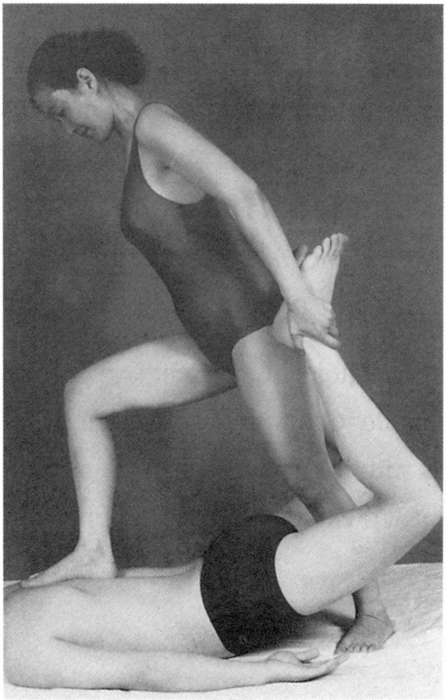

照片 (Photo) 157

圖示 (Fig.) 115

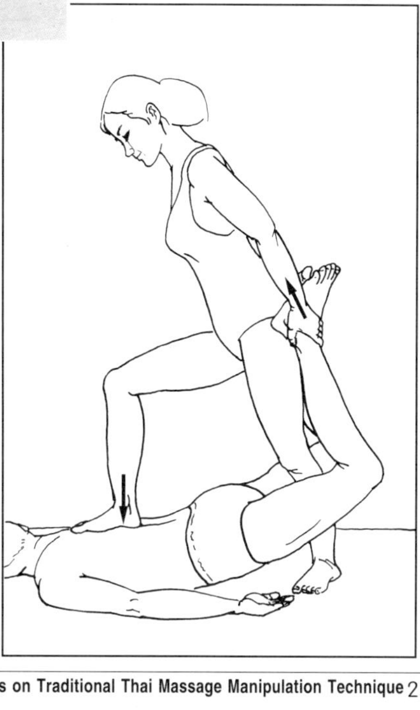

107 交替提拉法：

體位同上。按摩者一手握被按摩者腕關節，另一手握對側踝關節，雙手交替向上提拉（見照片**158**、**159**和圖示**116A**、**116B**），反復操作**2－4**次。一側完畢更換另一側。

Alternate lifting and pulling method:

In same position. The massagist holds the patient's wrist joint with one hand and the opposite ankle joint with the other hand and lifts and pulls upward alternately with both hands (see Photos 158, 159 and Figs. 116A , 116B). Repeat the manipulation 2-4 times. Do one side, then the other.

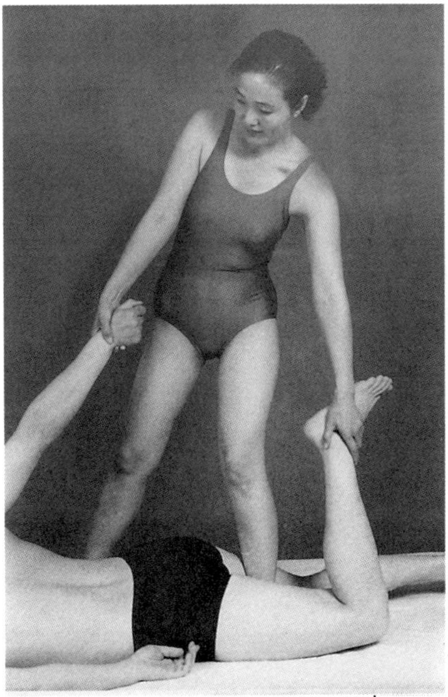

照片 (Photo) 158

圖示 (Fig.) 116A

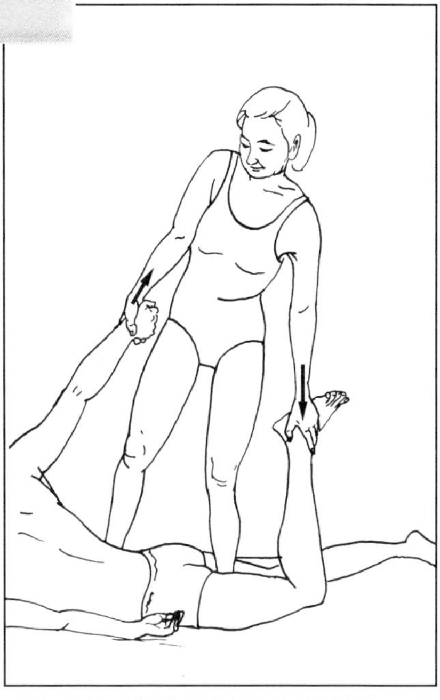

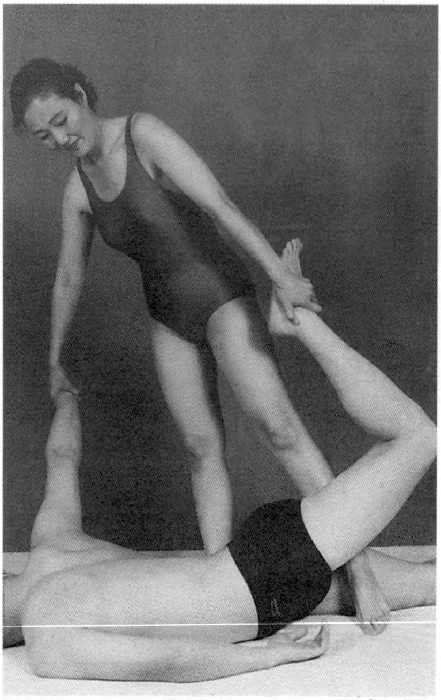

照片 (Photo) 159

圖示 (Fig.) 116B

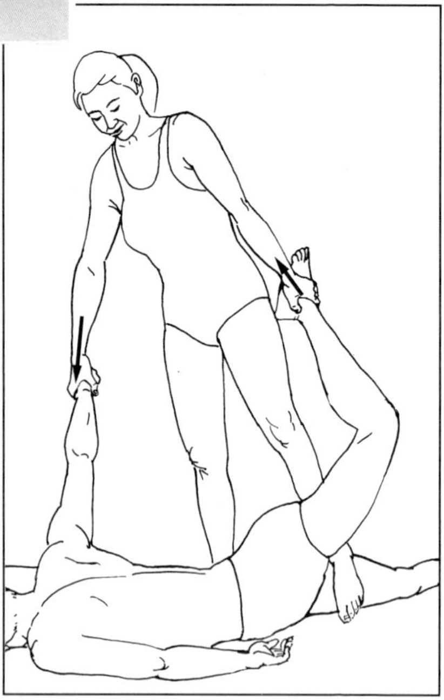

108 指揉頸部肌群：

被按摩者略側臥位，一下肢屈髖屈膝，按摩者跪坐於一側，一手拇指掌指及指間關節伸直，以指端為着力點，按揉頸部肌群，反復操作**2－4**次（見照片**160**、**161**和圖示**117A**、**117B**）。

Digital-rubbing neck muscles:

The patient lies slightly sideways and bends the hip and knee of a lower limb. The massagist kneels by the side of the patient and stretches joints between palm and thumb and finger joints straight; with the force of finger tips, presses and rubs neck muscles. Repeat the manipulation 2-4 times (see Photos 160, 161 and Figs.117A, 117B).

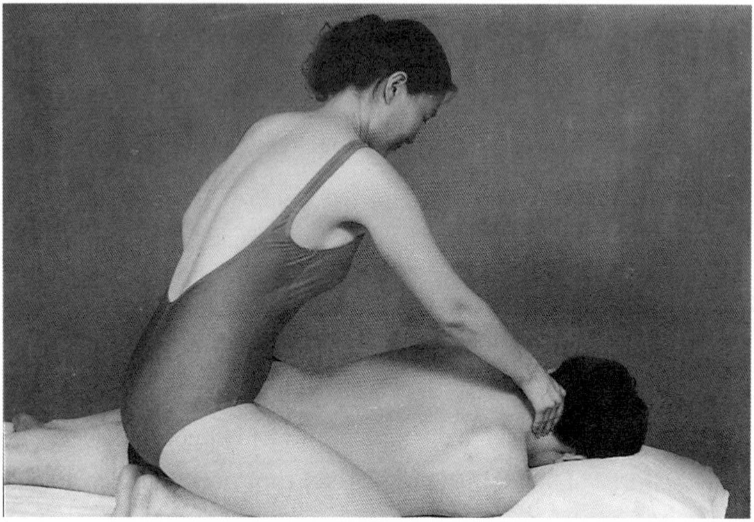

照片 (Photo) 160

圖示 (Fig.) 117A

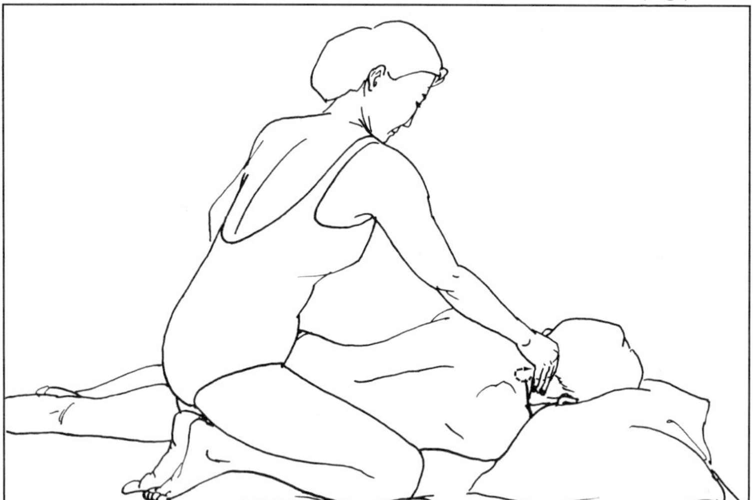

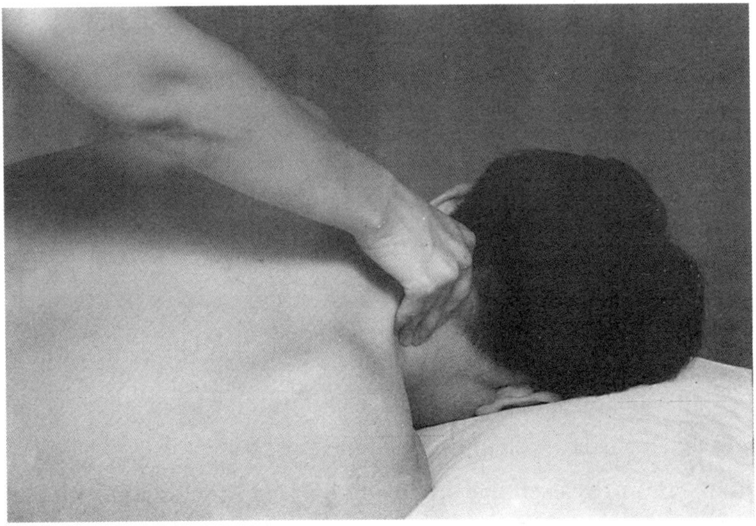

照片 (Photo) 161

圖示 (Fig.) 117B

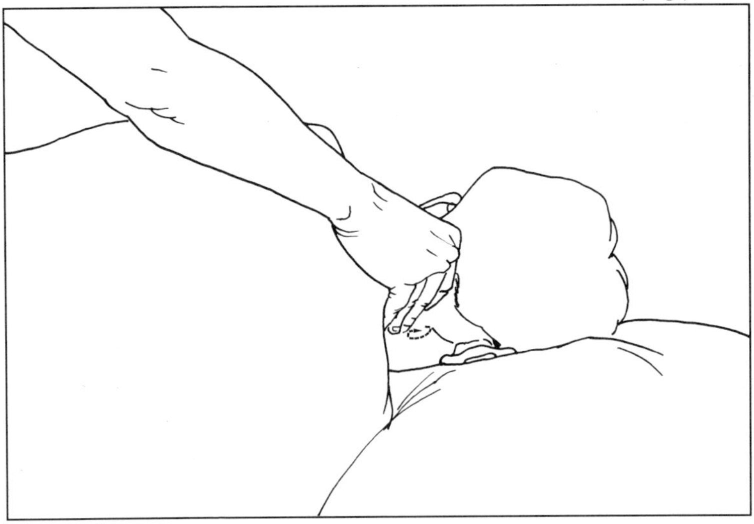

109 點按上肢後側肌群：

體位同上。按摩者一手握住被按摩者腕關節，以另一手拇指指端為着力點，從其肩部沿上肢後內側緣（見照片**162**和圖示**118A**）由近心端點按至遠心端（見照片**163**和圖示**118B**），反復操作**2－4**次。一側完畢更換另一側。

Pointing and pressing rear muscles of upper limb:

In same position. The massagist holds the patient's wrist joint with one hand and with the force of the thumb tip of the other hand, points and presses along the inside back of upper arm from the shoulder (see Photo 162 and Fig. 118A) from the near center to far center (see Photo 163 and Fig. 118B). Repeat the manipulation 2-4 times. Do one side, then the other.

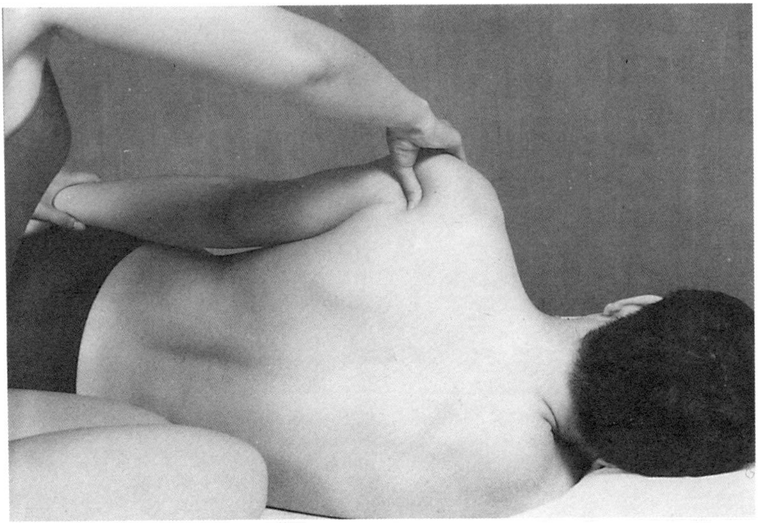

照片 (Photo) 162

圖示 (Fig.) 118A

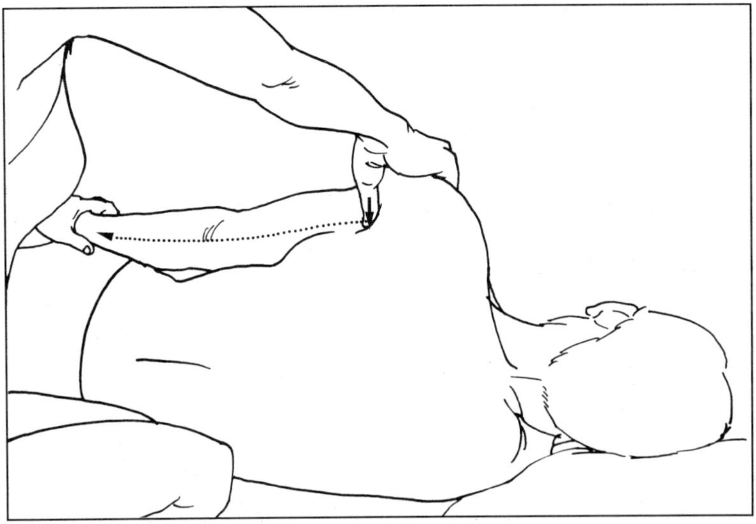

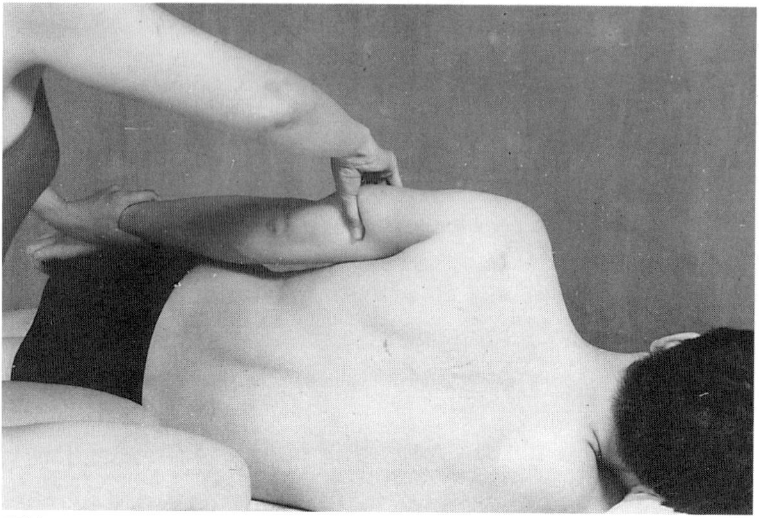

照片 (Photo) 163

圖示 (Fig.) 118B

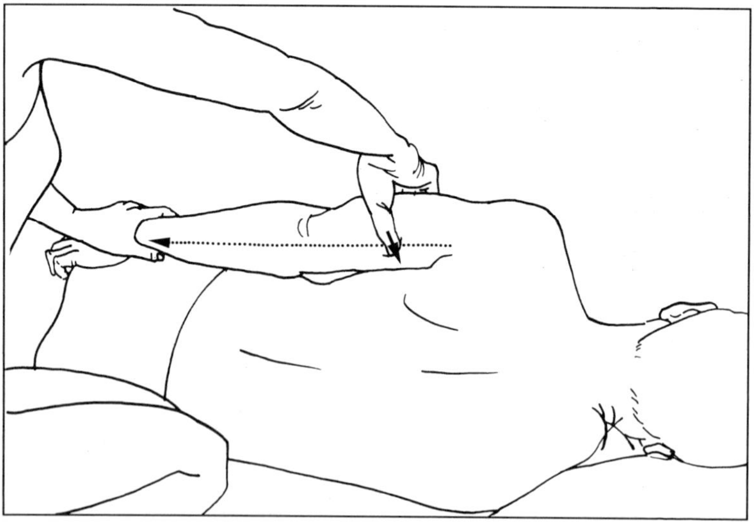

110 指揉後背法：

體位同上。按摩者以雙手拇指指腹着力，從被按摩者頸後部，沿斜方肌、菱形肌肌纖維走行（見照片**164**和圖示**119A**），按揉至肩胛骨及上肢後側（見照片**165**和圖示**119B**），反復操作**2－4**次。一側完畢更換另一側。

Digital-rubbing back method:

In same position. With the force of both thumb insides, the massagist presses and rubs from the back of patient's neck, along the rhombic muscle and rhomboid muscle tissue (see Photo 164 and Fig. 119A) to the shoulder blade and the back of upper arm (see Photo 165 and Fig. 119B). Repeat the manipulation 2-4 times. Do one side, then the other.

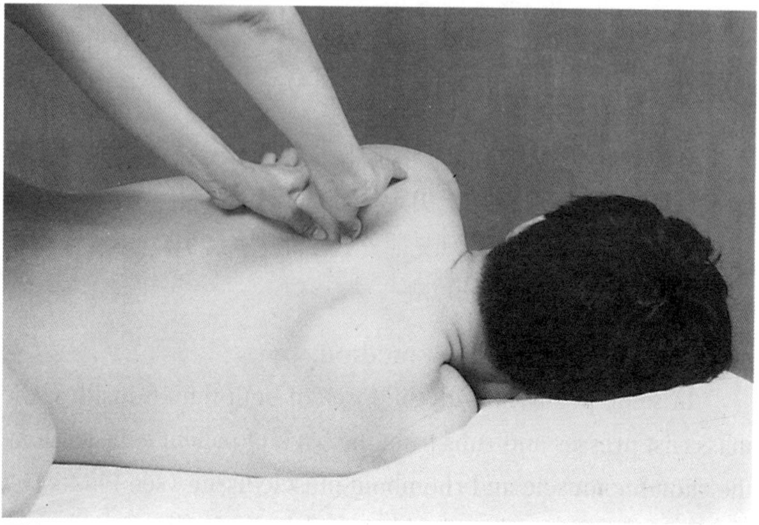
照片 (Photo) 164

圖示 (Fig.) 119A
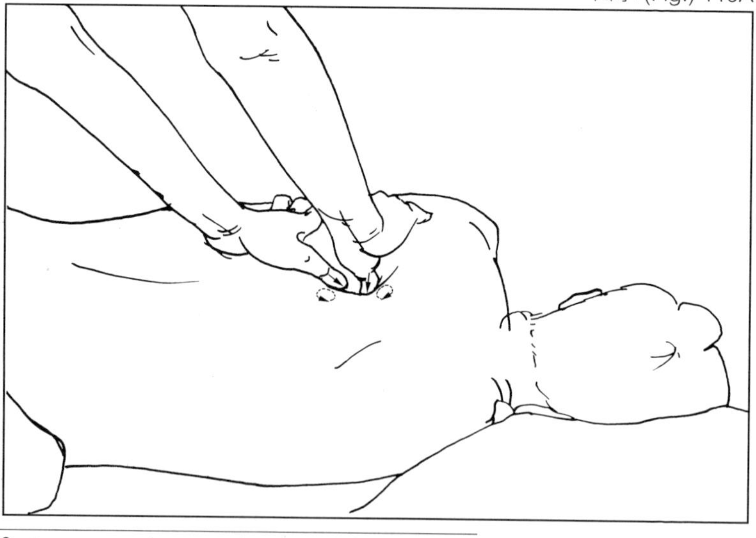

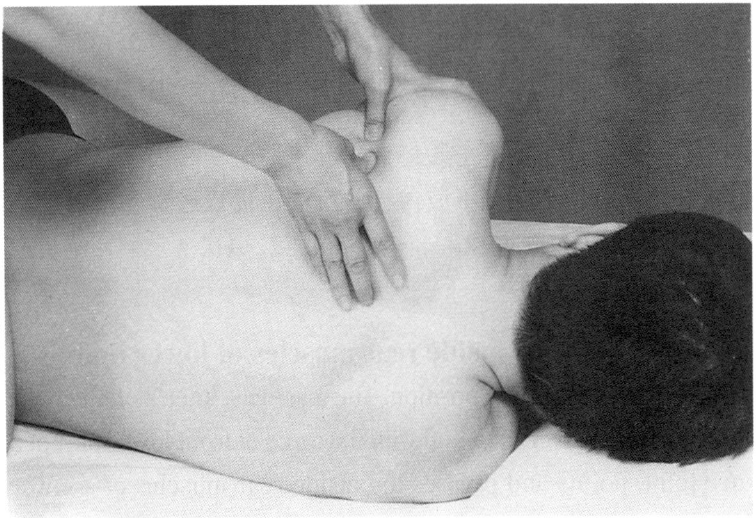

照片 (Photo) 165

圖示 (Fig.) 119B

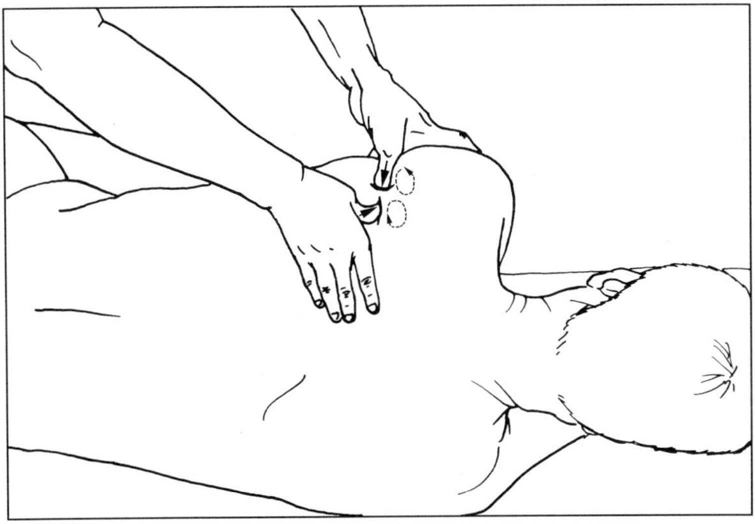

111 膝點下肢內後側肌群：

被按摩者體位不變，按摩者跪其下肢背側，以一側膝關節前下方為着力點，點按下肢內後側肌群，從近心端點按至遠心端（見照片**166**和圖示**120**），反復操作**2－4**次。一側完畢更換另一側。

Knee-pointing inside rear muscles of lower limb:

The patient in same position. The massagist kneels on the back of the patient's lower limb and with the force of front lower part of a knee joint, points and presses the inside rear muscles of a lower limb from near center to far center (see Photo 166 and Fig. 120). Repeat the manipulation 2-4 times. Do one side, then the other.

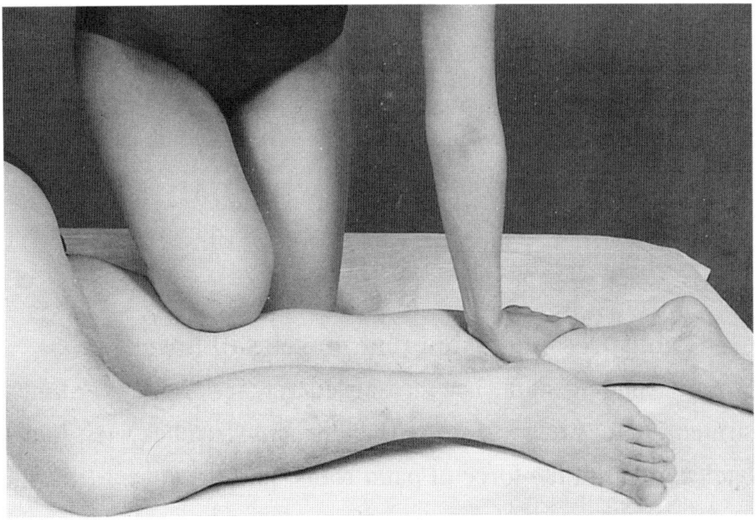

照片 (Photo) 166

圖示 (Fig.) 120

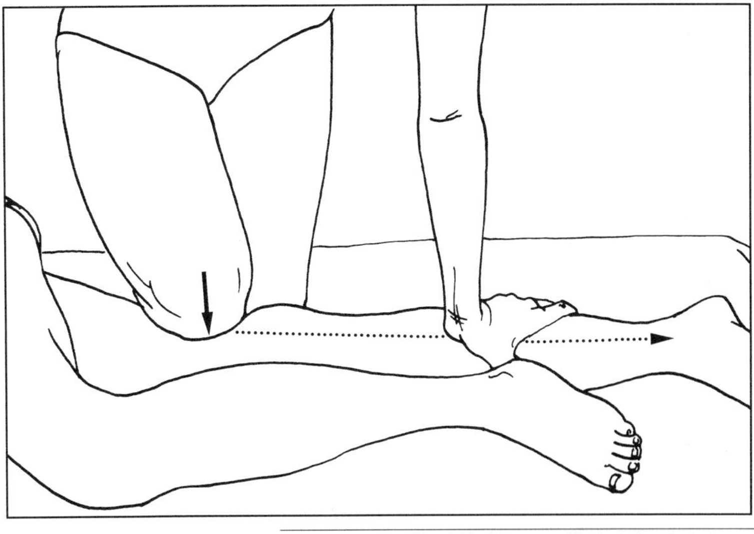

112 掌按下肢內後側肌群：

體位同上。按摩者雙上肢伸直，雙手重疊，腕關節背伸，以掌根為着力點，同時向下用力，從被按摩者下肢近端，沿內後側肌群按壓至遠心端（見照片167和圖示121），反復操作2－4次，一側完畢更換另一側。

Palm-pressing inside rear muscles of lower limb:

In same position. The massagist stretches both upper limbs straight, places one hand on the other and stretches wrist joints backward; with the force of palm roots, presses downward with force simultaneously from the patient's near end of lower limb, along the inside rear muscles to the far center (see Photo 167 and Fig. 121). Repeat the manipulation 2-4 times. Do one side, then the other.

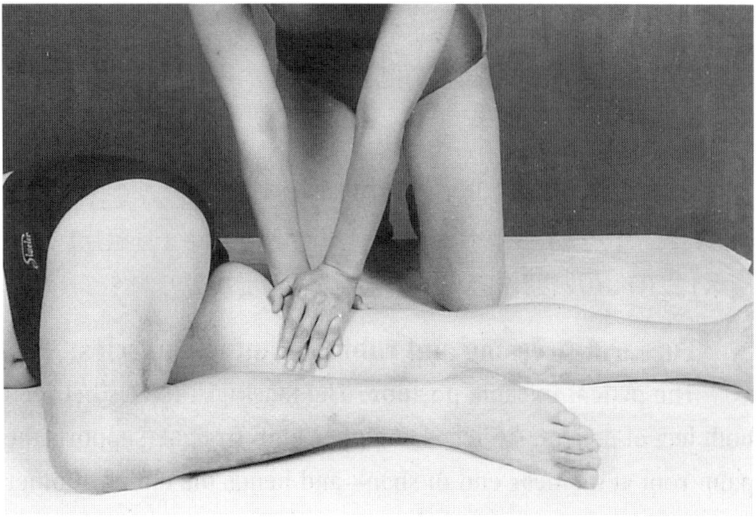

照片 (Photo) 167

圖示 (Fig.) 121

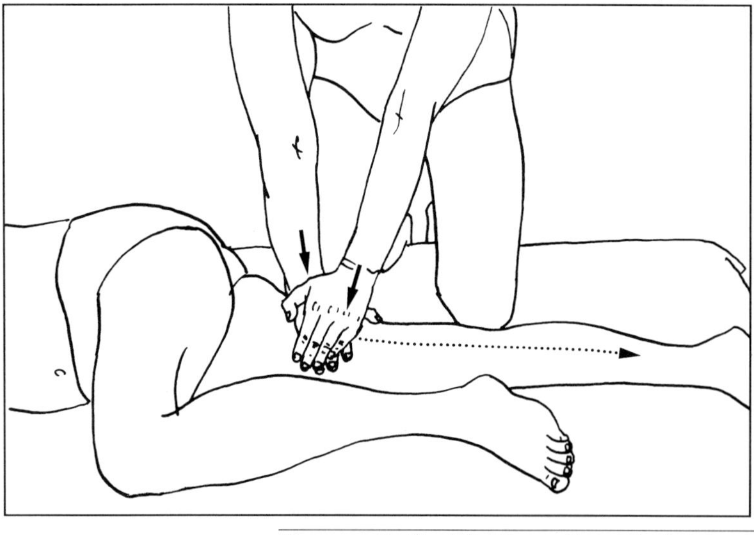

113 前臂按揉臀部肌群：

被按摩者體位同上。按摩者跪坐其雙足間，一上肢伸直，掌根撐扶於小腿近端，另一上肢屈肘，以前臂為着力點（見照片**168**和圖示**122A**），按揉臀部肌群至膝關節外側（見照片**169**和圖示**122B**），反復操作**2－4**次。一側完畢更換另一側。

Forearm-pressing and rubbing buttock muscles:

The patient in same position. The massagist kneels between both feet of patient, stretches an upper limb straight, supports the palm root at the near end of shank and bends the elbow of other upper arm; with the force of forearm (see Photo 168 and Fig. 122A), presses and rubs the muscles of buttocks to the outside of knee joint (see Photo 169 and Fig. 122B). Repeat the manipulation 2-4 times. Do one side, then the other.

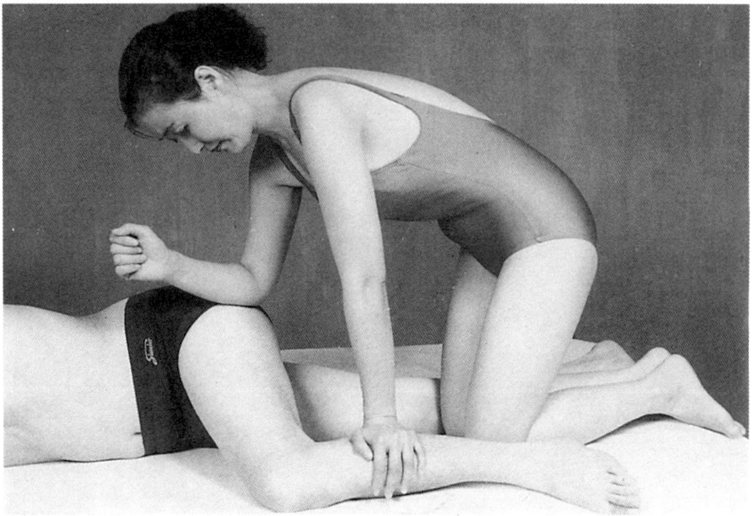

照片 (Photo) 168

圖示 (Fig.) 122A

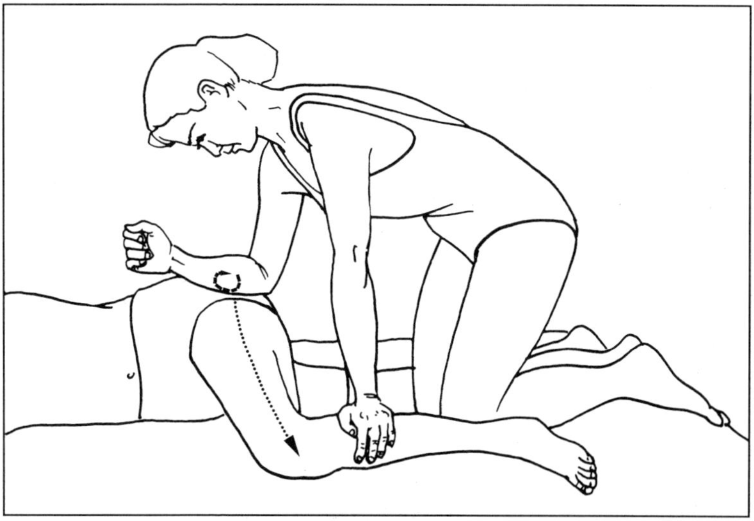

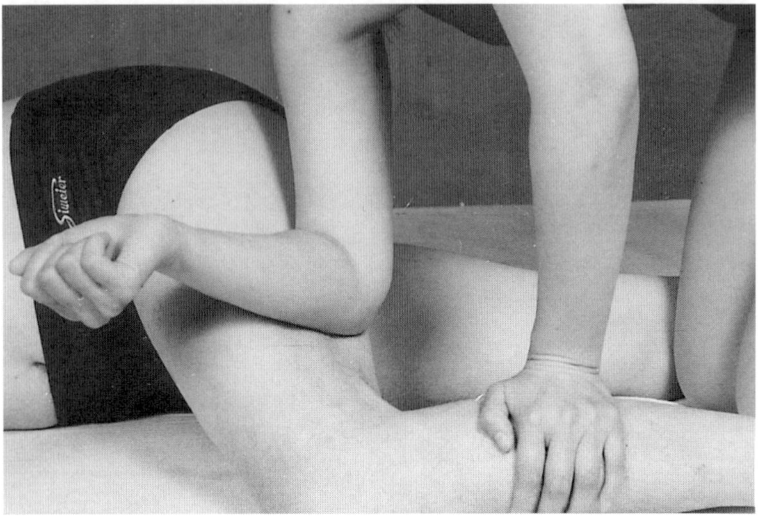

照片 (Photo) 169

圖示 (Fig.) 122B

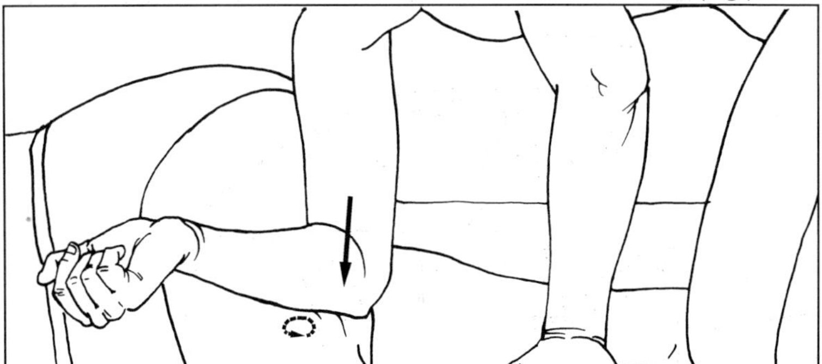

114 牽拉大腿前方肌群：

被按摩者側臥，一下肢屈髖屈膝位；按摩者坐其足側，一腳蹬被按摩者膝關節後上方，使其足背伸並勾於按摩者膝關節內側，雙手2、3、4、5指併攏，置於被按摩者下肢近端前方，以屈指之力向後外方牽拉其大腿前側肌群至膝關節處（見照片170和圖示123）。反復操作2－4次。一側完畢更換另一側。

Drawing front muscles of thigh:

The patient lies sideways and bends the hip and knee of a lower limb. The massagist sits by the side of the patient's foot, stamps on the upper back part of the patient's knee joint with a foot so that the foot of the patient stretches backward and hooks the inside of the massagist's knee joint, closes together the 2nd, 3rd, 4th and 5th fingers of both hands and places them on the front of lower limb near end of the patient; with the force of bent fingers, draws the front muscles of thigh backward and outward to the knee joint (see Photo 170 and Fig. 123). Repeat the manipulation 2-4 times. Do one side, then the other.

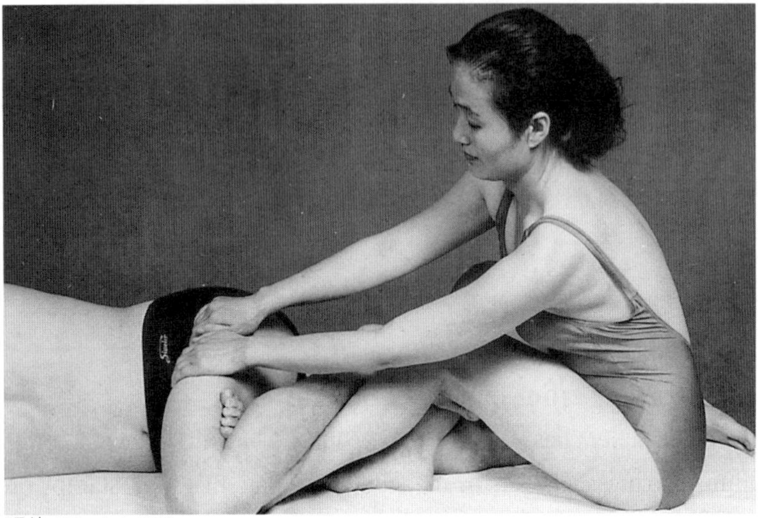

照片 (Photo) 170

圖示 (Fig.) 123

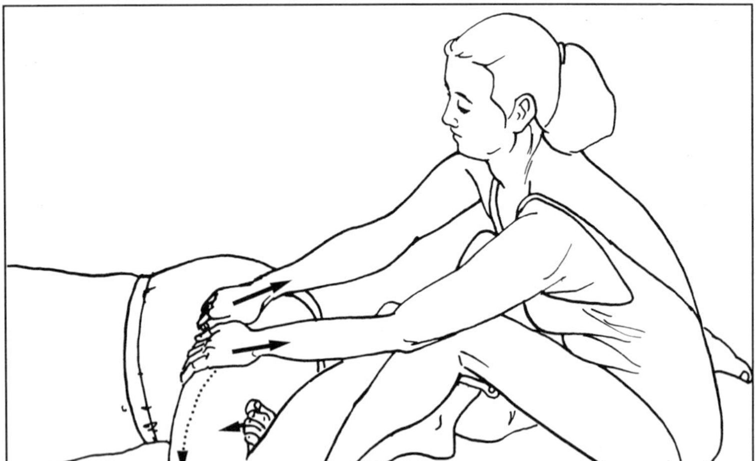

115 牽拉小腿後方肌群：

體位同上。按摩者雙手2、3、4、5指併攏，置於被按摩者小腿後方，以屈指之力，向外側牽拉小腿後方肌群至踝關節處（見照片171和圖示124），反復操作2－4次。一側完畢更換另一側。

Drawing rear muscles of shank:

In same position. The massagist closes together the 2nd, 3rd, 4th and 5th fingers of both hands and places them on the back of the patient's shank; with the force of bent fingers, draws the rear muscles of shank outward to the ankle joint (see Photo 171 and Fig. 124). Repeat the manipulation 2-4 times. Do one side, then the other.

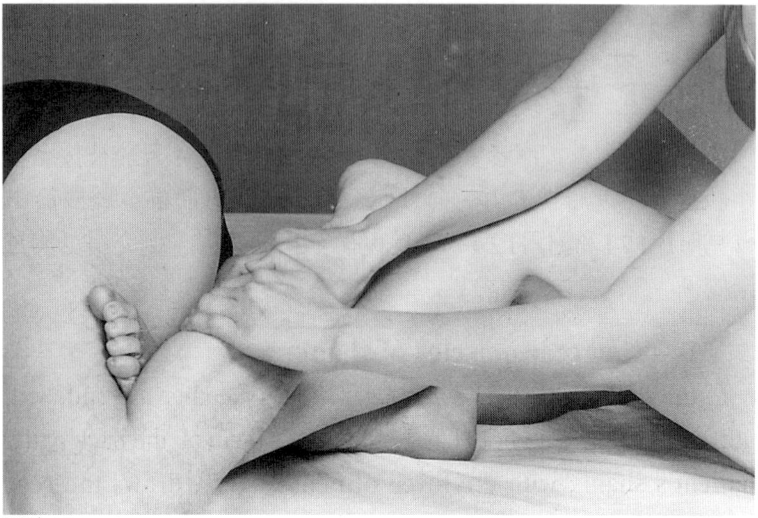
照片 (Photo) 171

圖示 (Fig.) 124

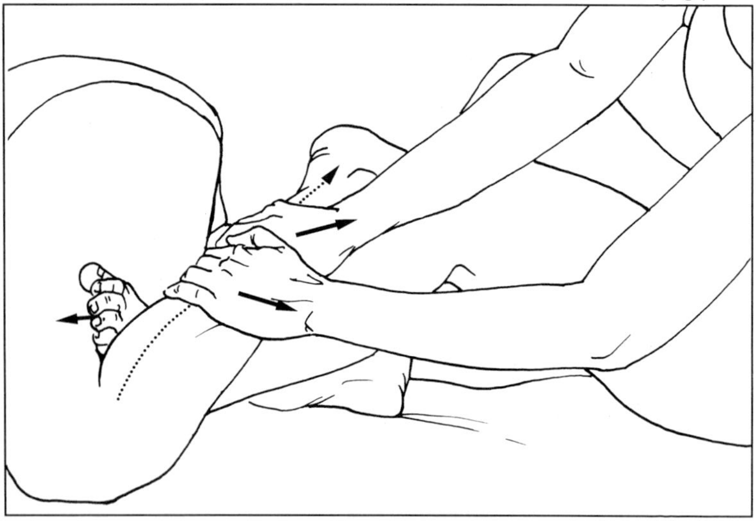

116 踩踏大腿後方肌群：

體位同上。按摩者一手握被按摩者踝關節，雙足置其臀橫溝處，以踩踏之力，從其大腿近端後側（見照片**172**和圖示**125A**）踩踏至膕窩處（見照片**173**和圖示**125B**），反復操作**2－4**次。一側完畢更換另一側。

Stamping rear muscles of thigh:

In same position. The massagist holds the patient's ankle joint with one hand and places both feet on the cross-groove on the buttocks; with the force of stamping, stamps from the back of thigh near end (see Photo 172 and Fig. 125A) to the hollow of knee (see Photo 173 and Fig. 125B). Repeat the manipulation 2-4 times. Do one side, then the other.

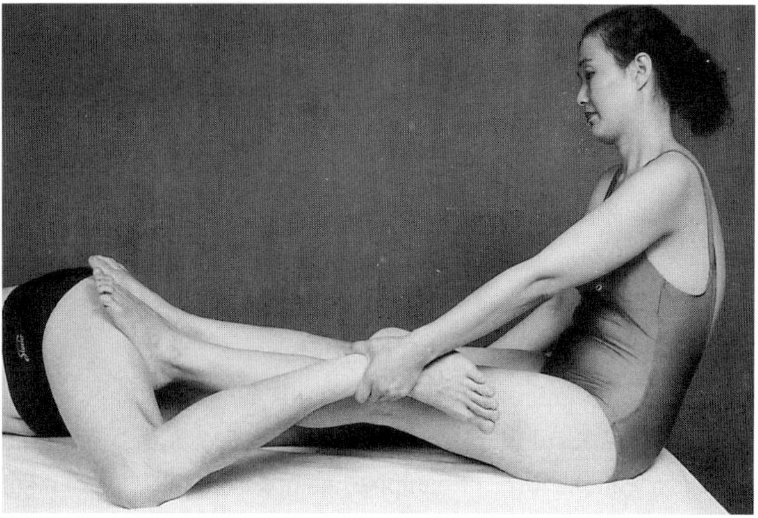

照片 (Photo) 172

圖示 (Fig.) 125A

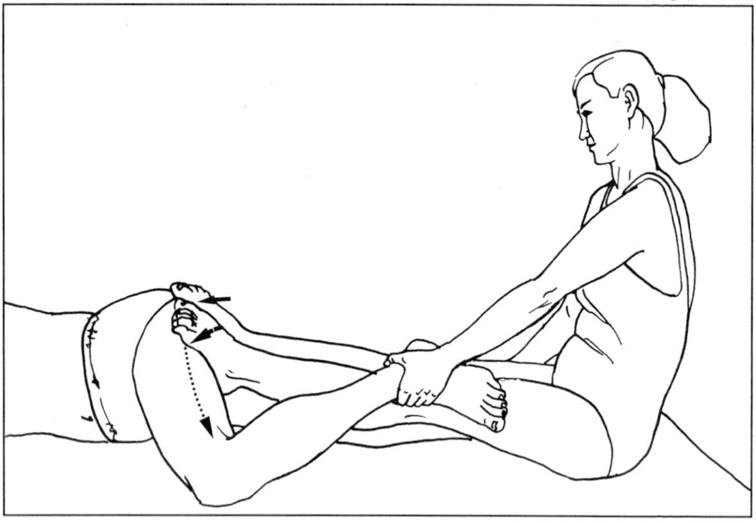

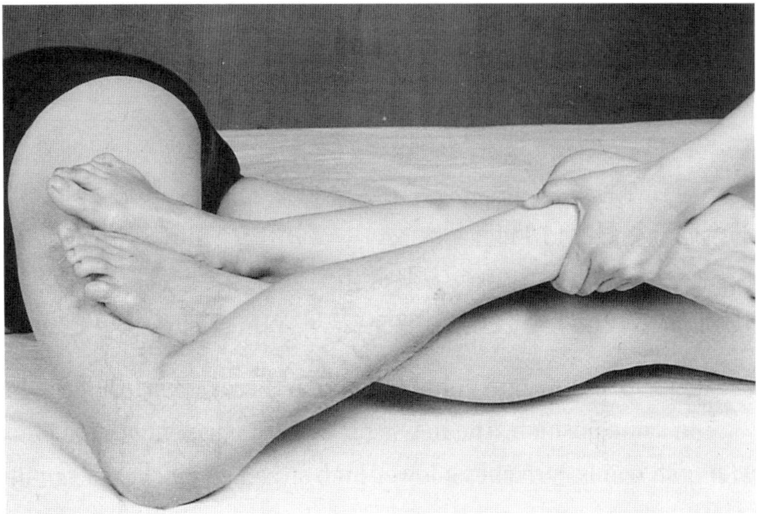

照片 (Photo) 173

圖示 (Fig.) 125B

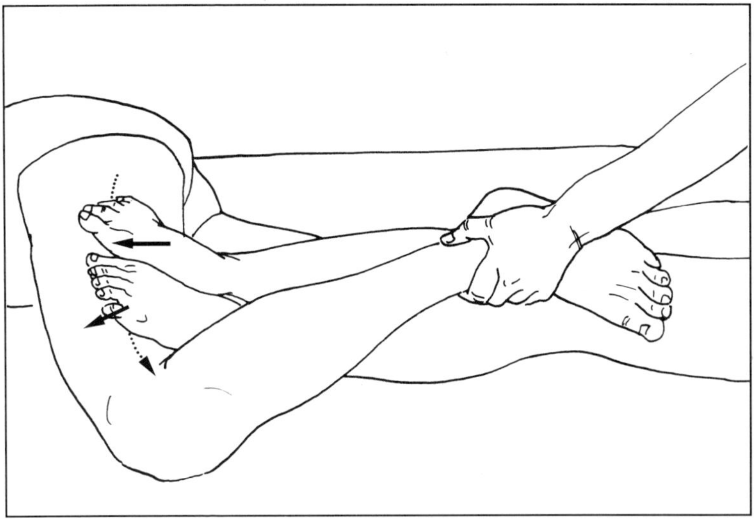

117 足按揉大腿前後方肌群：

體位同上。按摩者雙手握被按摩者踝關節，一下肢伸直，踝關節背伸將足背勾於被按摩者大腿前方，另一足蹬於其同水平的後側（見照片**174**和圖示**126A**），利用雙踝背伸，跖屈前足及搖動之力，按揉大腿前後方肌群，從近心端至膕窩處（見照片**175**和圖示**126B**），反復操作**2－4**次。一側完畢更換另一側。

Foot-pressing and rubbing front and rear muscles of thigh:

In same position. The massagist holds the patient's ankle joint with both hands, stretches a lower limb straight, stretches the ankle joint backward to hook the front of the patient's thigh with the dorsum of foot and stamps the other foot on the back at the same level (see Photo 174 and Fig. 126A); with the force of stretching both ankles backward, bending the sole of front foot and shaking, presses and rubs the muscles at front and back of thigh from near center to the hollow of knee (see Photo 175 and Fig. 126B). Repeat the manipulation 2-4 times. Do one side, then the other.

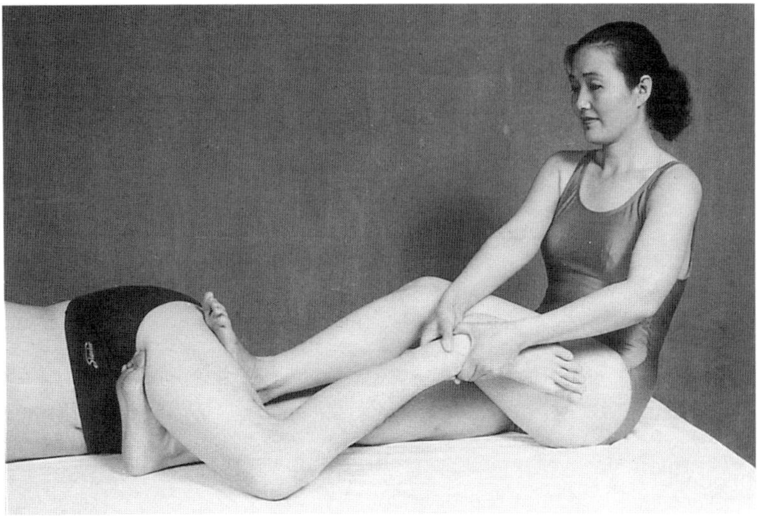
照片 (Photo) 174

圖示 (Fig.) 126A

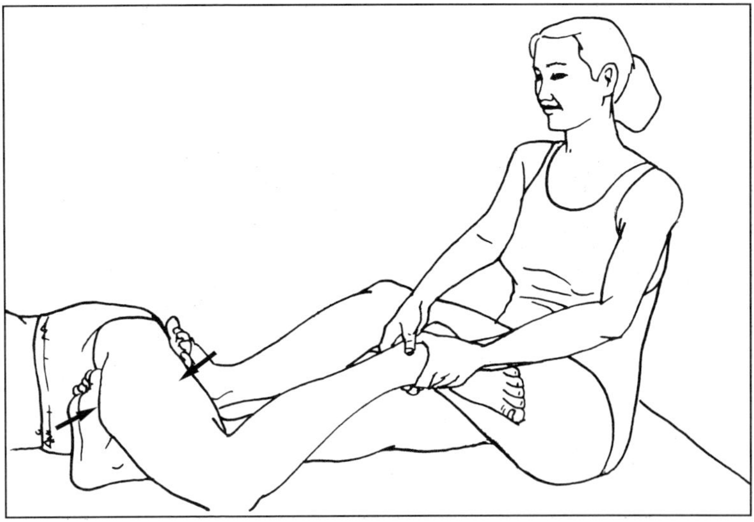

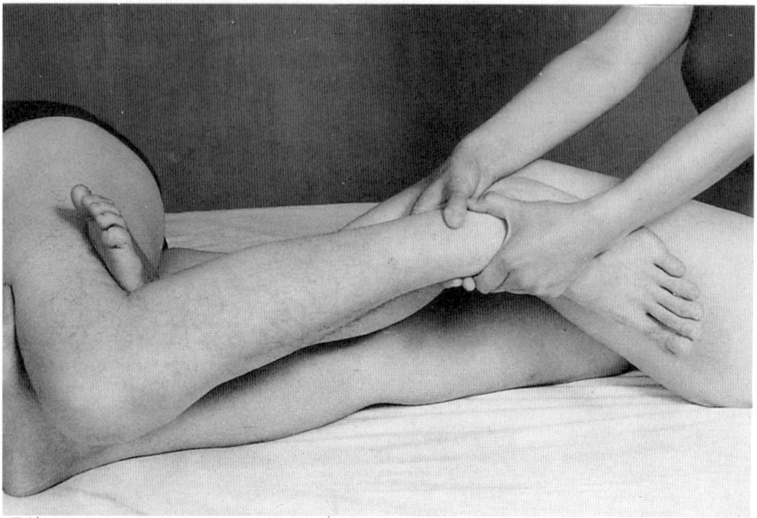

照片 (Photo) 175

圖示 (Fig.) 126B

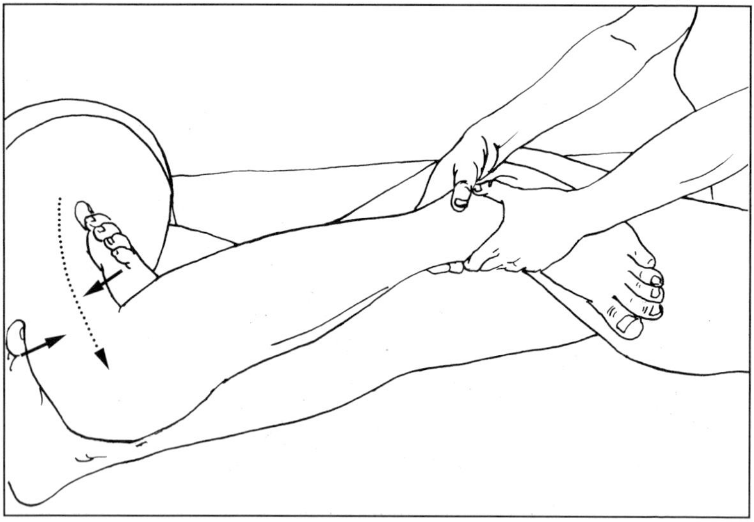

118 膝點小腿前外側肌群：

被按摩者俯臥位，一下肢內旋，膝關節屈曲，足背置於對側膕窩處，另一下肢屈膝；按摩者雙手分別扶按被按摩者臀部及前足背側，用膝關節前方點壓小腿前外側肌群，從近端至踝上方（見照片**176**和圖示**127**）。反復操作**2－4**次。一側完畢更換另一側。

Knee-pointing front outside muscles of shank:

The patient lies prone, revolves a lower limb inward, bends the knee joint, places the dorsum of foot in the opposite hollow of knee and bends the other lower limb. The massagist holds the patient's buttocks and the dorsum of front foot respectively with both hands and points and presses the front outside muscles of shank with knee joint from near end to the upper of ankle (see Photo 176 and Fig. 127). Repeat the manipulation 2-4 times. Do one side, then the other.

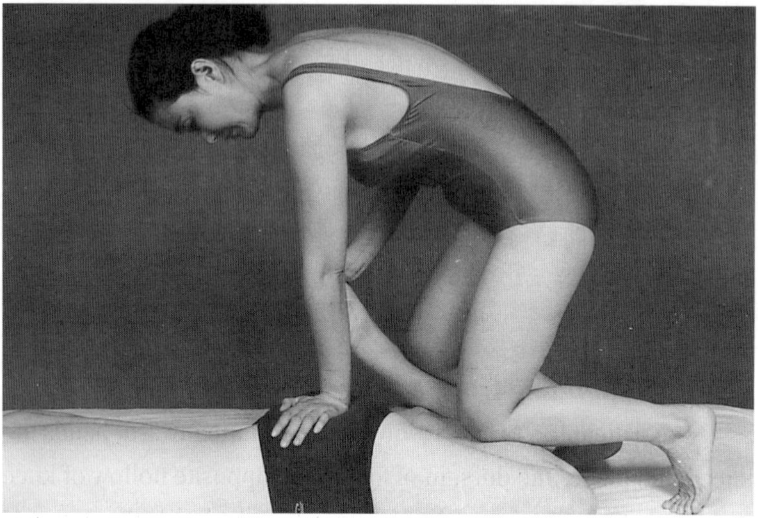

照片 (Photo) 176

圖示 (Fig.) 127

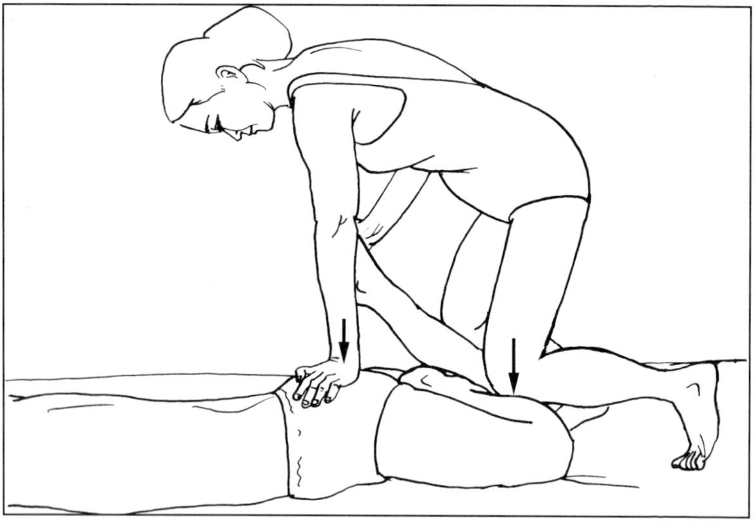

119 屈膝伸髖法：

體位同上。按摩者一手扶按被按摩者前足背側，另一手提扶膝關節前方，雙上肢交錯上下用力，使其被動屈膝伸髖（見照片177和圖示128），反復操作2－4次。一側完畢更換另一側。

Knee bending and hip stretching method:

In same position. The massagist holds the patient's dorsum of front foot with one hand and holds the front of the knee joint with the other hand; with the force of lifting and lowering both upper limbs alternately, makes the patient bend knee and stretch hip passively (see Photo 177 and Fig. 128). Repeat the manipulation 2-4 times. Do one side, then the other.

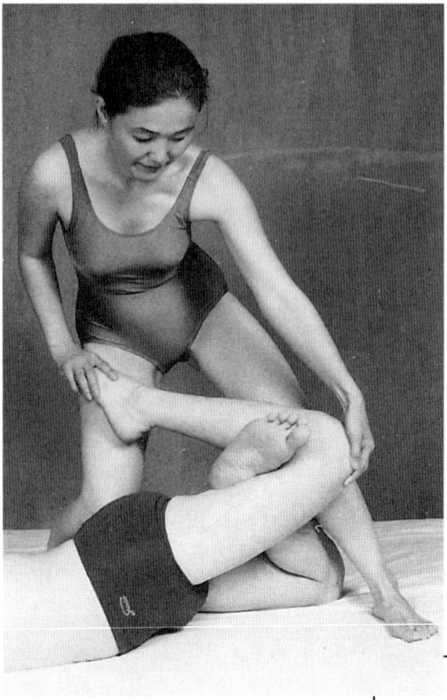

照片 (Photo) 177

圖示 (Fig.) 128

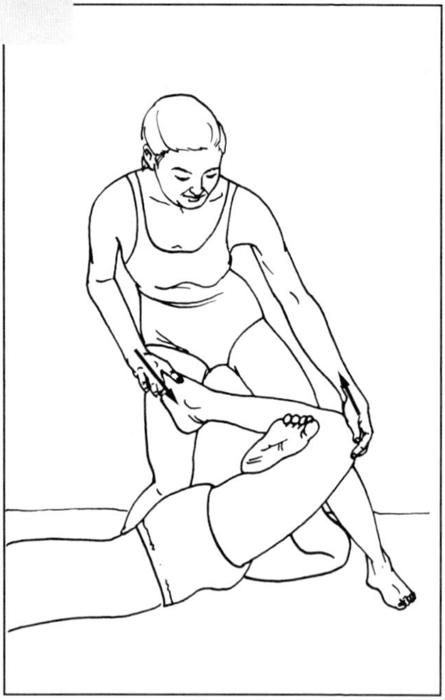

120 牽拉側屈法：

被按摩者側臥位，按摩者立其後，以一下肢小腿前側頂按被按摩者大腿近心端後側，而雙手緊握其右腕關節向遠心端牽拉（見照片**178**和圖示**129**），反復操作**2－4**次。一側完畢更換另一側。

Drawing and bending sideways method:

The patient lies sideways. The massagist stands behind the patient, steps on and presses the patient's back of thigh near center with the front of a lower limb shank and grasps the right wrist joint with both hands and draws it to the far center (see Photo 178 and Fig. 129). Repeat the manipulation 2-4 times. Do one side, then the other.

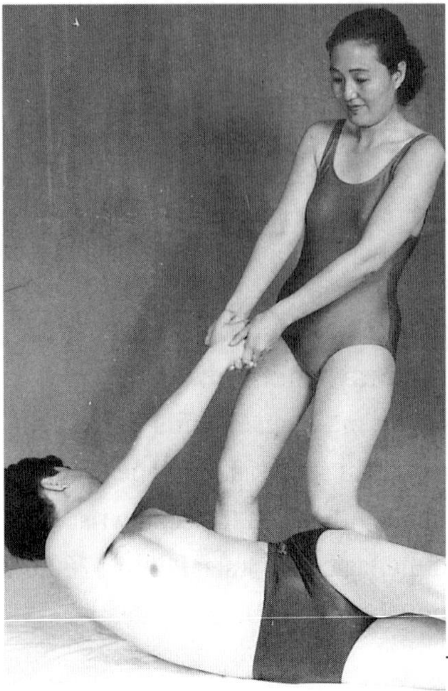

照片 (Photo) 178

圖示 (Fig.) 129

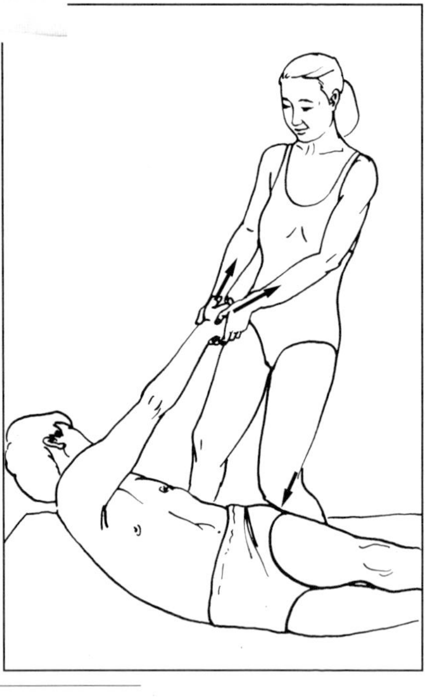

121 頂臀伸髖法：

被按摩者側臥位；按摩者屈髖屈膝，用膝關節前方頂住被按摩者臀部，雙手同時向後牽拉膝關節及下肢近端前方，使其被動伸髖（見照片179和圖示130）。反復操作2－4次。一側完畢更換另一側。

Stepping on buttocks and stretching hip method:

The patient lies sideways. The massagist bends hip and knee, steps on the patient's buttocks with the front of knee joint and draws the knee joint and the front of lower limb near end backward at the same time with both hands so that the patient stretches the hip passively (see Photo 179 and Fig. 130). Repeat the manipulation 2-4 times. Do one side, then the other.

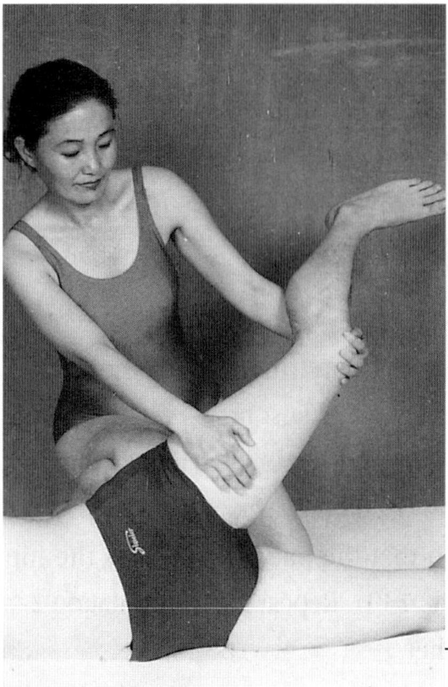

照片 (Photo) 179

圖示 (Fig.) 130

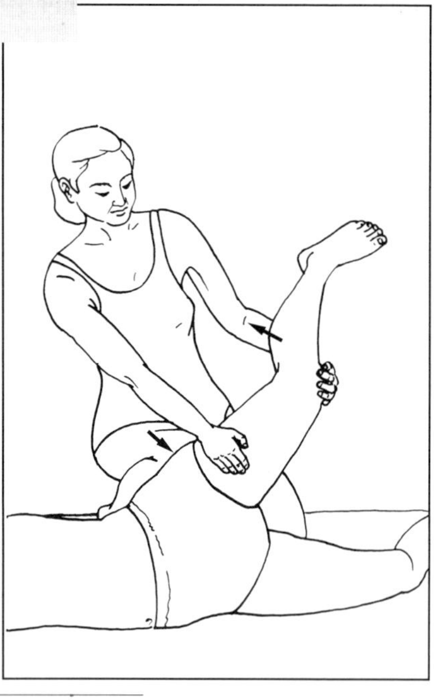

122 脊柱背伸法：

被按摩者俯臥位，按摩者立於床上，一足置於被按摩者臀部，一足在其兩下肢之間，雙手同時握住其雙腕關節，以腰部後伸之力向上提拉（見照片**180**和圖示**131**），反復操作**2－4**次。注意用力適中，避免造成肩關節損傷。

Stretching spine backward method:

The patient lies prone. The massagist stands on the bed, places one foot on the patient's buttocks and the other foot between both lower limbs and at the same time grasps both wrist joints with both hands; with the force of stretching the waist backward, lifts them upward (see Photo 180 and Fig. 131). Repeat the manipulation 2-4 times. Note, use moderate force to avoid injury to shoulder joint.

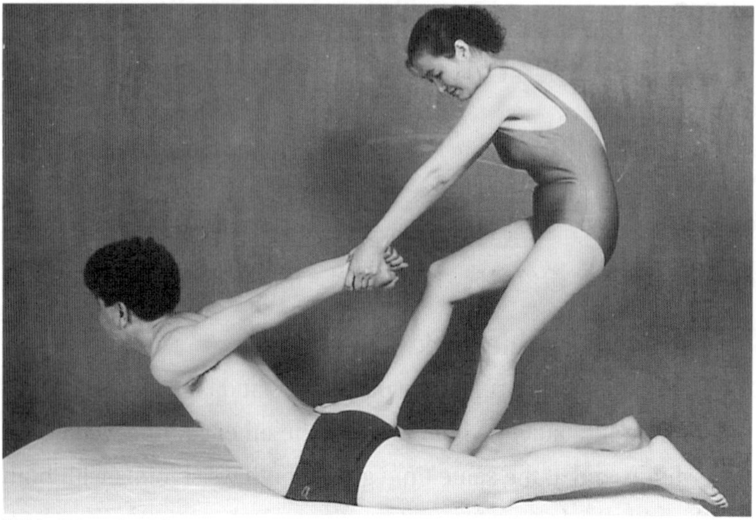

照片 (Photo) 180

圖示 (Fig.) 131

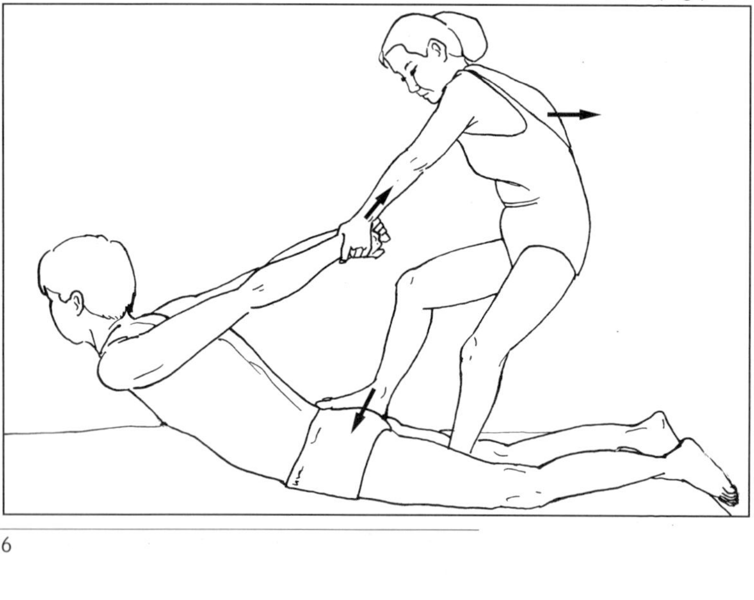

123 指揉大腿前方肌群：

被按摩者仰臥位，雙足分開與肩同寬；按摩者立於被按摩者足側，令其雙足蹬在自己的腹股溝處，利用腰部前屈，用雙手拇指指腹按揉腹股溝及大腿前內肌群（見照片181和圖示132），反復操作2次。

Digital-rubbing front muscles of thigh:

The patient lies flat on back with both feet apart the width of the shoulder. The massagist stands at the side of patient's foot so that both feet of the patient step on the massagist's groin; by bending waist forward, presses and rubs the groin and the front inside muscles of thigh with both thumb tips (see Photo 181 and Fig. 132). Repeat the manipulation twice.

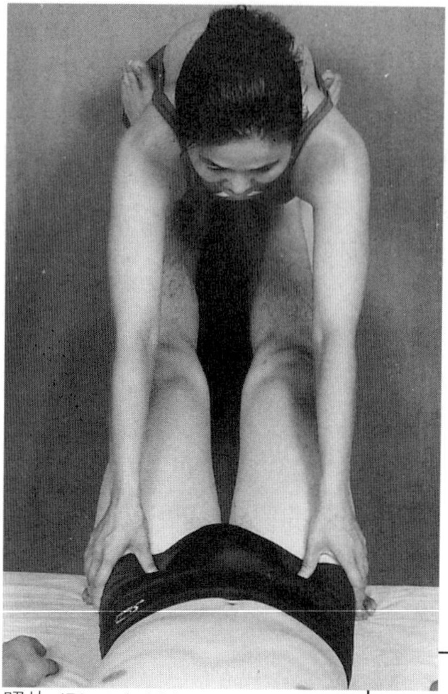

照片 (Photo) 181

圖示 (Fig.) 132

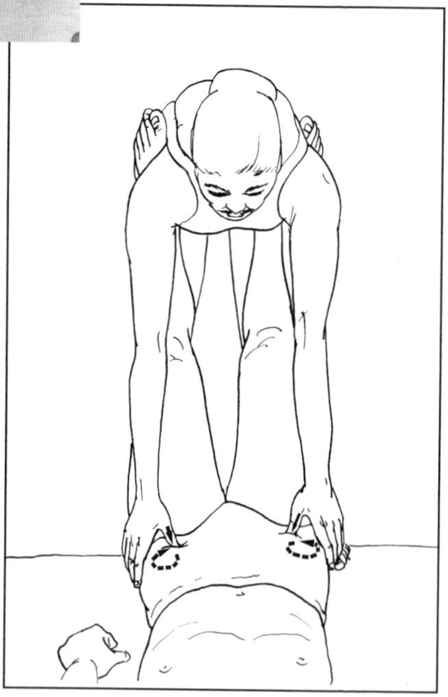

124 推按大腿前內側肌群：

體位同上。按摩者雙上肢伸直，腕關節背伸，手掌置於被按摩者腹股溝處，以推按之力，使其下肢前內肌群後旋至膝關節處（見照片182和圖示133），反復操作2－4次。

Pushing and pressing front inside muscles of thigh:

In same position. The massagist stretches both upper arms straight, stretches the wrist joints backward and places palms on the patient's groin; with the force of pushing and pressing, makes the patient's inner front muscles of lower limbs revolve backward to the knee joints (see Photo 182 and Fig. 133). Repeat the manipulation 2-4 times.

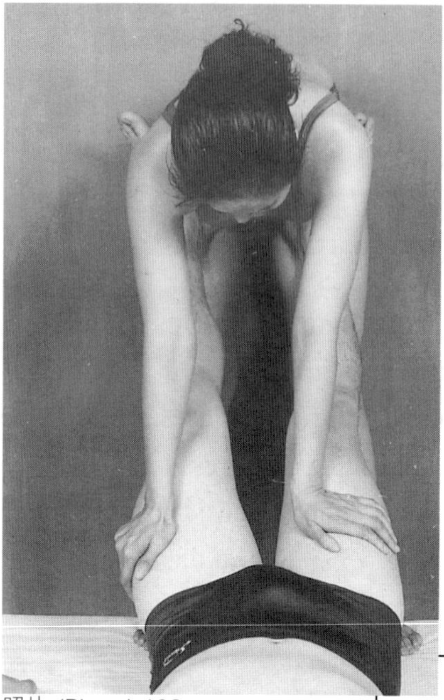

照片 (Photo) 182

圖示 (Fig.) 133

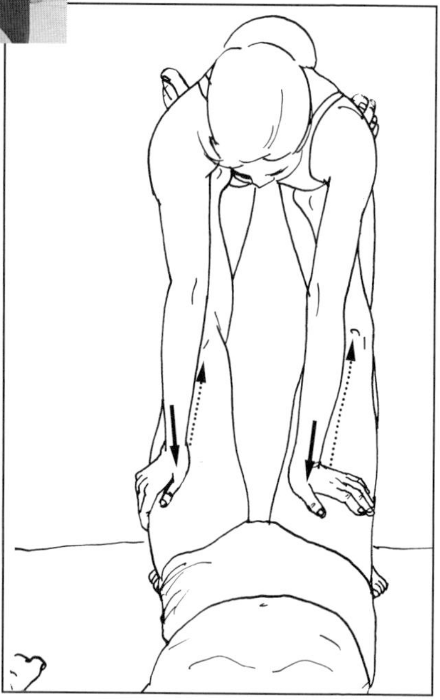

125 指叩下肢內側肌群：

被按摩者仰臥位，雙足下肢抬高**90**度，足背伸，雙上肢伸直，手扶膝關節處；按摩者立於被按摩者足側，兩手拇指置於其涌泉穴處（見照片**183**和圖示**134A**），屈髖屈膝向下壓，用雙膝關節頂住被按摩者腰骶部，使其臀部抬起（見照片**184**和圖示**134B**），再改為雙手五指併攏（見照片**185**和圖示**134C**），分別叩擊雙下肢內側肌群（見照片**186**和圖示**134D**）。

Digital-tapping inside muscles of lower limb:

The patient lies flat on back, raises both lower limbs at 90 degrees, stretches the feet backward, stretches both upper arms straight and holds the knee joints with hands. The massagist stands at the side of the patient's feet, places both thumbs on the patient's Yongquan acupoints (see Photo 183 and Fig. 134A), bends hip and knees to press downward and supports both ankle joints on the waist sacrum so that the patient raises the buttocks (see Photo 184 and Fig. 134B), and the massagist closes together five fingers of both hands (see Photo 185 and Fig. 134C) to tap the inside muscles of both lower limbs respectively (see Photo 186 and Fig. 134D).

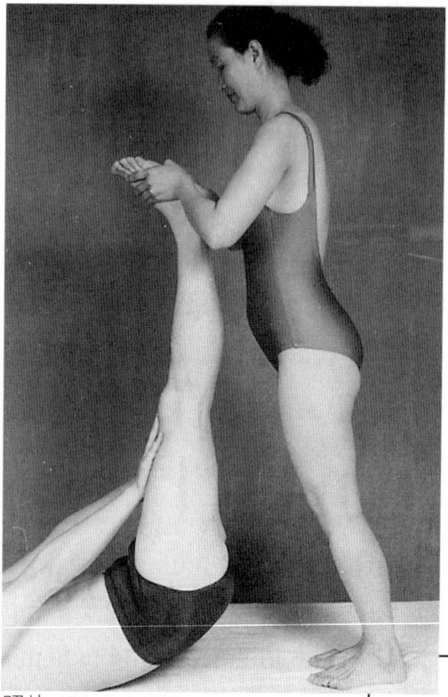

照片 (Photo) 183

圖示 (Fig.) 134A

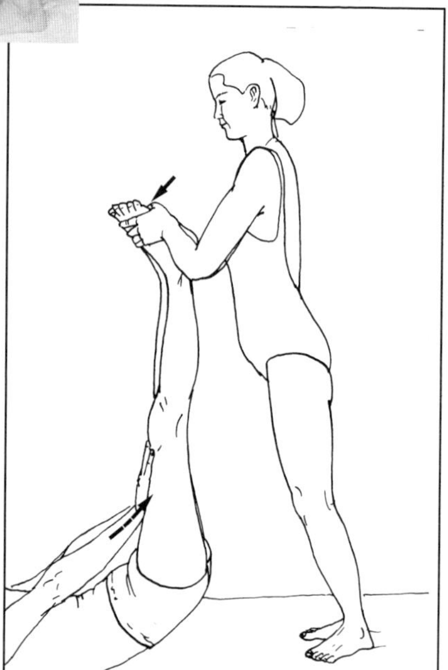

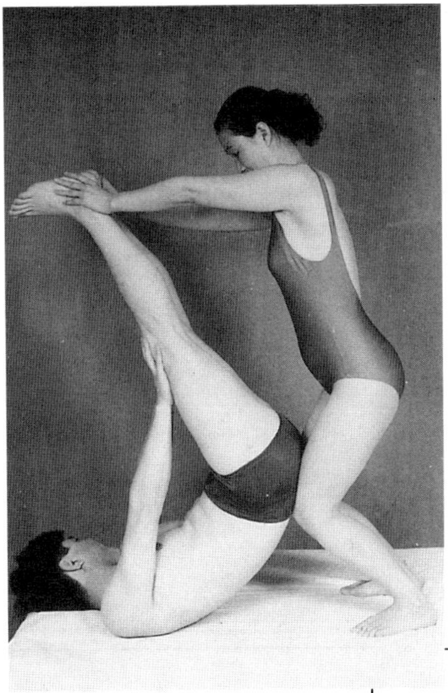

照片 (Photo) 184

圖示 (Fig.) 134B

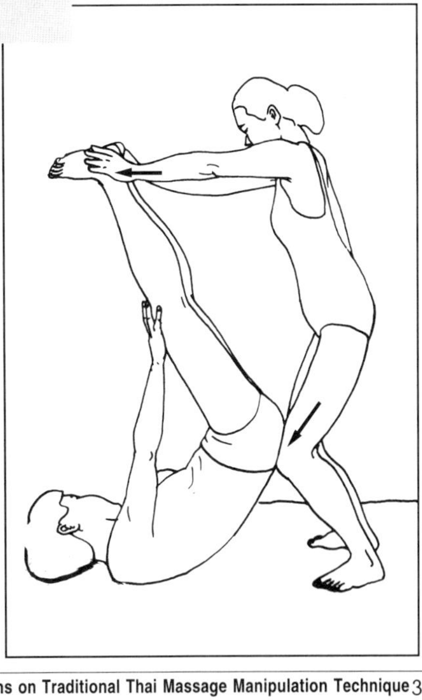

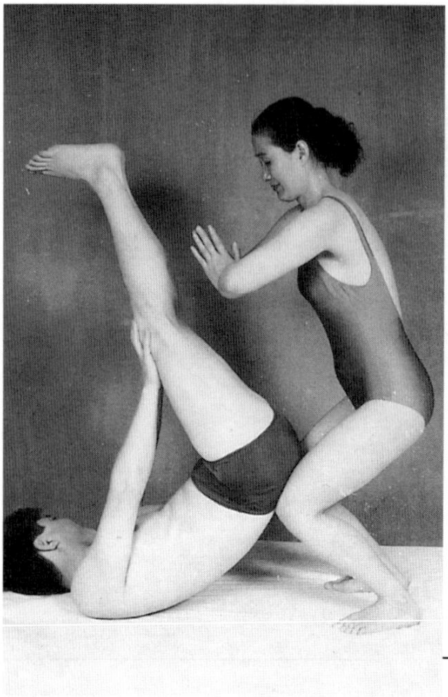

照片 (Photo) 185

圖示 (Fig.) 134C

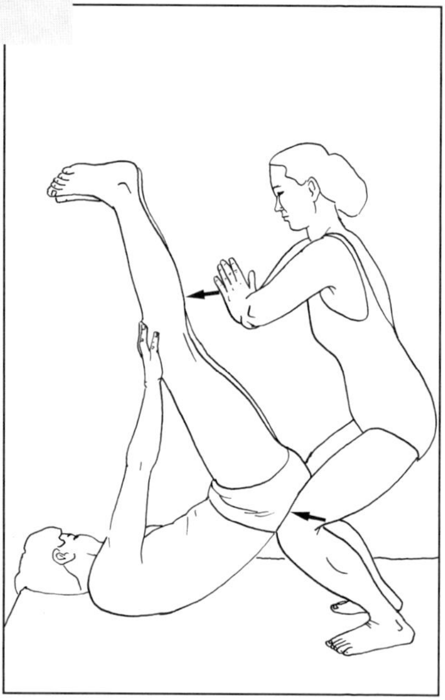

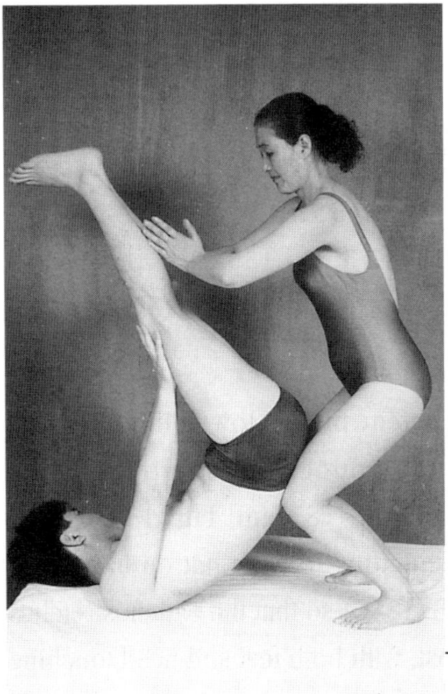
照片 (Photo) 186

圖示 (Fig.) 134D

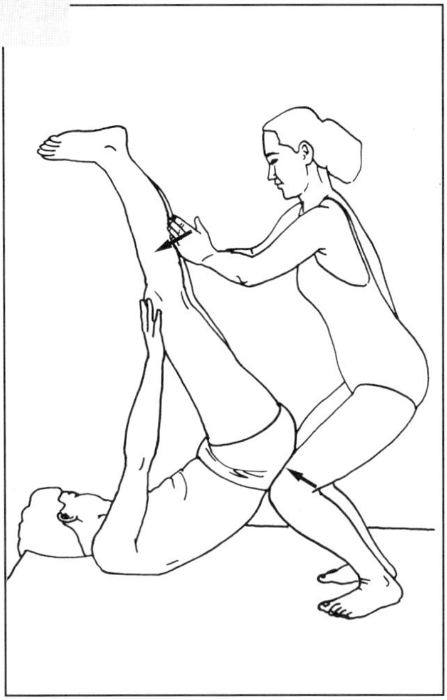

126 伸展脊柱法：

體位同上。被按摩者下肢置於按摩者肩部，而臀部位於按摩者膝關節的前方（見照片187和圖示135A）。按摩者由半蹲位改為仰臥位（見照片188、189和圖示135B、135C），使被按摩者極度背伸腰部，雙足及頭部着床（見照片190和圖示135D）。

Stretching spine method:

In same position. The patient places lower limbs on the massagist's shoulders, with the buttocks on the front of the massagist's knee joints (see Photo 187 and Fig. 135A). The massagist changes from half squatting to lying flat on back (see Photos 188, 189 and Figs. 135B, 135C) so that the patient stretches the waist backward to the utmost, with both feet and head touching the bed (see Photo 190 and Fig. 135D).

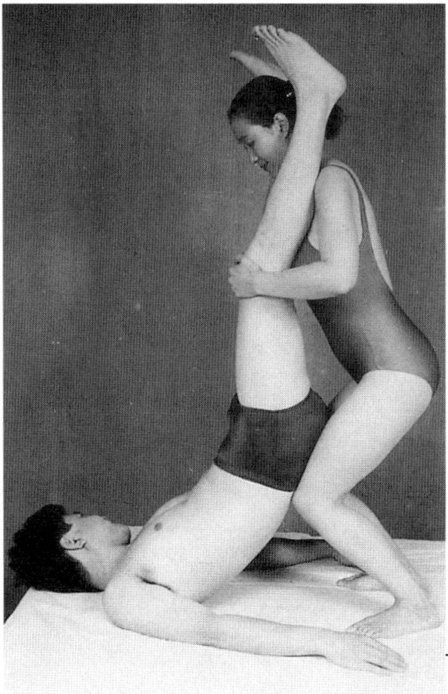

照片 (Photo) 187

圖示 (Fig.) 135A

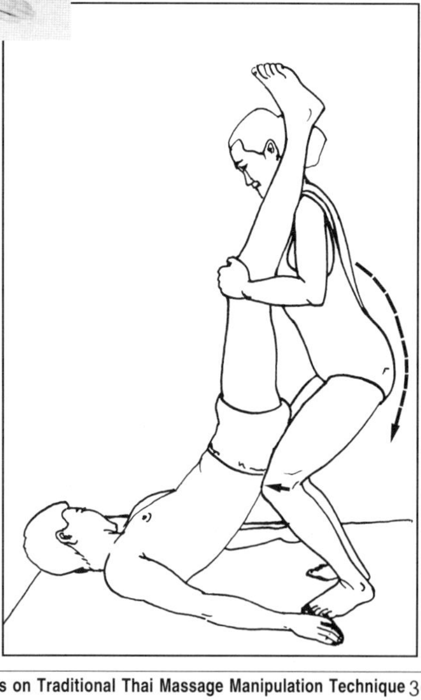

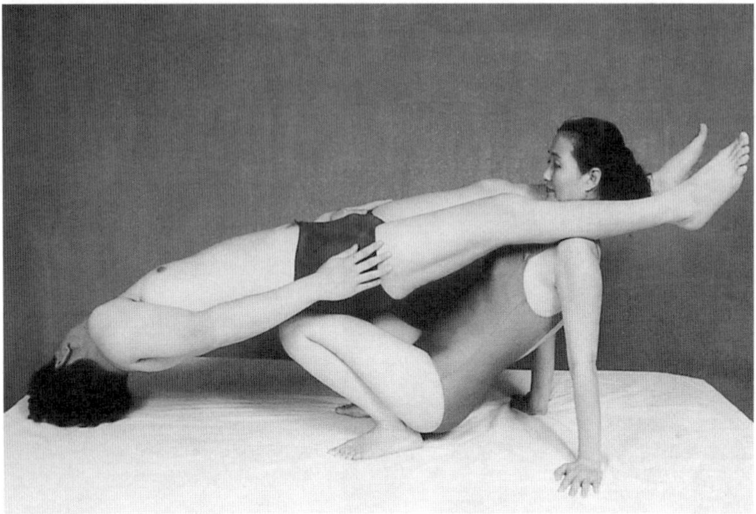

照片 (Photo) 188

圖示 (Fig.) 135B

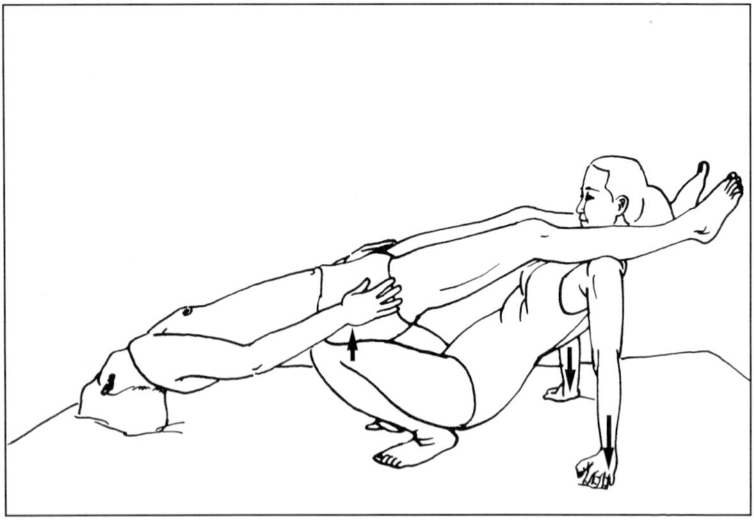

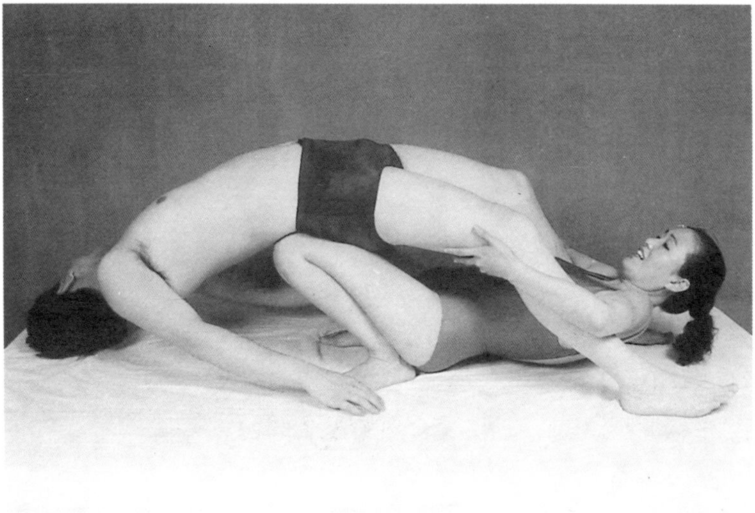

照片 (Photo) 189

圖示 (Fig.) 135C

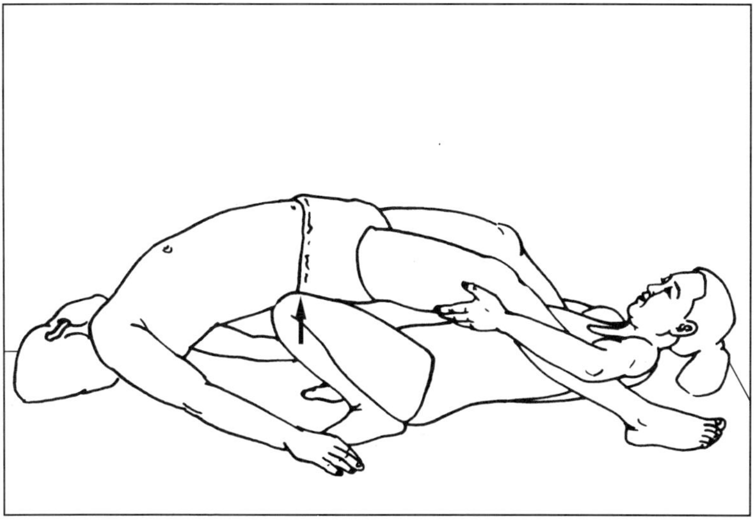

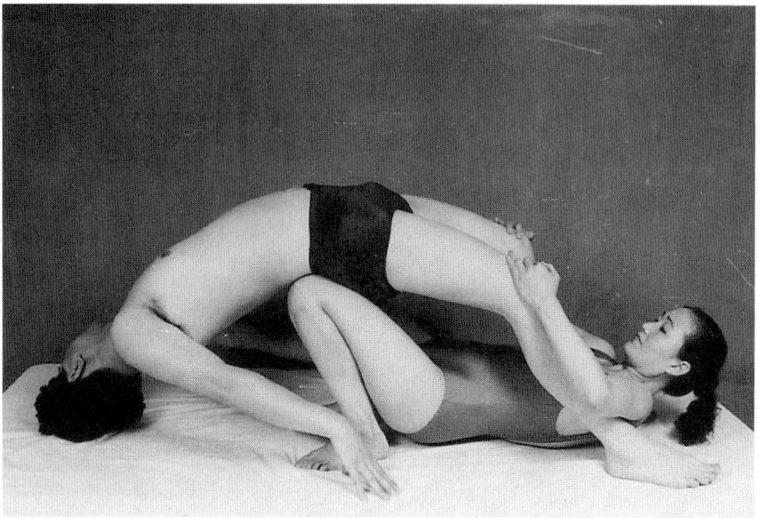

照片 (Photo) 190

圖示 (Fig.) 135D

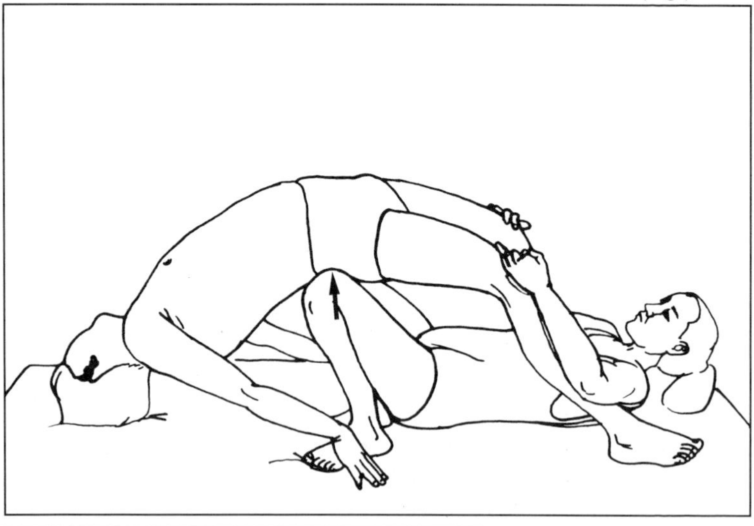

127 膝點大腿後方肌群：

被按摩者仰臥位，一下肢極度屈髖屈膝；按摩者站於其足側，雙手分別扶握其前足背側及膝關節處（見照片**191**和圖示**136A**），並用膝關節壓住其大腿後方肌群（見照片**192**和圖示**136B**），從膕窩處依次點壓至臀部，反復操作**2－4**次。一側完畢更換另一側。

Knee-pointing rear muscles of thigh:

The patient lies flat on back and bends the hip and knee of a lower limb to the utmost. The massagist stands at the side of patient's foot, holds the patient's dorsum of front foot and knee joint respectively with both hands (see Photo 191 and Fig. 136A) and presses the rear muscles of thigh with a knee joint (see Photo 192 and Fig. 136B) from the hollow of knee to buttocks in order. Repeat the manipulation 2-4 times. Do one side, then the other.

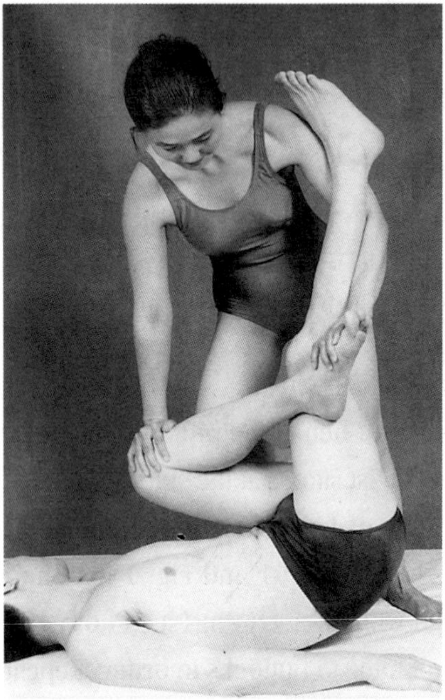

照片 (Photo) 191

圖示 (Fig.) 136A

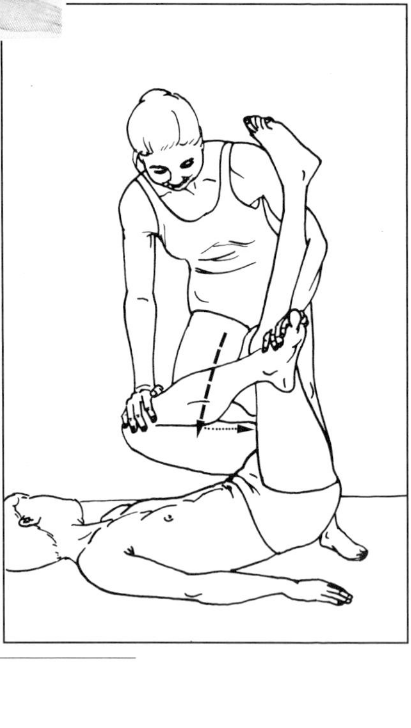

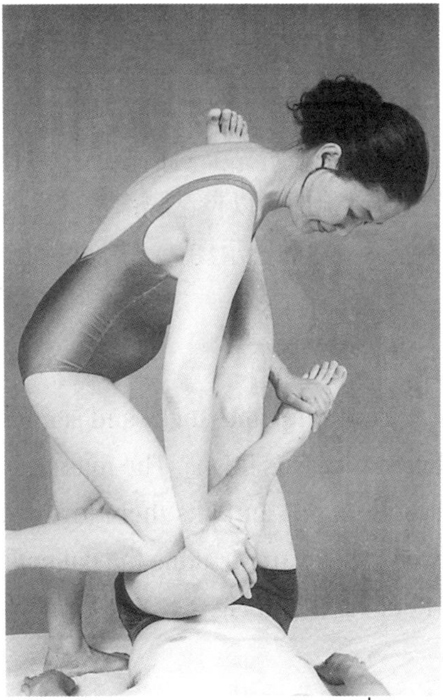
照片 (Photo) 192

圖示 (Fig.) 136B
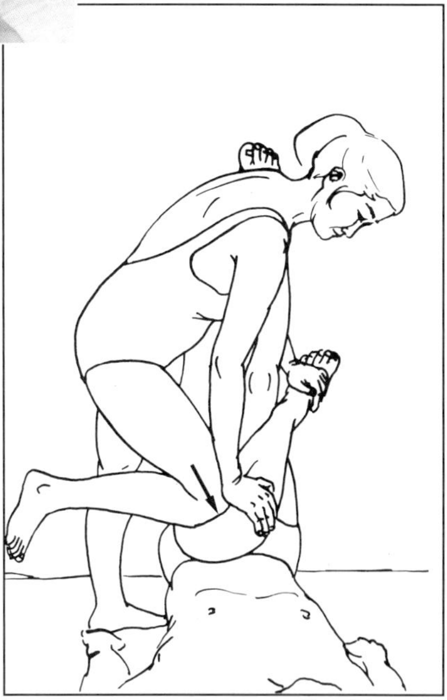

128 屈曲脊柱法：

被按摩者仰臥位，屈髖屈膝，雙足蹬於站立對面位的按摩者大腿前方；按摩者兩手緊握被按摩者腕部，以自己腰部後伸之力向前上拉起，使其上身前屈（見照片**193**和圖示**137**），反復操作**2－4**次。

Bending spine method:

The patient lies flat on back, bends hip and knees and stamps both feet on the front of standing massagist's thighs. The massagist grasps the patient's wrists with both hands and lifts them forward with the force of stretching the waist backward, making the patient's upper body bend forward (see Photo 193 and Fig. 137). Repeat the manipulation 2-4 times.

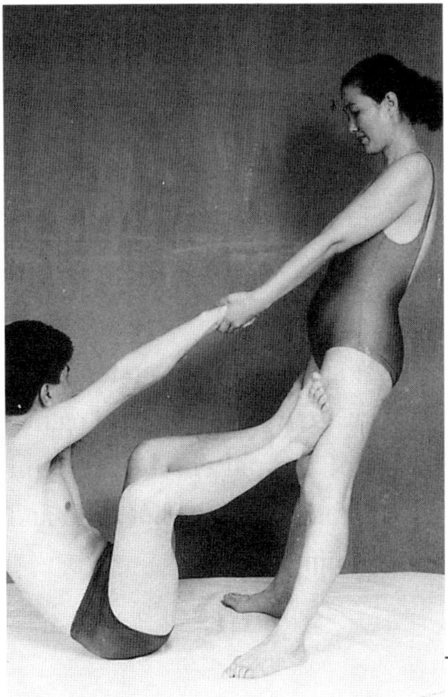

照片 (Photo) 193

圖示 (Fig.) 137

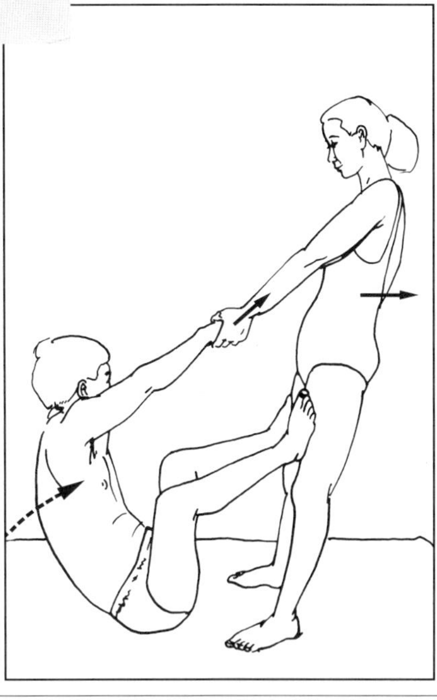

129 屈髖法：

體位同上。按摩者雙上肢伸直，腕關節背伸，以手掌為着力點，腰部前屈向下按壓被按摩者膝關節前方，以加強其屈髖之角度 （見照片**194**和圖示**138**），反復操作**2－4**次。

Bending hip method:

In same position. The massagist stretches both upper limbs straight and stretches wrist joints backward; with the force of palms, bends the waist to press the front of the patient's knee joint downward to enlarge the angle of bending hips (see Photo 194 and Fig. 138). Repeat the manipulation 2-4 times.

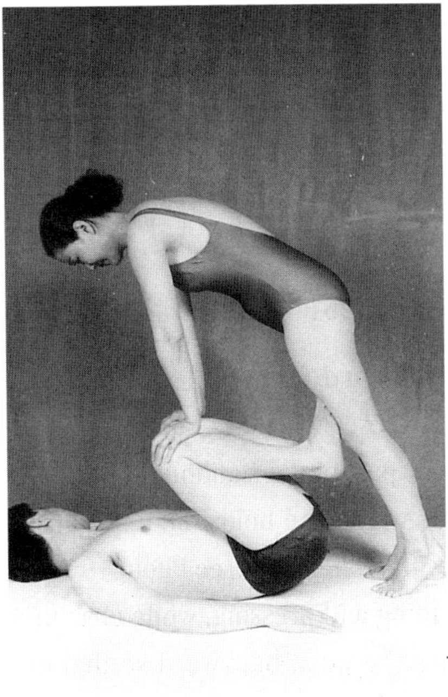

照片 (Photo) 194

圖示 (Fig.) 138

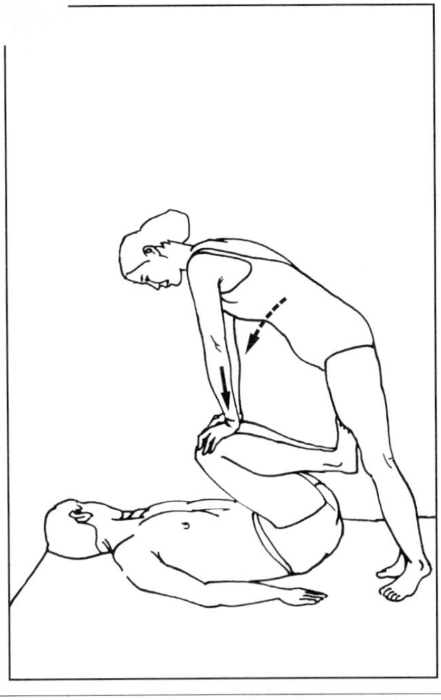

130 屈膝背伸法：

被按摩者仰臥位，雙下肢併攏，雙足分別置於站立位的按摩者膝關節上方。按摩者雙手屈腕握按被按摩者膝關節的前上方（見照片**195**和圖示**139A**），邊行握按之力，邊改半蹲位，並同時腰部背伸，使其肩部着床（見照片**196**和圖示**139B**）。

Stretching bent-knee backward method:

The patient lies flat on back, closes together both lower limbs and places both feet on the upper part of the standing massagist's knee joints. The massagist bends wrists and holds the upper front part of the patient's knee joints with both hands (see Photo 195 and Fig. 139A); with the force of holding and pressing, while changing into half squatting and stretches the waist backward so that the patient's shoulders touches the bed (see Photo 196 and Fig. 139B).

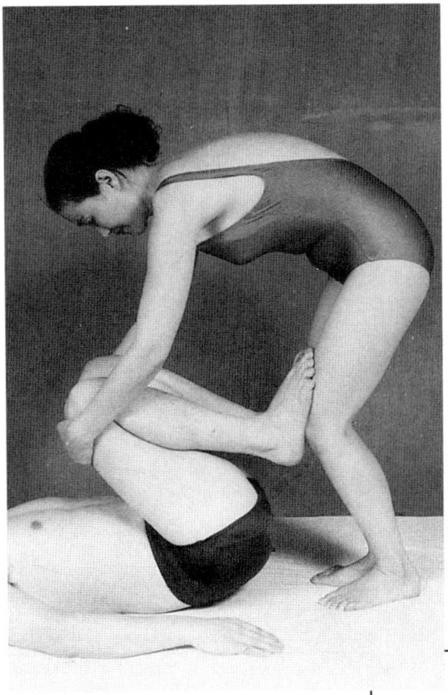

照片 (Photo) 195

圖示 (Fig.) 139A

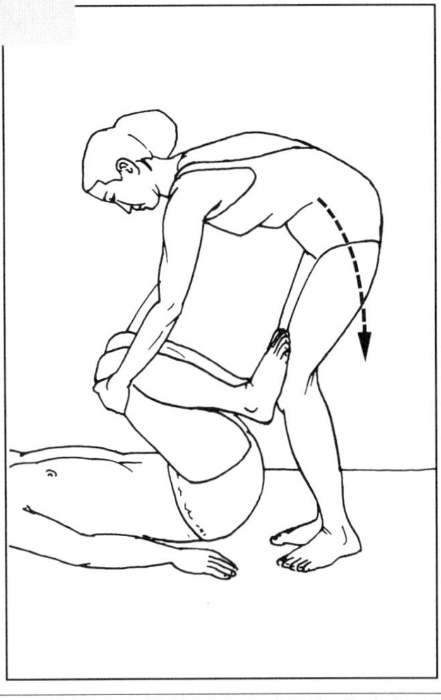

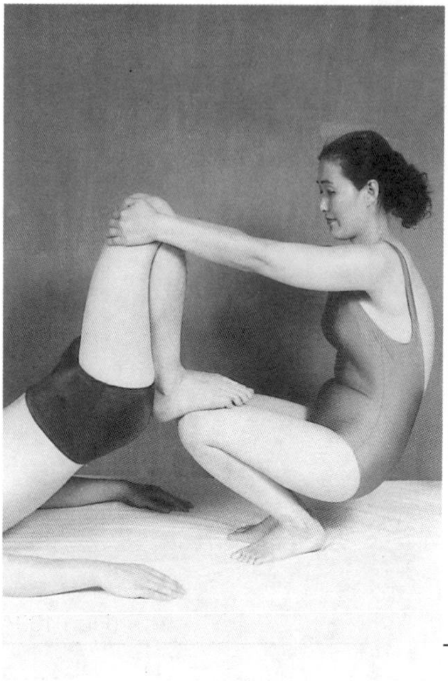

照片 (Photo) 196

圖示 (Fig.) 139B

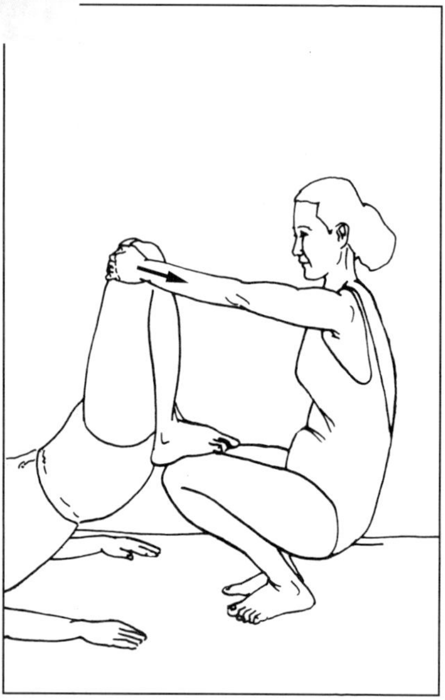

131 屈膝外旋法：

被按摩者仰臥位，右下肢伸直，左下肢外旋屈膝**90**度（**4**字試驗動作）。按摩者站立位，一足在被按摩者的軀幹部，一足在其臀部；一手握其足跟部，前臂向前壓足跖側，使足背伸，而一手握被按摩者另一足前部，使其保持**4**字式試驗姿勢（見照片**197**和圖示**140**）。一側完畢更換另一側。

Revolving bent-knee outward method:

The patient lies flat on back, stretches the right lower limb straight and revolves the left lower limb outward at 90 degrees (the shape of figure 4 experimental movement). The massagist stands with a foot at the side of patient's body and the other at the buttocks and holds the patient's heel with one hand and presses the sole forward with the front arm making the foot stretch backward; holds the front part of other foot of the patient with the other hand in the shape of figure 4 experimental posture (see Photo 197 and Fig. 140). Do one side, then the other.

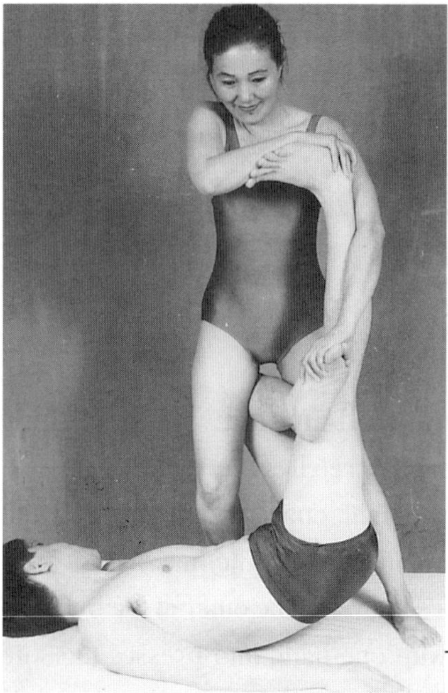
照片 (Photo) 197

圖示 (Fig.) 140
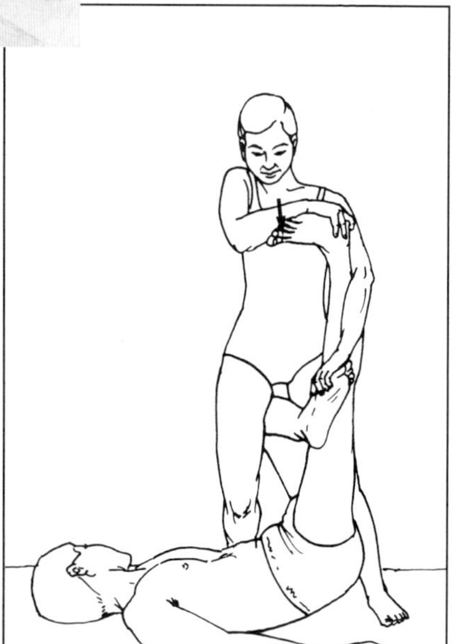

132 屈腰點壓法：

被按摩者仰臥位，雙足置於坐位的按摩者膝關節後方，兩人雙手緊握，借按摩者腰部後伸之力，使被按摩者上身屈曲，並拉起（見照片**198**和圖示**141A**），變按摩者為仰臥位，而被按摩者改坐位（見照片**199**和圖示**141B**）。借被按摩者前屈腰部時，按摩者在同時用雙前足部向其大腿內側後方肌群點壓，並適當變換點壓部位（見照片**200**和圖示**141C**），反復操作**2－4**次。

Bent-waist pointing and pressing method:

The patient lies flat on back and places both feet on the sitting massagist's back of knee joint. The two people grasp both hands. With the force of stretching the massagist's waist backward, make the patient bend the upper body and being pull up (see Photo 198 and Fig. 141A) so that the massagist lies flat on back and the patient sits (see Photo 199 and Fig. 141B). While the patient is bending the waist forward, the massagist points and presses the patient's rear inside muscles of thighs with both front feet and changes the part pointed and pressed properly (see Photo 200 and Fig. 141C). Repeat the manipulation 2-4 times.

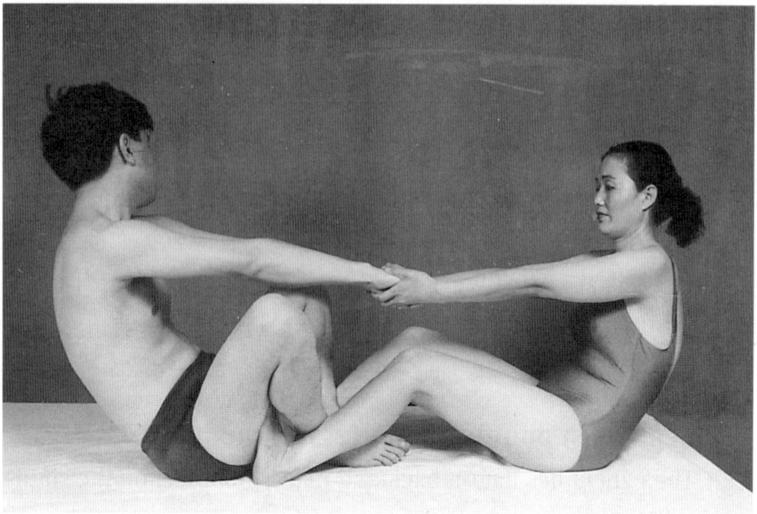
照片 (Photo) 198

圖示 (Fig.) 141A
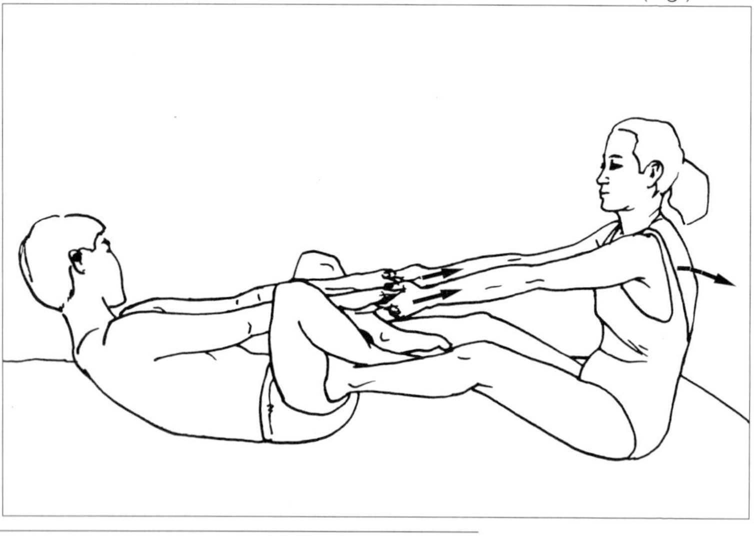

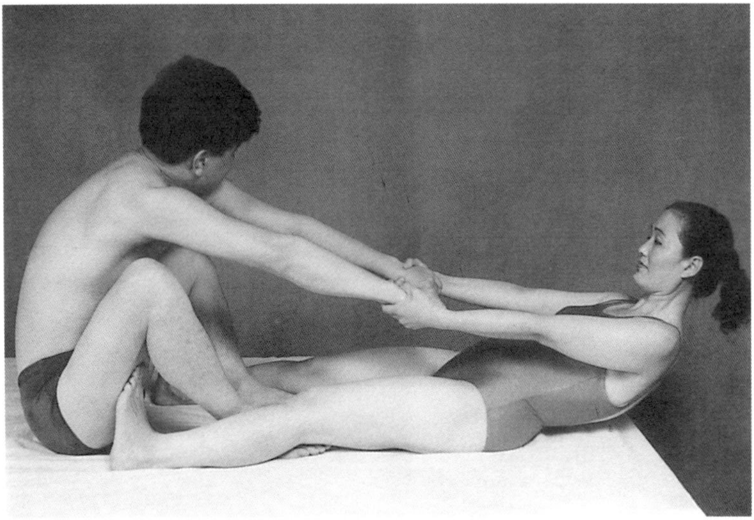

照片 (Photo) 199

圖示 (Fig.) 141B

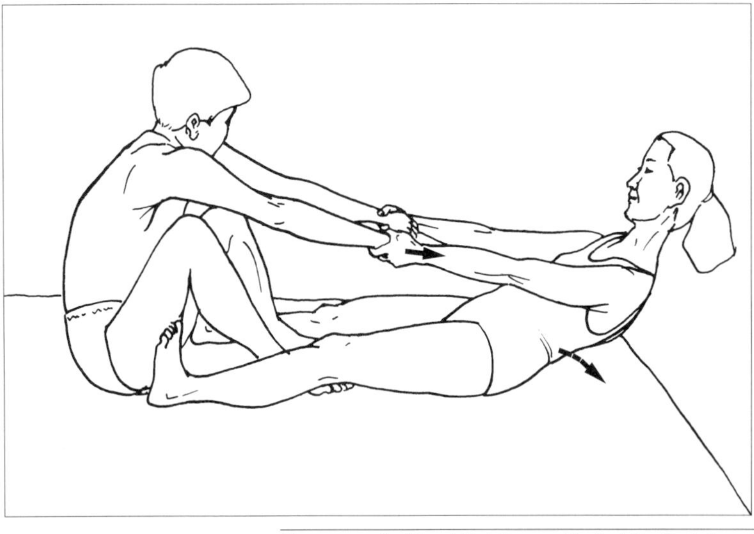

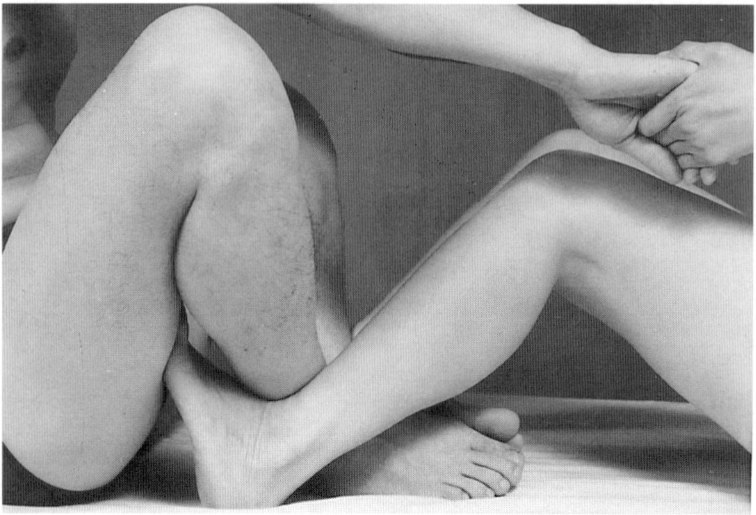

照片 (Photo) 200

圖示 (Fig.) 141C

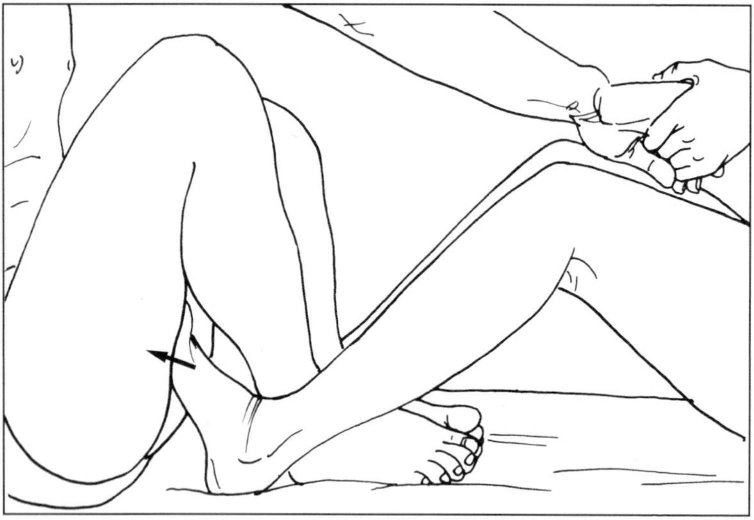

133 按壓大腿前方肌群：

被按摩者仰臥位，雙下肢略抬起，蹬在按摩者膕窩處；按摩者半蹲位，臀部坐被按摩者膝關節前下方，用雙手手掌按壓其大腿前方肌群，反復操作**2－4**次（見照片**201**和圖示**142**）。

Pressing front muscles of thigh:

The patient lies flat on back and slightly lifts both lower limbs to stamp on the hollow of massagist's knees. The massagist half squats with buttocks sitting on the patient's front lower part of knee joints, and presses the front muscles of thigh with both palms. Repeat the manipulation 2-4 times (see Photo 201 and Fig. 142).

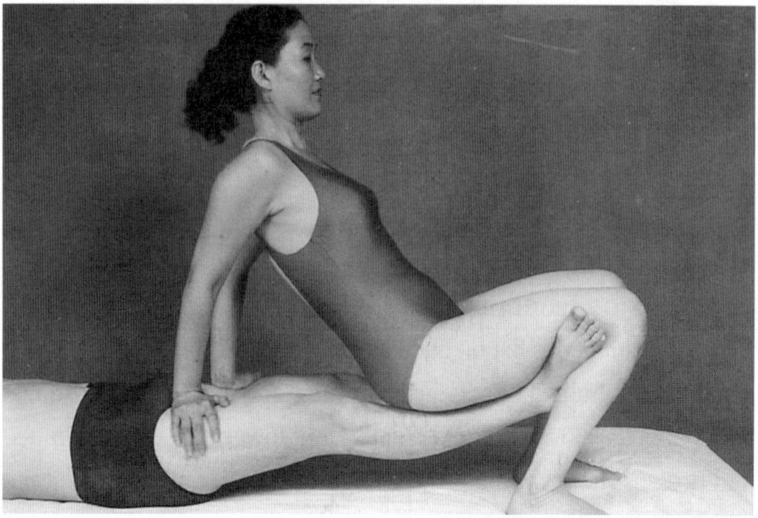
照片 (Photo) 201

圖示 (Fig.) 142

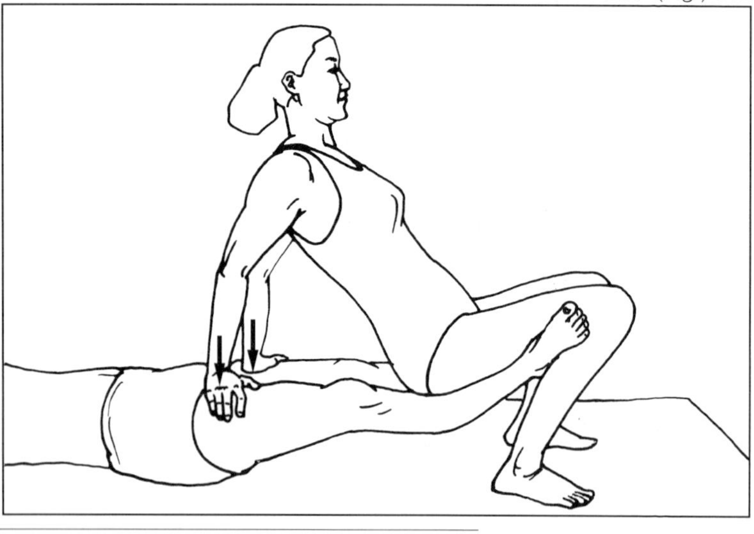

134 點按頭部諸穴：

被按摩者雙下肢外旋屈膝盤坐位，按摩者跪於身後，一手扶托其頭部，另一手拇指指端點按百會穴（見照片**202**和圖示**143**），然後改雙手五指點揉和彌漫點揉頭部（見照片**203**和圖示**144**）。

Pointing and pressing head acupoints:

The patient revolves both lower limbs outward and sits with bent knees and legs crossed. The massagist kneels behind the patient, supports the head with one hand, points and presses the Baihui acupoint with a thumb tip with the other hand (see Photo 202 and Fig. 143) and then points and rubs the whole head with five fingers of both hands (see Photo 203 and Fig. 144).

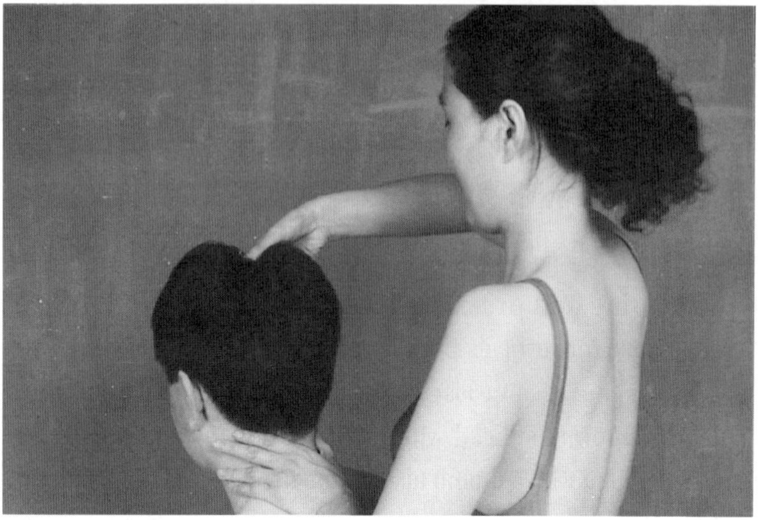
照片 (Photo) 202

圖示 (Fig.) 143
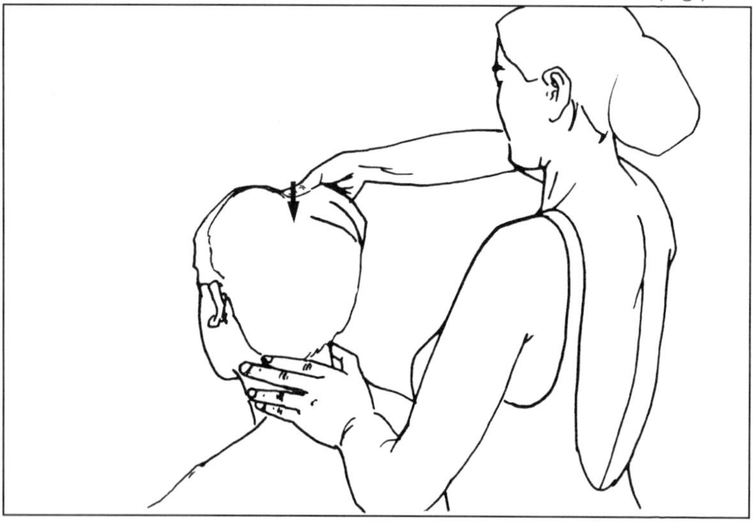

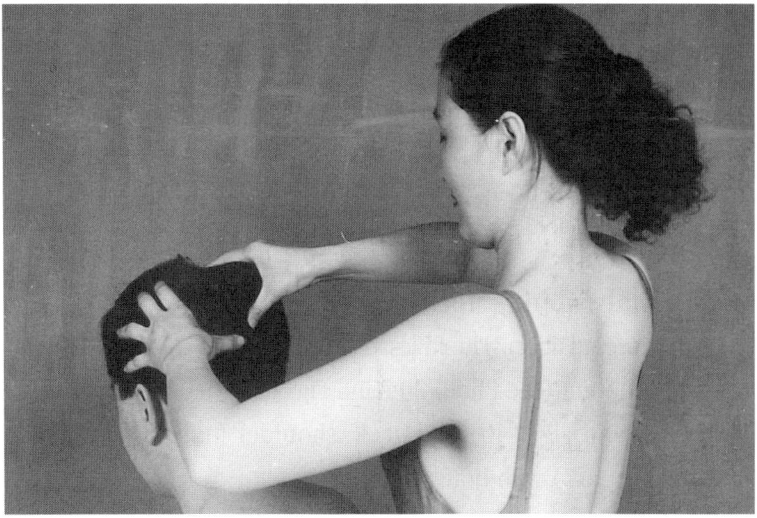
照片 (Photo) 203

圖示 (Fig.) 144
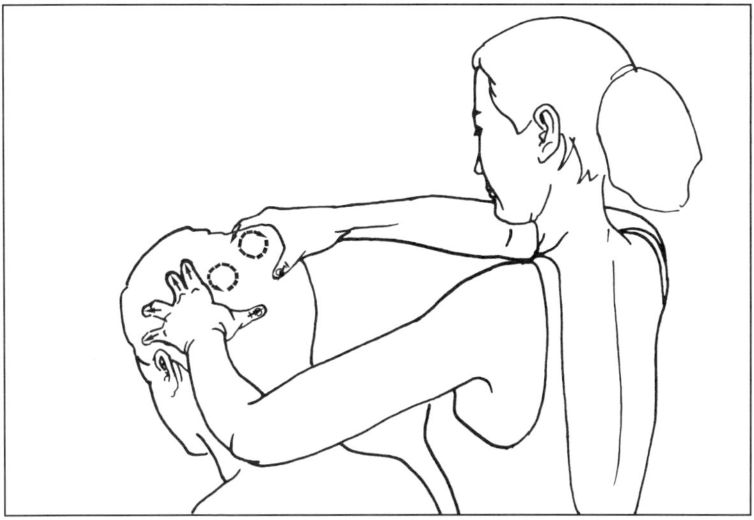

135 指揉頸肩部：

體位同上。按摩者雙手拇指按揉被按摩者風池穴（見照片**204**和圖示**145**）、項韌帶（見照片**205**和圖示**146**）及頸肩部肌群（見照片**206**和圖示**147**）。

Digital-rubbing neck and shoulders:

In same position. The massagist presses and rubs the patient's Fengchi acupoint (see Photo 204 and Fig. 145), nape ligament (see Photo 205 and Fig. 146) and neck, shoulder muscles (see Photo 206 and Fig. 147) with both thumbs.

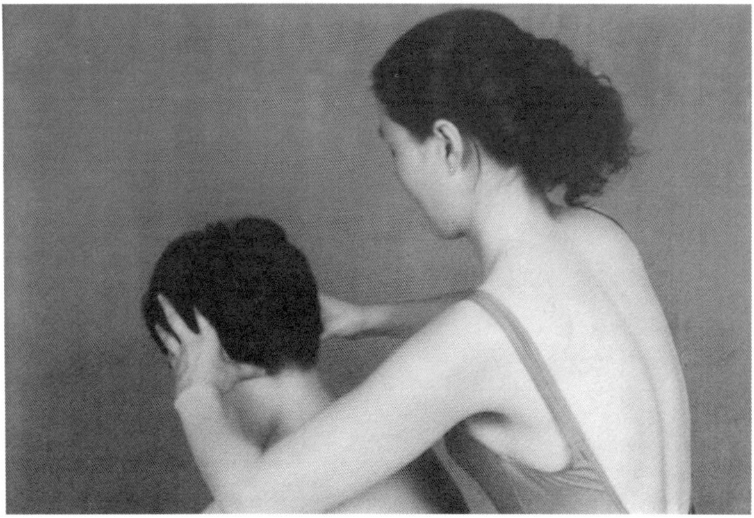

照片 (Photo) 204

圖示 (Fig.) 145

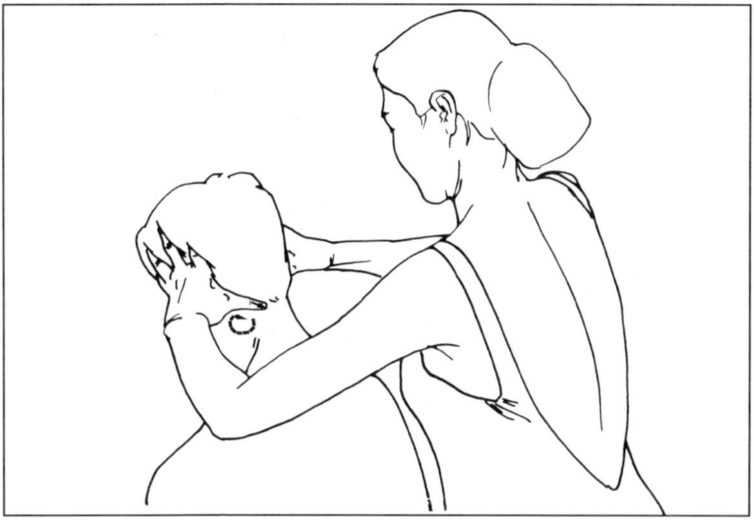

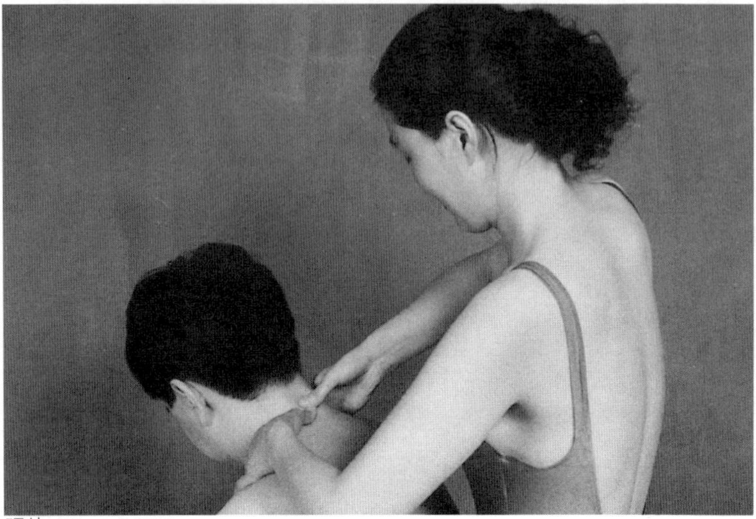
照片 (Photo) 205

圖示 (Fig.) 146
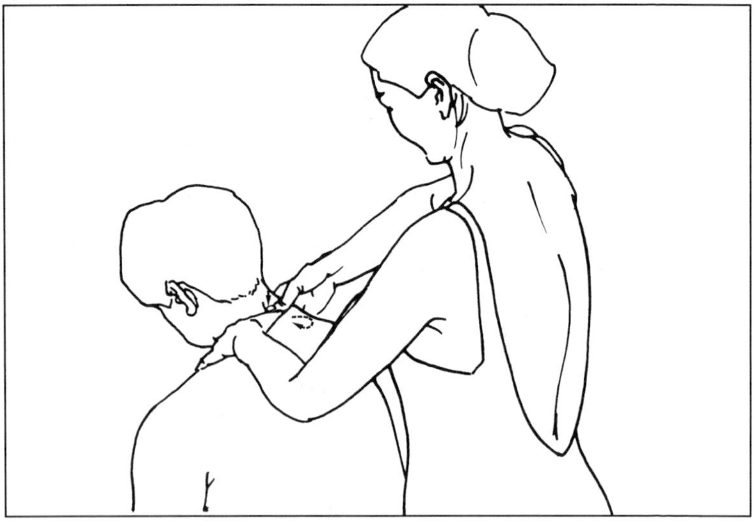

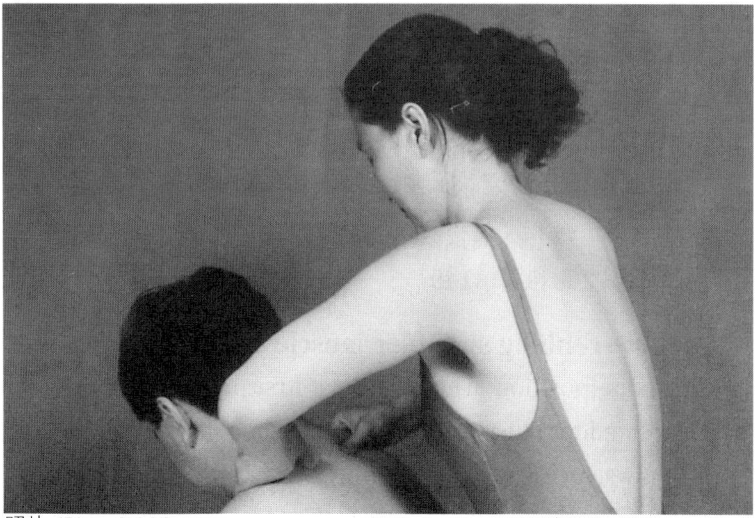
照片 (Photo) 206

圖示 (Fig.) 147

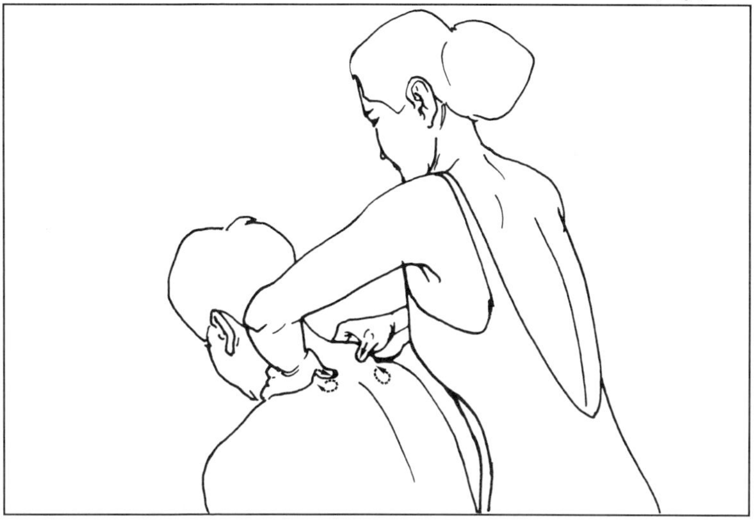

136 肘揉肩部肌群：

體位同上。按摩者先用雙肘按揉被按摩者肩部肌群或雙肘按壓一側肩部，邊按揉邊向外側移動，或兩側同時按壓亦可（見照片207和圖示148），然後改用鷹嘴部點按其夾脊穴，邊點揉，邊壓捋（見照片208和圖示149）。

Elbow-rubbing shoulder muscles:

In same position. The massagist first presses and rubs the patient's shoulder muscles or presses the shoulder at one side with both elbows, pressing and rubbing while moving outward, or presses the shoulders at both sides at the same time (see Photo 207 and Fig. 148); then presses the Jiaji acupoint with hawk beak part, rubbing while pressing and kneading (see Photo 208 and Fig. 149).

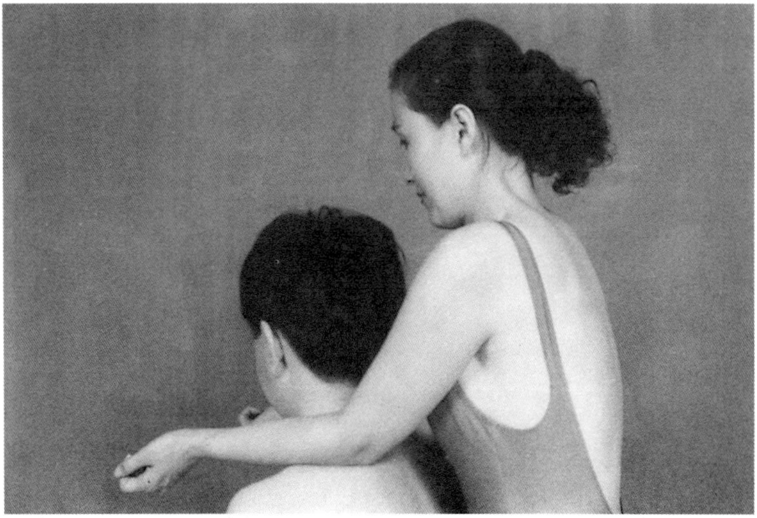
照片 (Photo) 207

圖示 (Fig.) 148

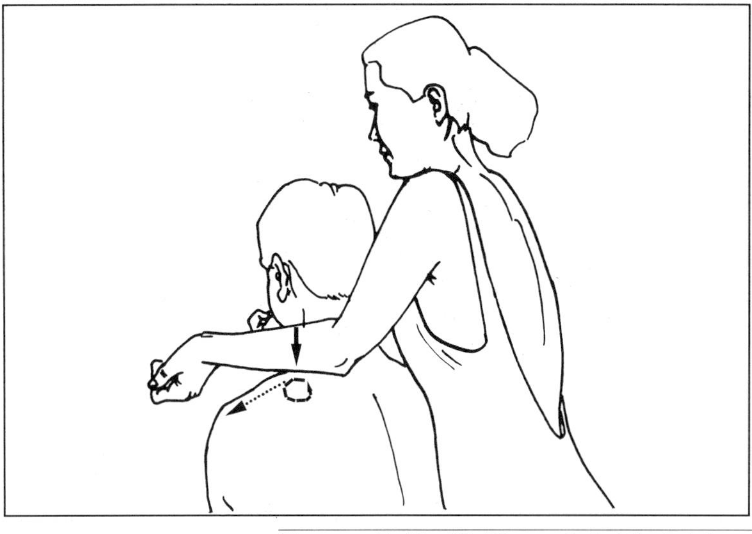

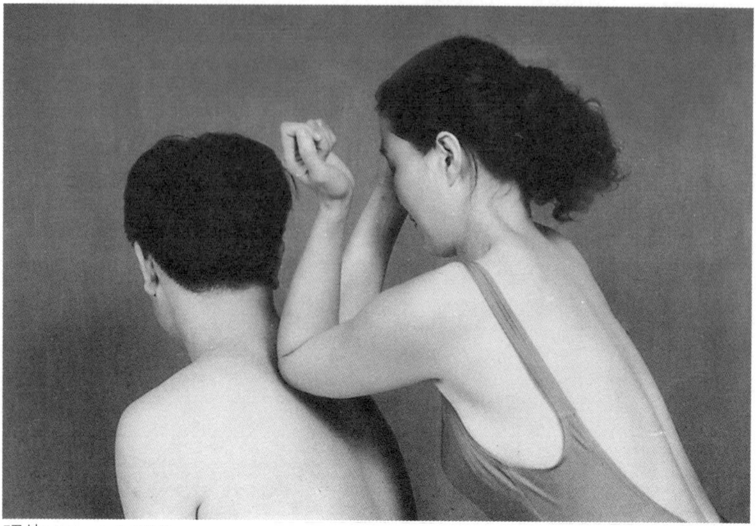

照片 (Photo) 208

圖示 (Fig.) 149

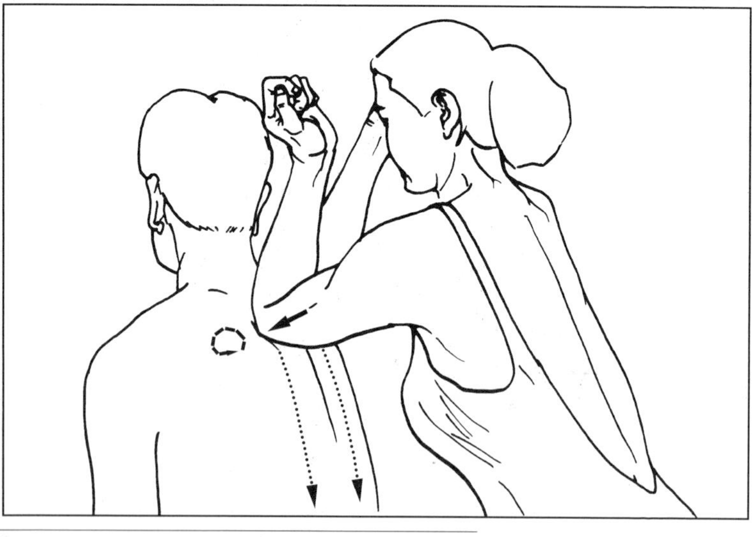

137 旋轉軀幹法：

被按摩者坐位，雙手五指交叉抱於後頭部。按摩者一下肢屈膝，跪於被按摩者身後，另一下肢置其前方，雙手從其腋下向前穿過緊握前臂（見照片**209**和圖示**150A**），使其軀幹向一側旋轉（見照片**210**和圖示**150B**），動作幅度由小到大。一側完畢更換另一側。

Revolving trunk method:

The patient sits and closes together the five fingers of both hands to hold the back of head. The massagist bends the knee of a lower limb and kneels behind the patient, places the other lower limb in front of the patient and grasps the forearms through armpits (see Photo 209 and Fig. 150A) so that the trunk revolves to one side (see Photo 210 and Fig. 150B). The movement should be from small to large. Do one side, then the other.

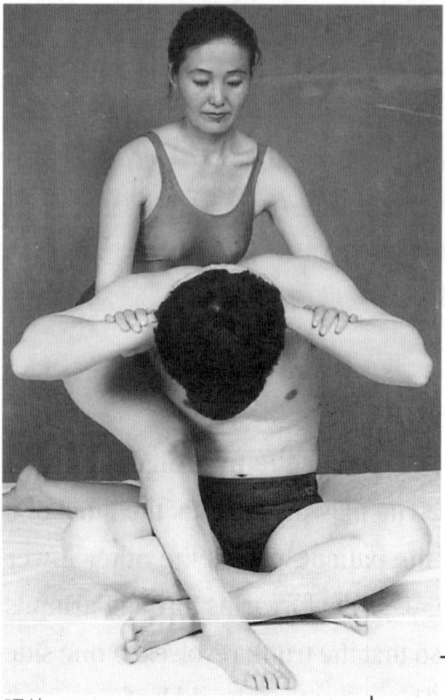

照片 (Photo) 209

圖示 (Fig.) 150A

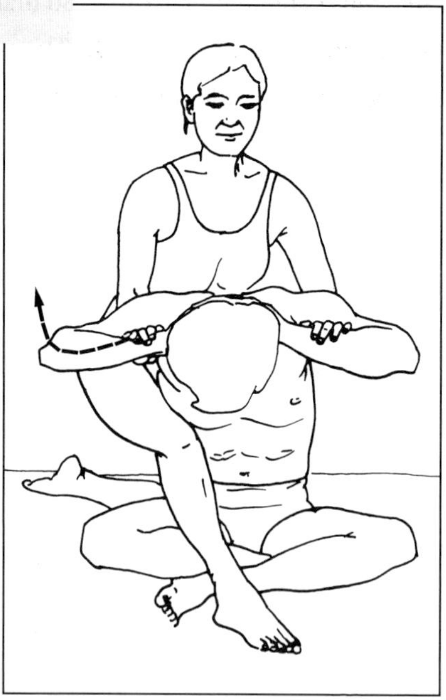

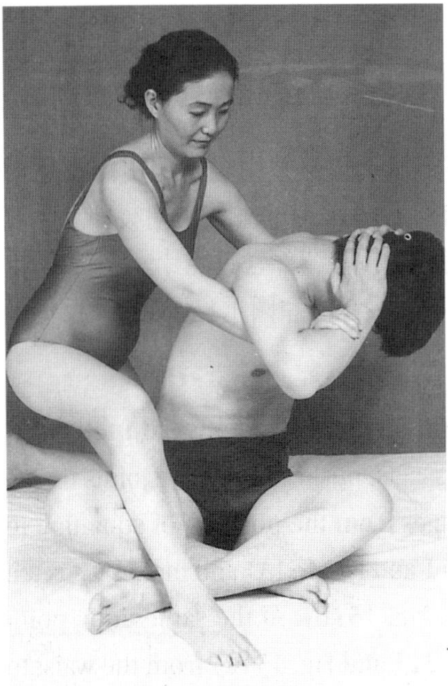

照片 (Photo) 210

圖示 (Fig.) 150B

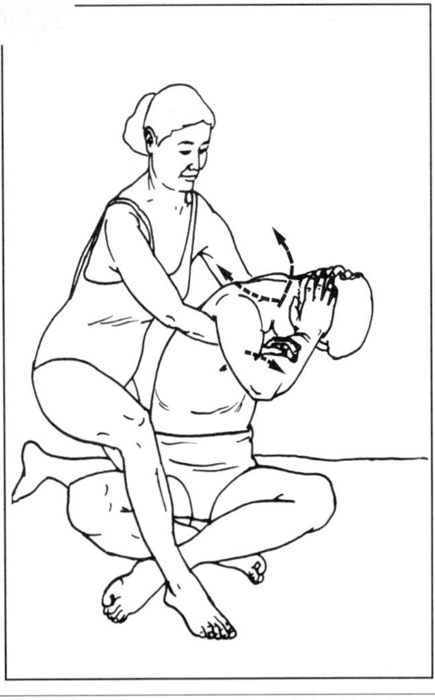

138 頂按後伸法：

體位同上。按摩者雙膝關節頂按被按摩者腰部由蹲位逐漸過渡到仰臥位（見照片211和圖示151A），並使其向後伸（見照片212和圖示151B），同時點按後背部（見照片213和圖示151C），從腰至上胸椎處（見照片214和圖示151D），反復操作2次。

Pushing on, pressing and stretching backward method:

In same position. The massagist pushes both knee joints on the patient's waist, gradually changes from the position of squatting to lying flat on back (see Photo 211 and Fig. 151A) and makes it stretch backward (see Photo 212 and Fig. 151B). At the same time, point and press the back (see Photo 213 and Fig. 151C) from the waist to the upper thoracic vertebra (see Photo 214 and Fig. 151D). Repeat the manipulation twice.

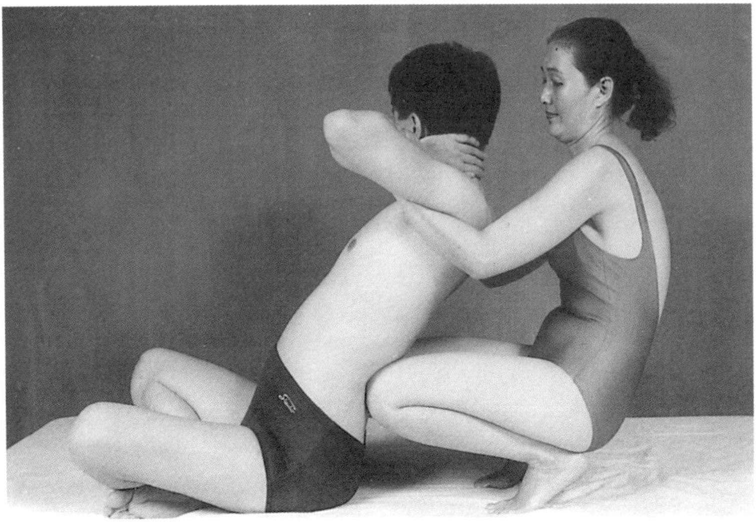

照片 (Photo) 211

圖示 (Fig.) 151A

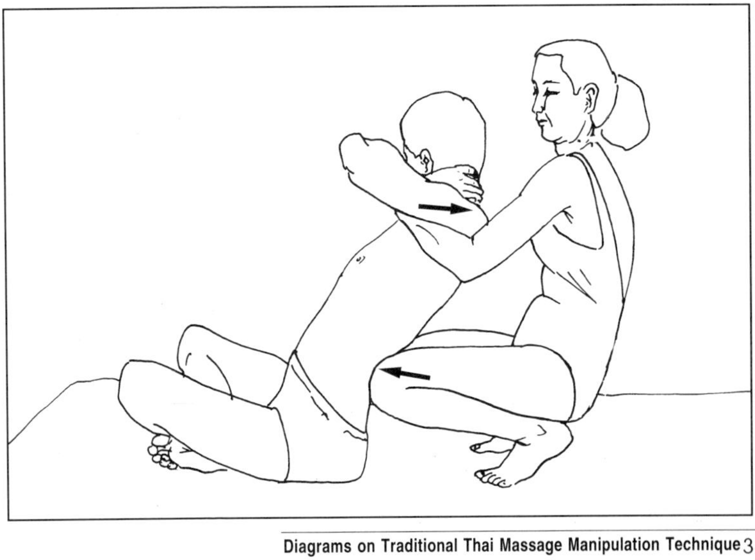

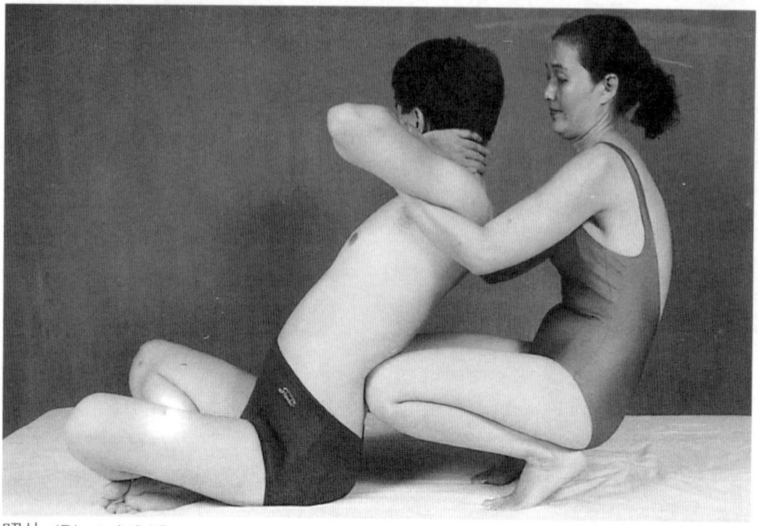
照片 (Photo) 212

圖示 (Fig.) 151B

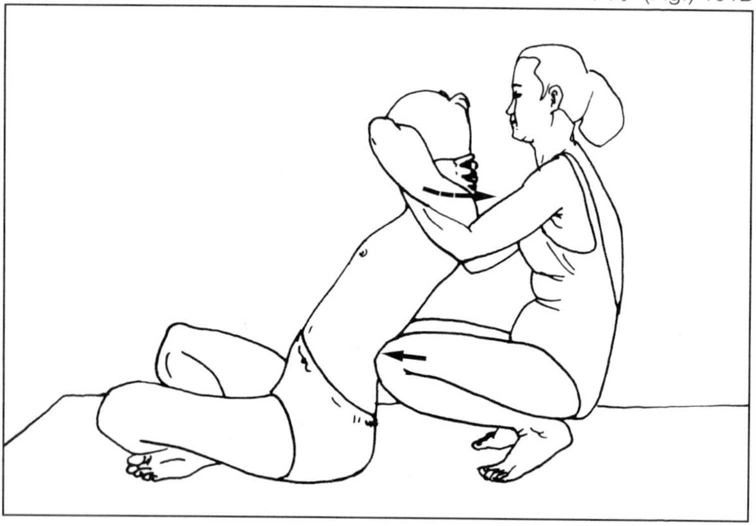

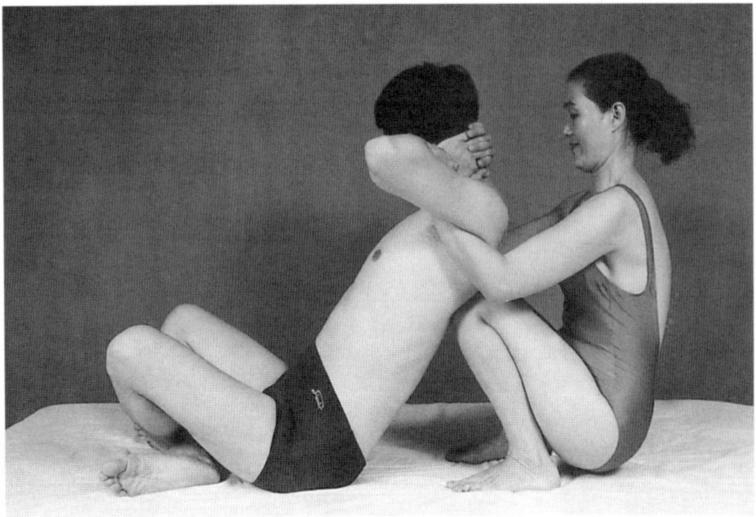

照片 (Photo) 213

圖示 (Fig.) 151C

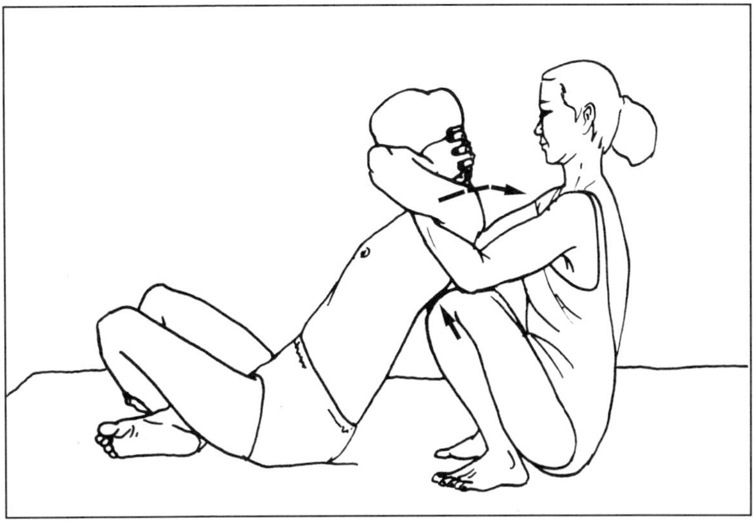

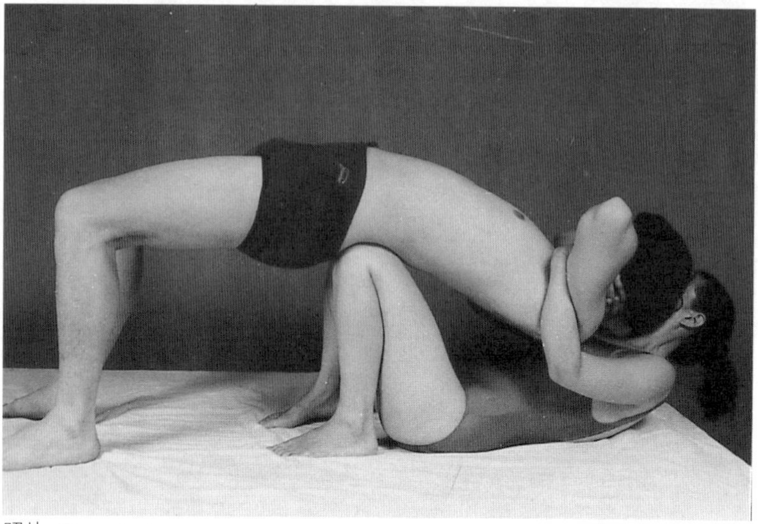
照片 (Photo) 214

圖示 (Fig.) 151D

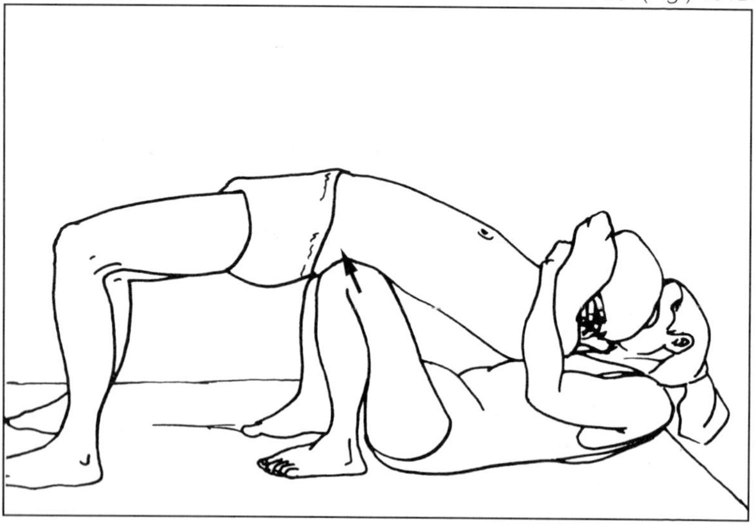

139 踩踏後拉法：

被按摩者坐位，雙上肢後伸，按摩者坐其後，雙下肢向前伸直，兩手緊握被按摩者後伸的雙上肢，並用腳踩其背部（見照片**215**和圖示**152A**），邊踩邊向後拉，由背部至腰部（見照片**216**和圖示**152B**），反復操作**2－4**次。

Stamping and pulling backward method:

The patient sits and stretches both upper limbs backward. The massagist sits behind, stretches both lower limbs straight, grasps both upper limbs of the patient with both hands and stamps on the back with feet (see Photo 215 and Fig. 152A), stamping while pulling backward from the back to the waist (see Photo 216 and Fig. 152B). Repeat the manipulation 2-4 times.

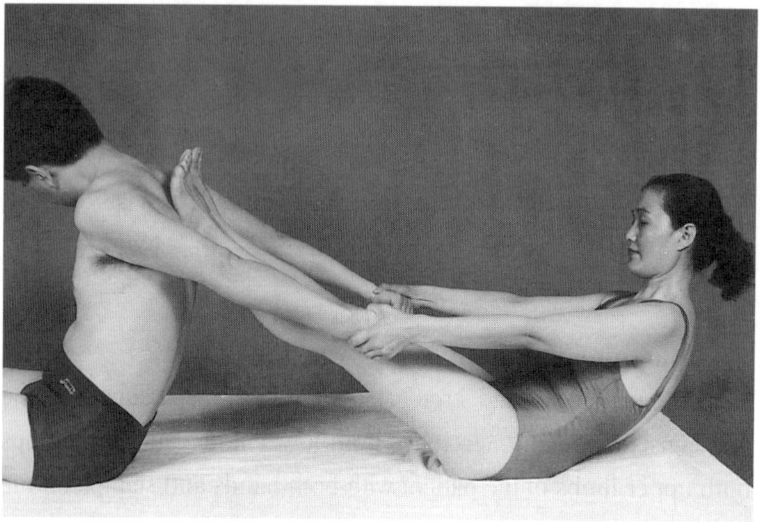
照片 (Photo) 215

圖示 (Fig.) 152A

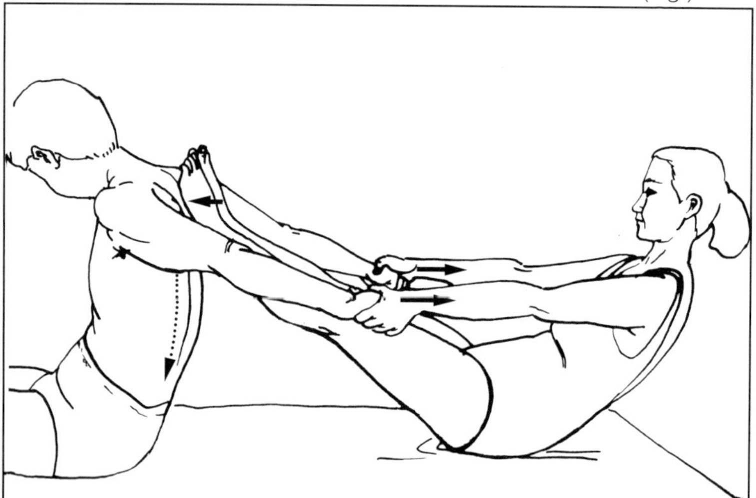

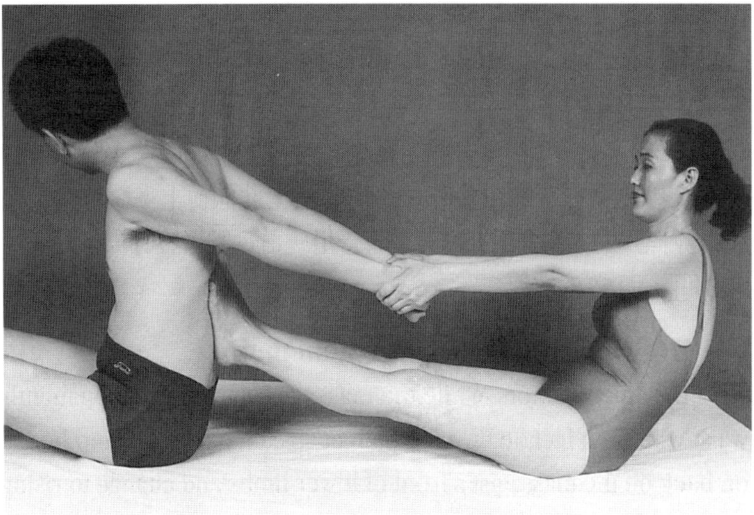

照片 (Photo) 216

圖示 (Fig.) 152B

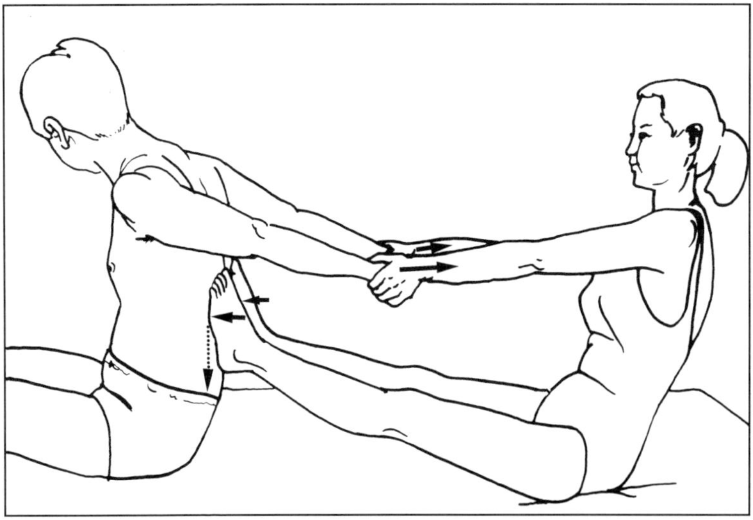

140 牽拉點背法：

體位同上。當按摩者雙足踩踏被按摩者腰部時，令其軀幹後伸成仰臥於自己下肢正前方，並使其雙上肢向前上舉，邊向上牽拉（見照片**217**和圖示**153A**），邊用雙前足點揉腰背部（見照片**218**和圖示**153B**）。

Drawing and pointing back method:

In same position. While the massagist stamps on the patient's waist with both feet, makes the patient stretch backward and lie flat on back on the massagist's front of lower limbs and change to rising both upper limbs upward, drawing upward (see Photo 217 and Fig. 153A) while pointing and rubbing the back of waist with both front feet (see Photo 218 and Fig. 153B).

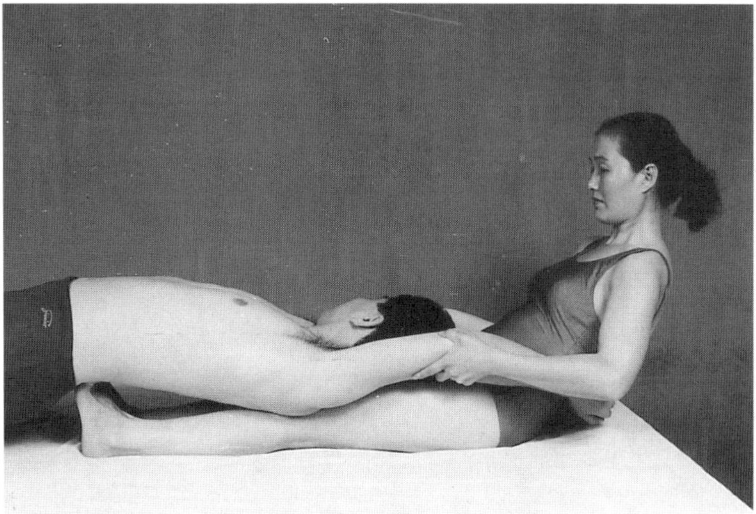
照片 (Photo) 217

圖示 (Fig.) 153A
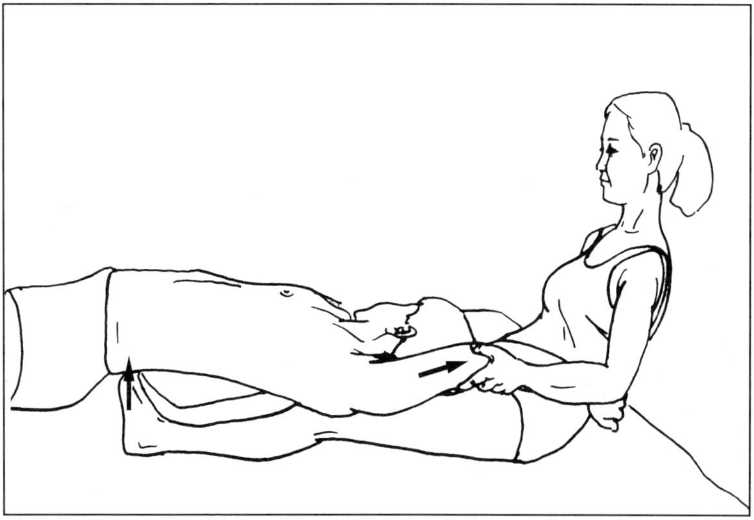

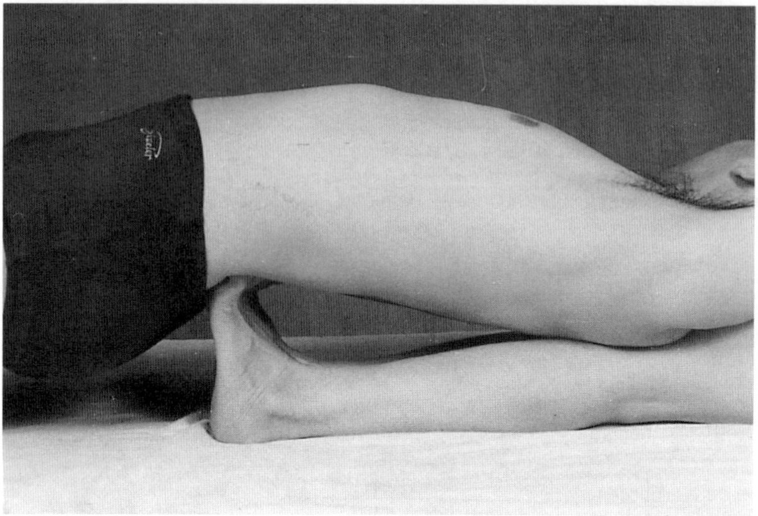

照片 (Photo) 218

圖示 (Fig.) 153B

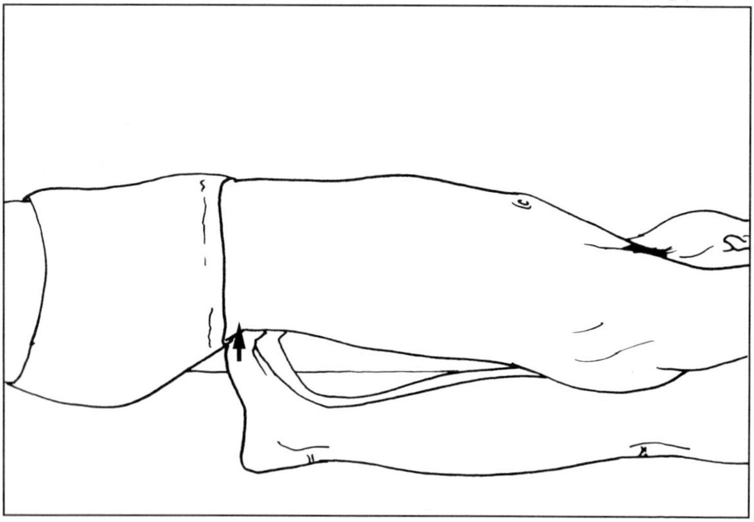

141 頂提法：

被按摩者雙下肢外旋，屈髖屈膝盤坐位，上肢五指交叉抱於後頭部；按摩者立其後，一下肢伸直，另一下肢略屈膝關節並向前頂住被按摩者胸椎棘突部位（見照片**219**和圖示**154**），先用雙手向後牽拉肘關節，然後改內收兩肘，向後上方提牽（見照片**220**和圖示**155**）。一側完畢更換另一側。

Pushing on and lifting method:

The patient revolves both lower limbs outward, bends hips and knees, sits with legs crossed and holds the back of head with five fingers crossed. The massagist stands behind, stretches a lower limb straight, slightly bends the knee joint of the other lower limb and pushes it on the protruding part of thoracic vertebra (see Photo 219 and Fig. 154); first draws the elbow joint of the patient backward with both hands and then pulls in both elbows to lift it backward and upward (see Photo 220 and Fig. 155). Do one side, then the other.

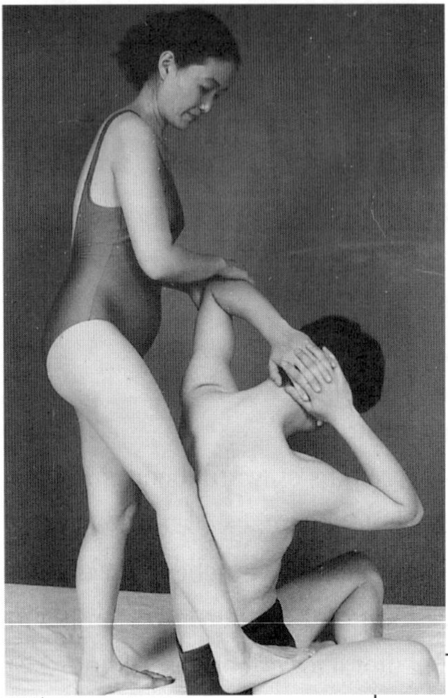

照片 (Photo) 219

圖示 (Fig.) 154

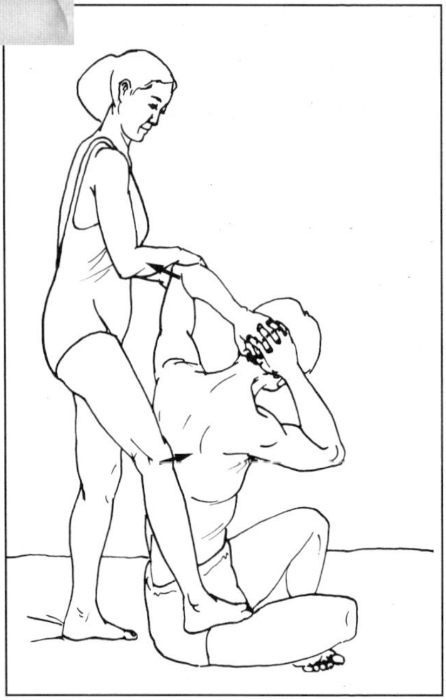

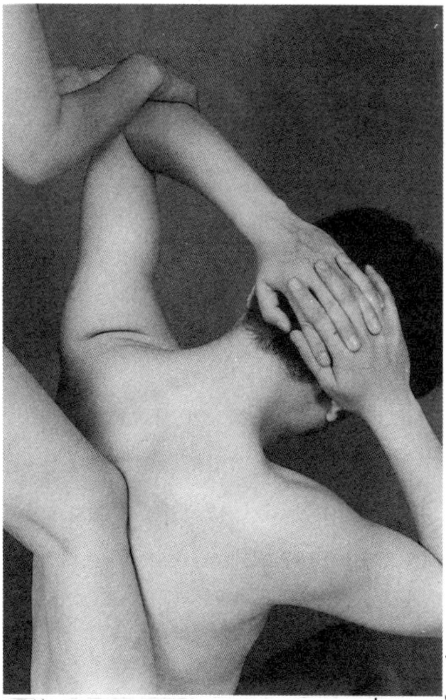

照片 (Photo) 220

圖示 (Fig.) 155

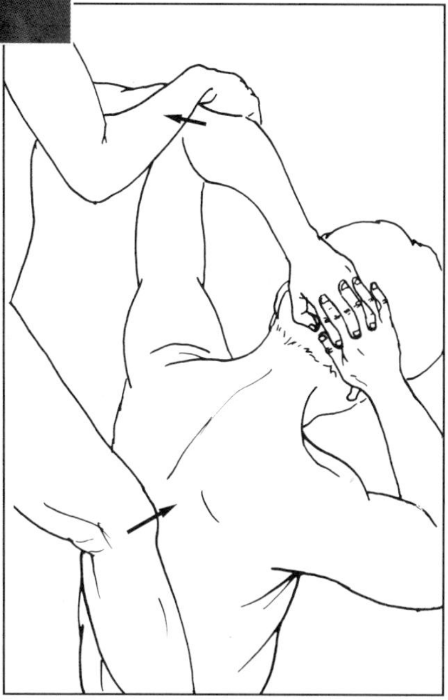

142 牽拉上肢前方肌群：

體位同上。按摩者一腳踩在被按摩者一側下肢的大腿近端，同時膝關節頂住其腰背部，一手提肘關節，另一手握住上臂（見照片**221**和圖示**156A**），將前方肌群向後方牽拉（見照片**222**和圖示**156B**）。一側完畢更換另一側。

Drawing front muscles of upper limb:

In same position. The massagist stamps on the patient's near end of thigh with the lower limb at one side, supports the back of waist with a knee joint, lifts an elbow joint with one hand, grasps the upper arm with the other hand (see Photo 221 and Fig. 156A) and draws the front muscles backward (see Photo 222 and Fig. 156B). Do one side, then the other.

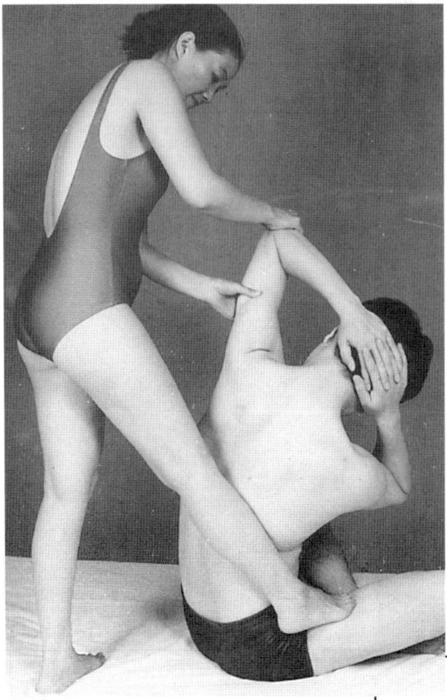

照片 (Photo) 221

圖示 (Fig.) 156A

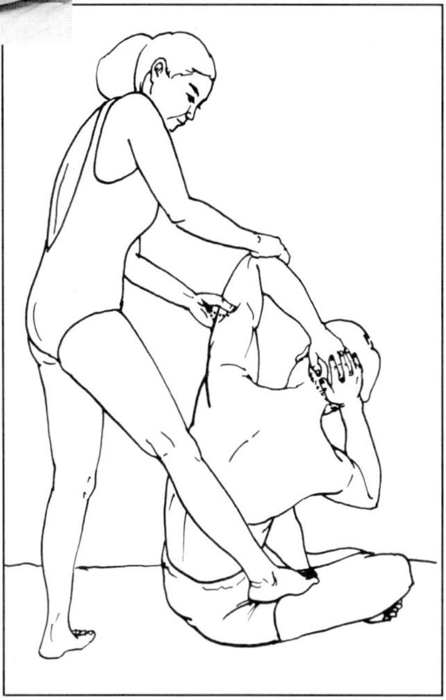

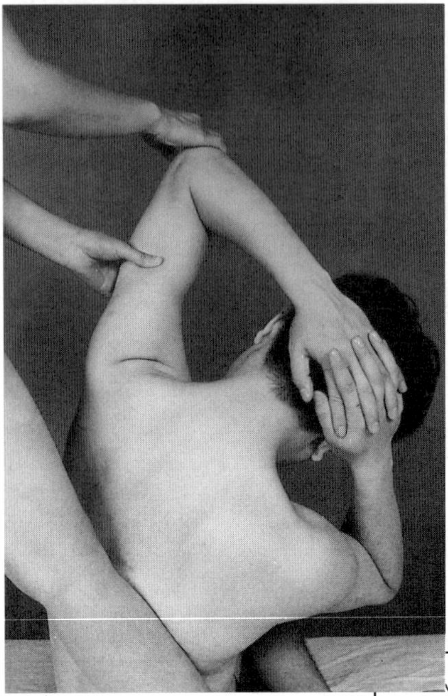

照片 (Photo) 222

圖示 (Fig.) 156B

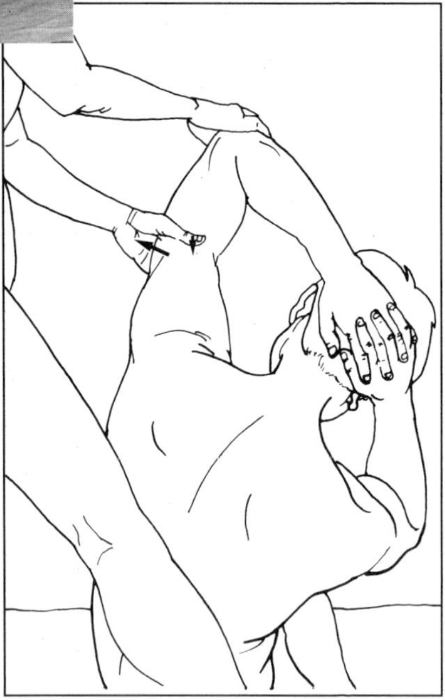

143 旋頸法：

被按摩者坐位，按摩者立於一側，一手扶托被按摩者頭頂，另一手扶托其下頜，雙手交錯旋轉用力做頭部旋轉活動（見照片223和圖示157）。一側完畢更換另一側，重復操作以上動作，注意旋轉幅度應在正常活動範圍內。

Revolving neck method:

The patient sits. The massagist stands at one side, holds the top of the patient's head with one hand and supports the lower jaw with the other hand. Revolve the head with both hands using force alternatively (see Photo 223 and Fig. 157). Do one side, then the other. Repeat the above manipulation. Note that the revolving should be of normal scope.

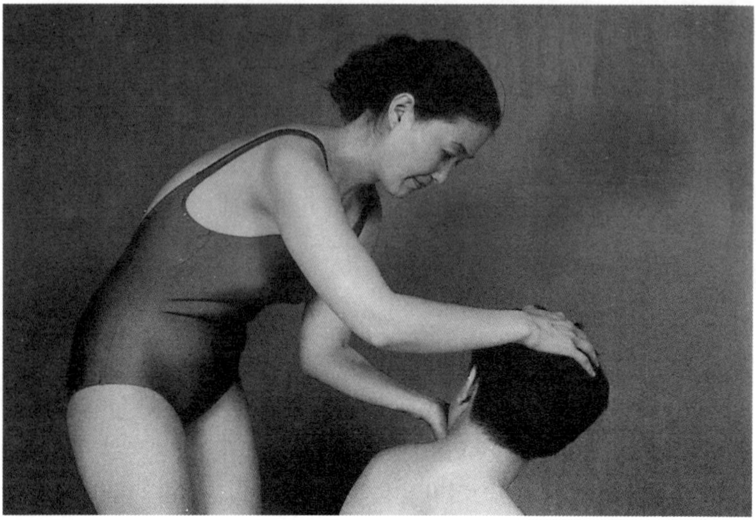

照片 (Photo) 223

圖示 (Fig.) 157

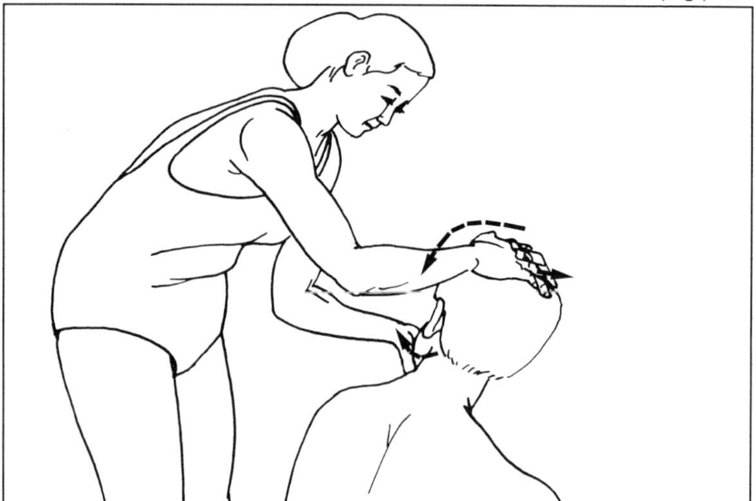

144 牽拉上肢法：

被按摩者仰臥位，雙上肢上舉屈肘，手掌部按床面。按摩者下肢外旋，屈髖屈膝盤坐其頭側（見照片**224**和圖示**158A**），兩手握被按摩者上肢近端（見照片**225**和圖示**158B**），向後牽拉至肘關節，再改雙手同時牽拉兩側上肢遠端，被按摩者由屈肘位變伸肘位（見照片**226**和圖示**159**）。

Drawing upper limb method:

The patient lies flat on back, lifts both upper limbs upward, bends elbows and places palms on the bed. The massagist revolves the lower limbs outward, bends hips and knees, kneels at the side of patient's head (see Photo 224 and Fig. 158A) and holds the near end of upper arms with both hands (see Photo 225 and Fig. 158B) to draw them backward to the elbow joints of the patient. Once again draws the far ends of both upper arms simultaneously with both hands. The patient changes his attitude from bent arms to straight arms (see Photo 226 and Fig. 159).

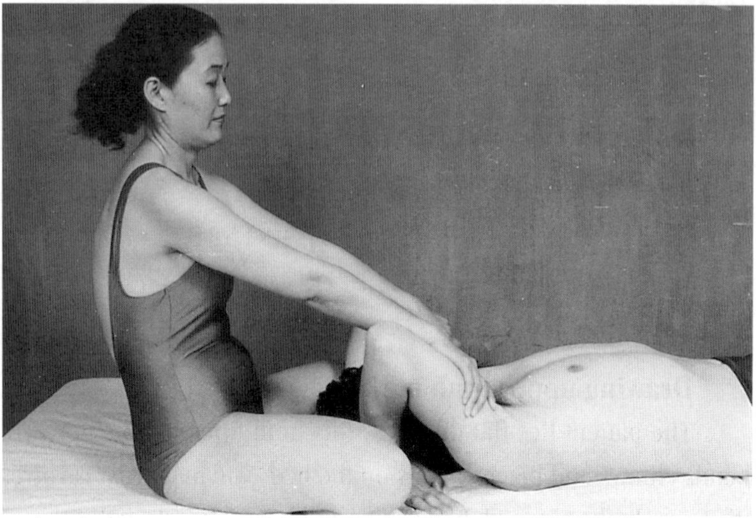

照片 (Photo) 224

圖示 (Fig.) 158A

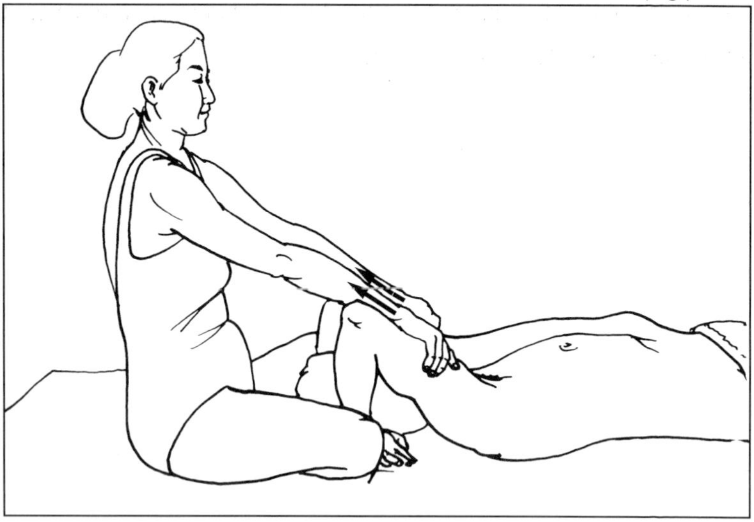

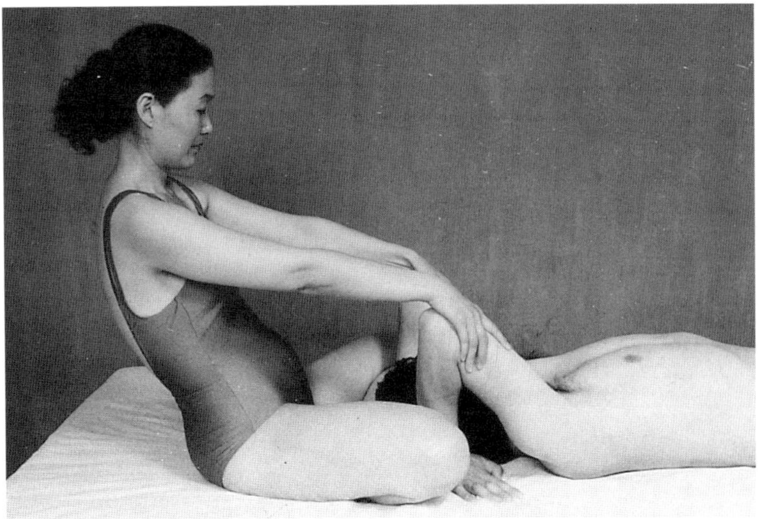

照片 (Photo) 225

圖示 (Fig.) 158B

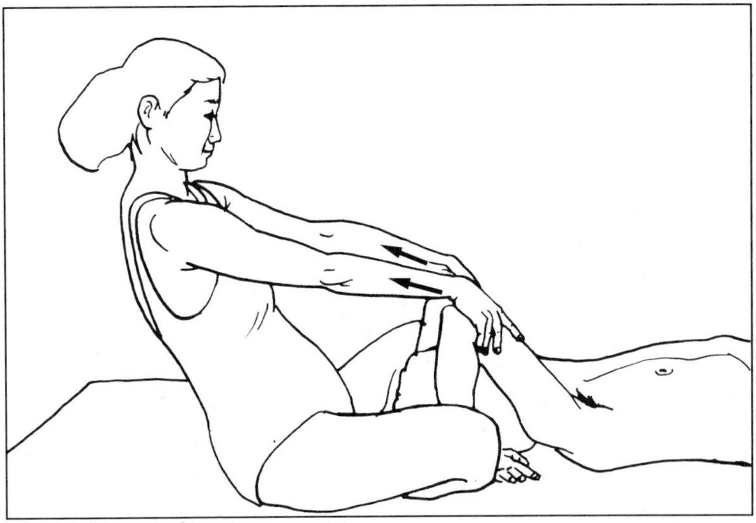

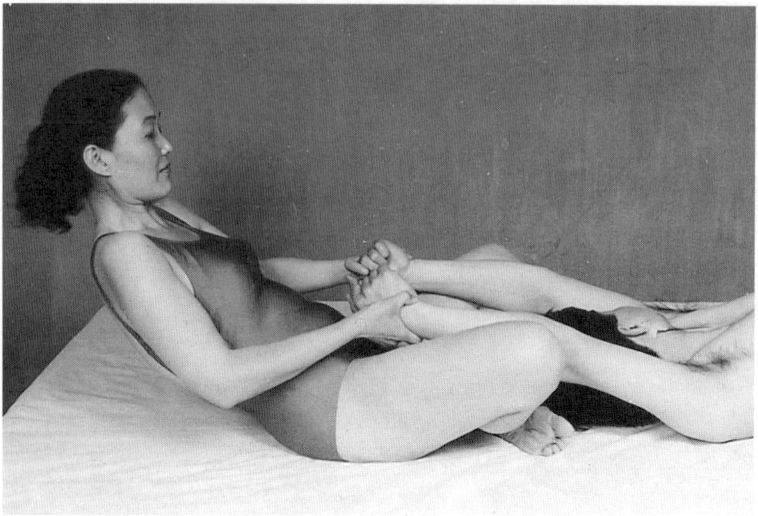
照片 (Photo) 226

圖示 (Fig.) 159
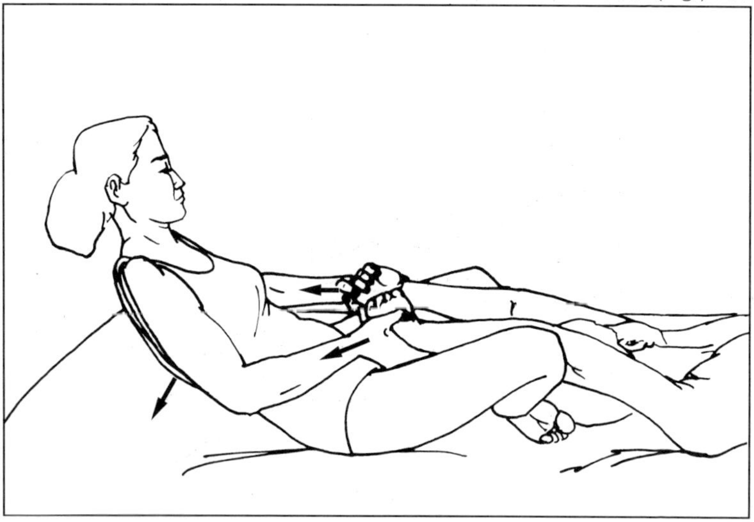